131 METHOD

ALSO BY CHALENE JOHNSON

Books
PUSH: 30 Days to Turbocharged Habits, a Bangin'
Body, and the Life You Deserve!

CDs/DVDs
Health and Fitness Series
Turbo Jam
ChaLean Extreme
Turbo Fire
PiYo

Podcast
The Chalene Show

***

131 METHOD

Your Personalized Nutrition Solution to Boost Metabolism, Restore Gut Health, and Lose Weight

CHALENE JOHNSON

HAY HOUSE, INC.

Carlsbad, California • New York City

London • Sydney • New Delhi

Published in the United States by: Hay House, Inc.: www.hayhouse.com®
• **Published in Australia by:** Hay House Australia Pty. Ltd.: www.hayhouse
.com.au • **Published in the United Kingdom by:** Hay House UK, Ltd.: www
.hayhouse.co.uk • **Published in India by:** Hay House Publishers India: www
.hayhouse.co.in

Indexer: Jay Kreider • *Cover and interior design:* Ashley Lima
Front-cover photo and lifestyle photography: Paul Von Rieter
Food and recipe photos: Aubrie Pick

Cataloging-in-Publication Data is on file at the Library of Congress

Hardcover ISBN: 978-1-4019-5678-3
e-book ISBN: 978-1-4019-5677-6
e-audio ISBN: 978-1-4019-5835-0

11 10 9 8 7 6 5 4 3 2
1st edition, April 2019

Printed in the United States of America

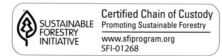

Certified Chain of Custody
SUSTAINABLE FORESTRY INITIATIVE
Promoting Sustainable Forestry
www.sfiprogram.org
SFI-01268

SFI label applies to the text stock

This book is dedicated to the superhot barista with all the tattoos; to our CFO, who ensures that my brilliant ideas don't bankrupt us; to my personal chef; and to the most caring, protective, and thoughtful friend, business partner, husband, and father I've ever met. Bret, thank you for allowing me to always chase my passions with reckless abandon and setting up all the orange cones along the way so no one gets hurt! Life is way more fun with you!

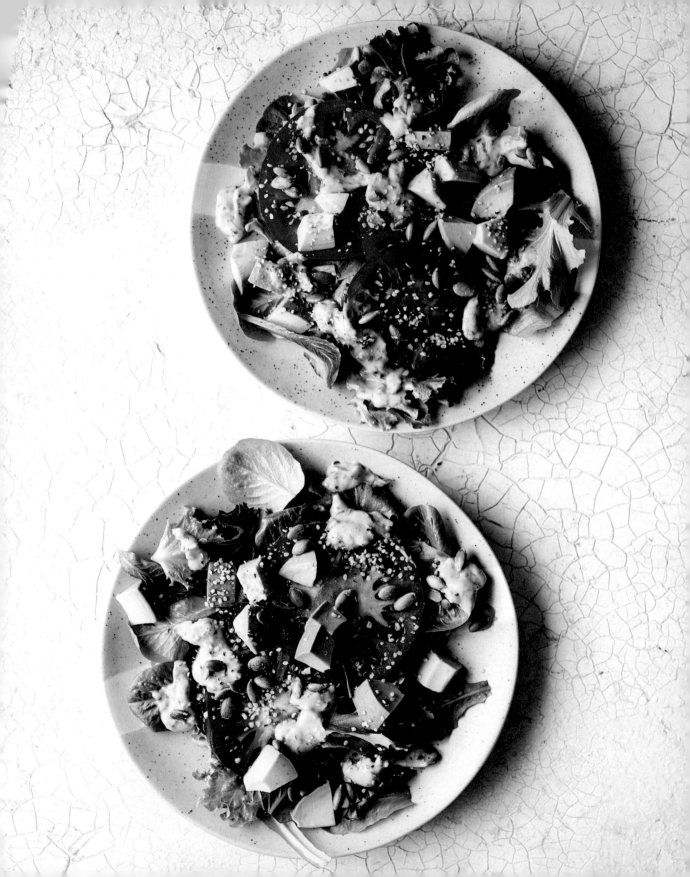

CONTENTS

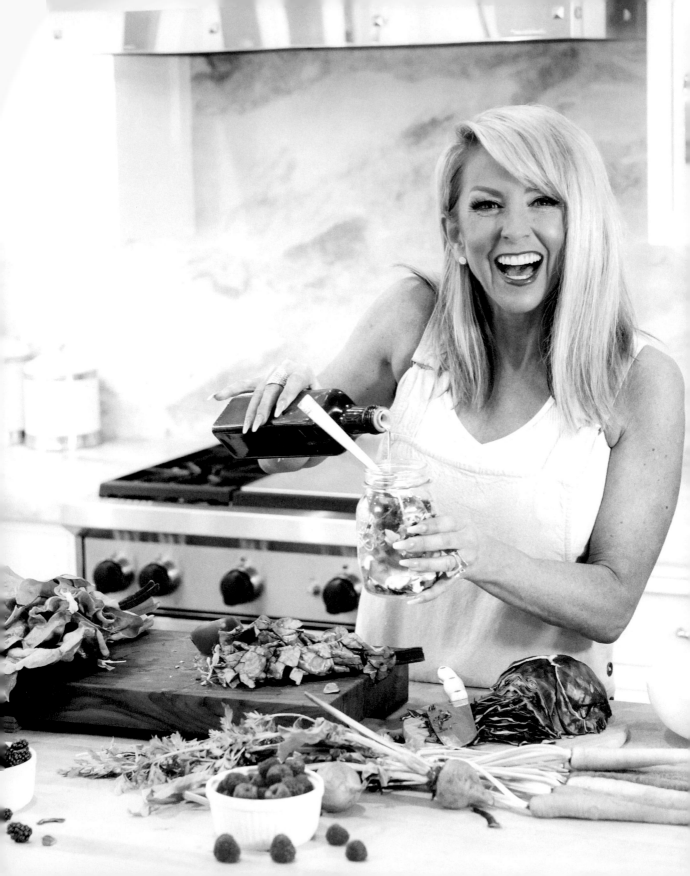

INTRODUCTION

What was I thinking? How could I have been so irresponsible, so trusting? Reflecting on the hypocrisy of it all stirs up a wave of emotions for me as feelings of regret and even anger start to bubble up. My close friend Dr. Mcayla likes to remind me that anger often masks more vulnerable feelings such as sadness, disappointment, or shame. (Sometimes it's a pain in the butt to have a friend who's a psychologist.)

EMOTION FUELS PASSION

Let me cut to the chase and get this off my chest. I need to start this book off with an apology. It is said that to whom much is given, much is expected. As a health and fitness expert for the past 25 years, I did not do my best to honor the role I was in. I can't go back and undo things I've done. If I said it, I meant it, even if I hadn't looked for science to substantiate my claims. My own health issues helped me to realize the depth of my responsibility as a leader in health and fitness, and how I had messed up.

My own health scare, followed by years of eye-opening, truth-seeking research and investigation, have brought me to a very different place mentally and physically than I was just three years ago. Have you ever noticed how ex-smokers are the folks most intolerant of smokers? Well, that's how I feel about the unhealthy health movement I was once a part of. It's why today I denounce my ways of the past, why I'm unaffected by the criticism and rejection by colleagues. I am fired up and devoted to seeking the truth and uncovering the greedy sabotaging way of the diet industry. I have spent the last three years of my professional career dedicated to making this right by you, debunking the bullshit, ignoring the trends, and getting the answers you deserve. Getting the answers *we* deserve.

As Eleanor Roosevelt said, "No one can make you feel inferior without your consent." If that's true, it means I volunteered to have the health and fitness industry make me feel like a failure for more than 25 years. That sucks. Who wants to feel like a victim? Not me! And that's why I wrote this book. I started this research because it was time to put an end to the stupidity and take back our health. We have to stop blindly following the misguided advice of fitness, nutrition, and so-called "wellness experts" who have marched us like soldiers onto the battlefield to wage an all-out war against our bodies. It's time for a rebellion.

Three years ago, as I was preparing to film my 200th (not an exaggeration) exercise video, I experienced a health scare that ended up creating a fork in the road of my life. The following months were fueled by the passion and emotion. But I also experienced a great deal of disappointment in myself. I was angry that I had ignored my common sense and willfully subjected my mind and body to dangerous extremes in diet, sleep, and exercise, all in the name of health. To make matters worse (as if I didn't feel bad enough already), I influenced a lot of people to follow my lead.

This is my opportunity to fix it.

That anger is gone today, replaced with pride. My passion is fueled by the confidence that comes with results: the proof! Today I have helped tens of thousands of people redefine and reclaim their health. I feel free, as if I've escaped the grips of a dangerous cult, ready to sneak back in the dead of night to rescue others!

Today I stand proudly as the trusted guide you deserve. This work is my labor of love. The 131 Method is how I make things right.

For decades, frankly, we've been brainwashed into believing that to achieve the perfect body, to lose weight, and be healthy, we simply need to eat fewer calories and exercise more. We believe magazine covers suggesting if we just cut that one thing (whether it's fat, carbs, or gluten), effortless weight loss and an Instagram-worthy physique is within our grasp. And it's not just the diet and fitness industry that's perpetuated these unhealthy, often conflicting ideas. Oftentimes this outdated and misguided information trickles down from the U.S. government and the medical establishment. I mean, when was the last time your health-care provider asked a few questions about your nutrition? *SO RARE!* We look for pills and potions to fix things—quickly. We've become obsessed with the notion that we must change, lift, sculpt, deprive, and pound our bodies into submission and lost all sight of health in the process.

And, despite our valiant efforts, we've never been unhealthier. Obesity has never been higher. According to the CDC, more than 70 percent of Americans are overweight and one-third of us are obese.[1] It doesn't take a brainiac to figure out that most of what we've been doing to lose weight and get healthy has completely backfired. Walk into an elementary school and it's hard to miss the generational impact of this nightmare. And how sad that when these dumb ideas don't work, we don't question their validity or ask if the advice we've been spoon-fed was scientifically substantiated. Nope, we just keep following along. We assume failure means we messed up. We should have tried harder. We blame ourselves when diets don't work.

Honestly, I struggle daily not to beat myself up that for years I ignored my own good sense when it came to so many beliefs around nutrition. Even as a health and fitness professional, I too accepted the ridiculous advice as legit simply because it was the predominant message. If enough really fit people are saying the same thing, isn't that all the proof we need? Uh . . . no.

I mean, the idea that any one diet or even any one fitness program will work for *everyone* makes about as much sense as one-size-fits-all skinny jeans. The notion that a 20-year-old man and a 60-year-old woman could expect optimal health by following the same plan defies logic. What was I thinking? Or rather, what were we *all* thinking?

As naturally curious and skeptical as I am, it bothers me to think I too was quick to accept common advice as fact. I can't help but feel regret that I never thought to question or research the validity of "expert" advice. Like most everyone else, I just accepted and often repeated the same thing all the other experts were saying, like *Eat every two to three hours. Never skip breakfast. Cut back on fat and eat more protein! Move more! Eat less. Look for zero-calorie snack packs. Down a bowl of oatmeal when you wake. Do more cardio. Only eat egg whites! Fat makes you fat. Drink this shake and eat this bar, but don't eat too much. Now move! Move more! Now add in some high-intensity, body-punishing cardio—and don't forget to stretch.* #nodaysoff

Most of what we hear from so-called health experts, weight loss companies, and even the U.S. government is based on well-intended guesswork blinded by profit-seeking entities, then repeated, regurgitated, and indoctrinated into our collective thinking. Who are we supposed to trust? Even our health-care system seems to want nothing to do with health. When most of our nation's medical costs are associated with diseases preventable though nutrition and lifestyle changes,[2] it seems ironic we refer to the management of sick people as a health-care system. (Don't get me started!)

Where do we turn when we want the truth? Who can we trust when food, diet, and fitness companies spend billions to promote flip-flopping fad diets and programs that contradict the message we were served last week?

Shoot, you'll hear these confusing voices just about everywhere, from social media to the five o'clock news. These ideas are so prevalent, so commonly cited, that eventually we ignore our common sense. We dismiss the fact that we're worse off and so too are most of our friends and family members. Not only do we choose to ignore the fact that something hasn't worked for us or anyone we know, but we make it worse by allowing this false information to form our beliefs.

I too ignored my own common sense and accepted many of these ideas as truth. As a health and fitness expert, I watched the people I was trying to help as they lost and gained the same weight over and over again. Every year they'd lose and gain, and then lose and gain—and gain and gain and gain. With rare exceptions, they always seemed to gain back *more* than what they'd initially lost.

I never thought to question the science behind the advice I was regurgitating. It felt safe to agree with the so-called experts. But here's the irony: I too was (and I am still today) known as a health and fitness expert. Millions of people look to me for guidance.

In fact, most late nights you can still flip on your TV and probably catch one of my fitness infomercials, like "Turbo Jam," "Turbo Fire," "ChaLean Extreme" or "PiYo." You'll hear me say, "You, too, can get these results in as little as 30 minutes a day while enjoying delicious meals like these." Now, to be clear, I would never *intentionally* mislead my audience, and many people *have* achieved outrageous results from my programs. I am very proud of those workouts. I believed what I was saying. I truly believed anyone could achieve those results if they followed the plan exactly. I just didn't believe it for me. I thought my metabolism must be defective.

PRACTICALLY FROM BIRTH WE ARE CONDITIONED TO BELIEVE WE ARE FLAWED.

The advice I was giving, the advice most all diet experts promote, just didn't work for me for a lot of reasons. To be clear, it wasn't that I was overweight. I just couldn't *lose* weight, and eventually just maintaining my weight turned into a tortured existence. Oh sure, I could point to many different reasons why this was going on, but eventually I settled on the explanation that I must have "bad genes." In reality my efforts just to maintain my weight had now become a full-time, all-consuming battle. I never set out to be a fitness or nutrition expert. I really had no clue the workouts I was creating in my living room would catch on in health clubs and eventually be transformed into infomercials seen by tens of millions of people around the world. I was just trying to solve my own problem, and now people were looking to me for the solution. By 2005, I was an internationally recognized health and fitness expert. I felt like the whole thing was snowballing and there was no way for me to stop it. My personal struggle with my metabolism only complicated things further. I was suffering from what is commonly known as imposter syndrome.

IMPOSTER SYNDROME: *a belief that you don't belong. A feeling of doubt or persistent fear of being exposed as a "fraud" despite experience and or evidence of one's credentials, competence, or experience. An individual doubts their accomplishments and has a persistent internalized fear of being exposed. Despite their credibility, the individual does not feel worthy of the identity and often attributes their success to luck or deception.*

CAN YOU RELATE?

Yup. That was me. I felt like what a financial adviser who secretly had to file for bankruptcy must feel like. I was embarrassed by my malfunctioning metabolism. Was I broken? I couldn't follow the advice I was giving to others because it didn't work for me. Somehow I missed the fact it wasn't working for *anyone*.

My first infomercial, "Turbo Jam," appeared on TV in 2005. And each year that my programs aired, I found myself exercising more, yet my metabolism got slower and slower. At this point I had given up on the idea that I might be able to lose a few pounds. I was too busy trying to figure out why my metabolism was working against me. Because I thought I couldn't afford to gain even a pound, I felt I had no choice but to eat less and try to exercise more, just to maintain. My workouts were getting longer and more punishing, lasting two to four hours most days. My body was tired. I knew I was overtraining. I couldn't sleep. I couldn't keep up this pace. Maybe I was eating too much? Out of options, I cut down on my calorie intake, stripped the fat from my diet, and adopted the strictest of habits. I wouldn't dare allow myself a cheat meal, let alone a cheat day. It was pretty brutal. Despite the crazy amount of discipline and time I sacrificed, I could justify it because at least I looked healthy. (Oh the irony!)

By this point I was in my mid-forties (I'm 50 today) and this relentless cycle was taking its toll. I pressed on and ignored all the signs of my diminishing health. To fit in extra workouts, I woke most days by 4:30 A.M. I couldn't sleep. I was tired all the time. I could no longer multitask or handle too much sound or commotion. I couldn't focus. I became painfully forgetful. My vocabulary suffered. I would walk into a room and not remember why I was there or get in my car and forget where I was going. I just didn't feel like myself. My joints were achy and swollen. Every day at 3 P.M. my head would start throbbing. My face was swollen, my stomach was bloated, and my hair was thinning. I woke most days feeling like I was 90 years old. Everything hurt. Despite my strict diet and exercise routine, my body fat started to creep up. I felt doughy and soft.

BUT I COULD BARELY STAY AWAKE.

My family doctor politely suggested what I was experiencing was "just a part of getting older." "Maybe you're going through menopause," he remarked. I was 46. But I wasn't buying that explanation. Something wasn't right. Certain I needed testing, I persuaded him to refer me to a neurologist.

And there I sat in the office of world-renowned neurologist Daniel Amen, anxiously awaiting the results of my brain scan and nutritional panel. I tried to reassure myself, *What do I have to worry about?* I had spent the past 25 years dedicated to the pursuit of health and fitness and helping others to do the same. I had a number one fitness TV infomercial. I had sold tens of millions of exercise DVDs and created fitness programs featured in health clubs around the globe! (Now, I'm not one to boast, but I had to remind myself that I had helped a lot of people. Surely I must have known what I'm doing!) Shoot, I had taught Kelly Ripa and Michael Strahan how to do a three-person plank on live TV!

I exercised every day and my diet was "clean." Girl, you're tripping, I thought to myself.

Dr. Amen's pensive expression, followed by a series of peculiar questions, foreshadowed the dire news to come. "Now, just to be clear . . . You mentioned you exercise regularly? And can we talk about your diet for a moment? And may I ask if you have had chemotherapy or if you're a habitual IV drug user now or in the past?"

Huh? I thought he must have someone else's results.

My face must have given away my defensive thoughts. He quipped, "There's no denying you *look* healthy, but your test results tell us a different story."

Spread across his desk were my results—measures of what was really going on inside my body. My nutritional panel showed I was deficient in nearly every essential nutrient. My inflammatory markers were through the roof, and my brain health, by his assessment, required immediate intervention. The SPECT scan (which shows brain function) revealed a rather severe case of decreased perfusion (low blood flow) to critical areas of my brain. The room suddenly felt like it was closing in on me. He asked again if I had a recent bout of chemotherapy or a history of drug and/or alcohol abuse.

"No!" I answered.

Sensing my anxiety he explained that the dimpled appearance on the surface of my brain revealed a pattern often associated with toxicity or a brain infection. He added that most often this pattern is seen after certain chemotherapy treatments, in cases of severe chronic dehydration, and in drug addicts and alcoholics. None of these conditions were the cause of my diminished cognitive function. I was about to find out how my nutrition and lifestyle choices had resulted in this damage.

The good news was that I finally had some answers to explain my brain fog, irritability, and forgetfulness. The bad news was that I was on the fast track to early-onset Alzheimer's disease.

Fame as a health and fitness expert, a low body fat percentage, and the number of likes on my last Instagram post were suddenly irrelevant. I had just been given a failing grade.

I spent the next hour in his office as he explained what I was up against and how my lifestyle choices may have contributed. I maintained my smile and positive disposition, then walked to the parking lot, sat in my car, and sobbed.

I LITERALLY CRIED MY LASH STRIPS RIGHT OFF!

The tears weren't for me; they were for my kids, Brock and Cierra. How could I have done this? How could I not have known the damage I was doing? And how had my choices impacted their health, their future? I let it all out, then vowed from that day forward everything would be different. I was going to get to the bottom of this, study the research, follow the advice of the world's most knowledgeable experts, and heal myself.

Thus began my three-year quest to figure out where, what, and how this had happened. And if it happened to me, what about the millions of other people who had been listening to the same experts? How is it we know more about the body, food, nutrition, and exercise than ever before, yet obesity rates continue to rise all over the world? We have apps to count our steps and tell us if what we're eating is "good" or "bad" for us. We can buy fat-free chocolate, gluten-free pasta, and sugar-free cocktails, yet diabetes, heart disease, and other illnesses with dietary links are at epidemic proportions. Unhealthy diet contributes to approximately 678,000 deaths each year in the United States from nutrition-related diseases, such as heart disease, cancer, and type 2 diabetes.[3]

I now know that in my case, much of the damage was caused by dietary and lifestyle choices I believed were healthy. Ironically, the foods I was eating in an attempt to keep my calorie count low were actually contributing to a condition known as gut permeability, or "leaky gut." The irritation created by stress, over-exercising, and eating such fake foods as articial sweeteners and fat-free, low-fat, and zero-calorie versions of anything I could find had resulted in low-grade gut inflammation, which thins the intestinal walls. This results in malabsorption, a slower metabolism, imbalanced hormones, weight gain, and countless other negative effects.

The last three years of my life have been devoted to an intense study of our biology, nutrition, and the real science of weight loss. What I learned forced me to question everything I once believed to be true—what I had been feeding my family and myself, and the advice I was sharing with the people who trusted me. The fact is, not only had I fallen prey to the diet and fitness dogma, but I had been a part of the problem . . . on a global scale. Ouch.

Armed with my research, interviews, and the advice of top experts, I was able to successfully balance my hormones, heal my gut, reverse the damage to my brain, master my metabolism, and get healthy from the inside out. First, I assembled a team of true health experts consisting of more than ten registered dieticians, integrative and functional medical doctors, and the top researchers in metabolism and gut health. I set out to determine which health issues could create a domino effect. Next, we prioritized these issues. Finally, I identified one powerful health objective and created a nutritional plan to achieve that while allowing for personalization. I followed the plan for three weeks, to mimic the natural cycle of seasonal phasing our ancestors experienced. I then followed those three weeks with one week of fasting and refueling, to rest and rebuild the strength of my digestive system (which happens to be responsible for 70 to 80 percent of your immune function). Let me recap that formula . . .

I GET ASKED ALL THE TIME WHAT 131 MEANS . . . NOW YOU KNOW!

- 1 Health Objective
- 3 Weeks of Diet Phasing
- 1 Week to Fast and Refuel

The results were nothing less than astonishing. In June of 2017 I returned to the Amen Clinic to retest. This time my nutrition panel revealed nearly zero deficiencies. I had reversed nearly all disease factors, balanced my hormones, healed my gut and my brain, and reclaimed my health. I did this not with a pill or magic potion but by following the customizable framework of the 131 Method.

Dr. Amen beamed as he presented my follow-up results. He remarked that my brain was now "aging in reverse." He has since proudly shared my results on his PBS special and on *The Dr. Oz Show*, to name just a few.

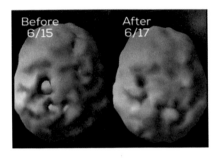

The image above is a side-by-side comparison of my brain using SPECT imaging. The image on the left was in June of 2015. Large divots, and white areas represent regions of the brain where I was receiving little to no blood flow. The image on the right is from exactly two years later following the 131 Method detailed in this book.

Today I don't just look healthy, I am healthy. I have no brain fog. Headaches are rare, as is bloating, soreness, and fatigue. I never count calories or deprive myself of foods I want to eat. I'm consuming things I once thought I had to give up for good. The mystery of weight loss is gone. I now know what it feels like to effortlessly maintain my weight. Now my workouts are for me! I choose activities that make me feel restored and strong. By eating more and exercising less, my body is getting better results! My cognitive function continues to improve and I can't say that I've ever had this much energy. My skin looks better and my body feels, well . . . young. At 50, I have a regular cycle, and none of the premenopausal symptoms I once experienced. I feel better today than I have in my entire life. I finally know what it feels like to feel good.

ALL OF THIS IS POSSIBLE FOR YOU TOO!

The moment I started this quest, I made a commitment to share my discoveries. This journey was the catalyst for *131 Method*. I want this for you!

Today I'm on a mission to set the story straight and share with you what you deserve to know—the truth.

You are way too smart to waste precious time on another dumb diet. *131 Method* will teach you how to be healthy from the inside out.

You won't need to question the validity of what you read in this book. *131 Method* isn't based on what I think, anecdotal finding, or what I've heard others say. *131 Method* includes the most current, credible, scientifically validated, and Nobel award–winning research on autophagy and metabolism. Together with a team of experts this method was tested and perfected over and over and over again. More than 25,000 people took part in the testing and personalization of this program before we officially released it to the public in March. This book includes the findings of experts: specialized doctors, top researchers, and registered dietitians. When it comes to hormones, leaky gut, inflammation, nutrition, weight loss, and metabolism, they know their stuff.

ALWAYS BE OPEN TO NEW SCIENCE!

If there's one thing I've learned after several years of immersing myself in the science of human health and metabolism, it's that we have a lot to learn. If we are to avoid falling into the trap of blind acceptance again, we must at every turn be willing to rethink our beliefs as science-based discoveries improve.

When it comes to gut health, metabolism, the brain, and how connected these all are to our overall health, there is still so much we have to learn. With that in mind, step one on this path to your new life is to keep an open mind. Clinging to a diet identity or an inflexible belief is a recipe for disaster. When we know better, we must do better.

131 Method isn't a book about getting skinny. *131 Method* is about being smart and getting healthy.

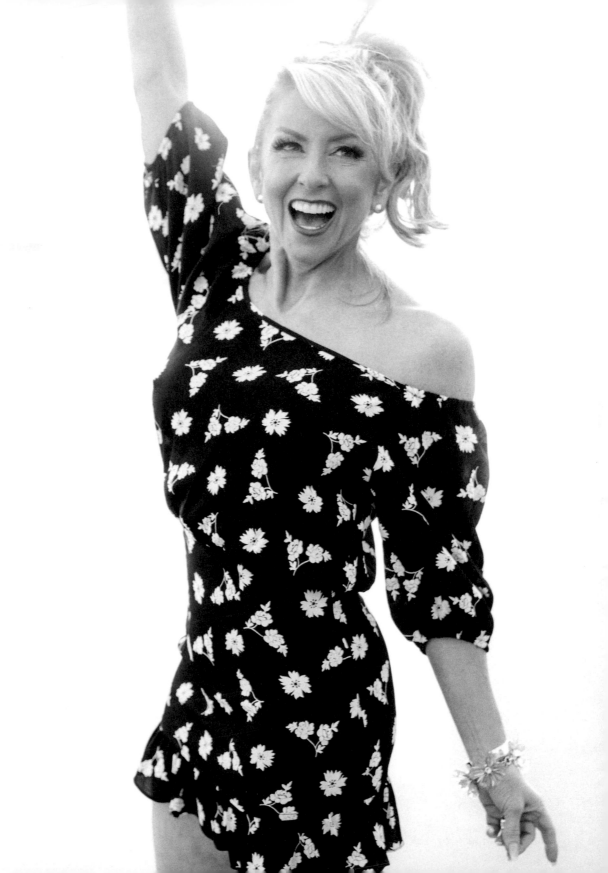

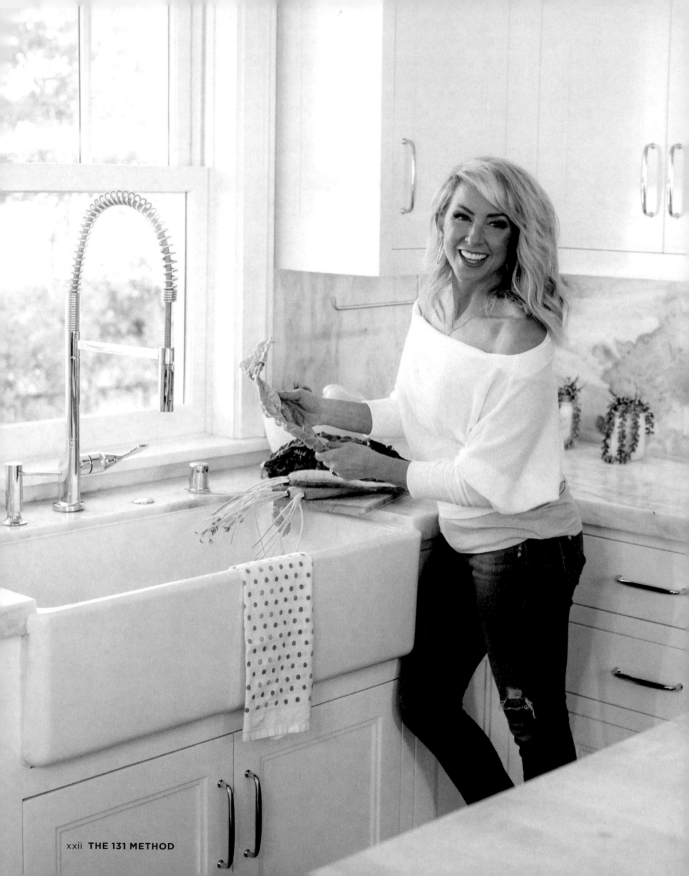

PART I

ERASING FALSE BELIEFS AND UNDERSTANDING YOUR BIOLOGY

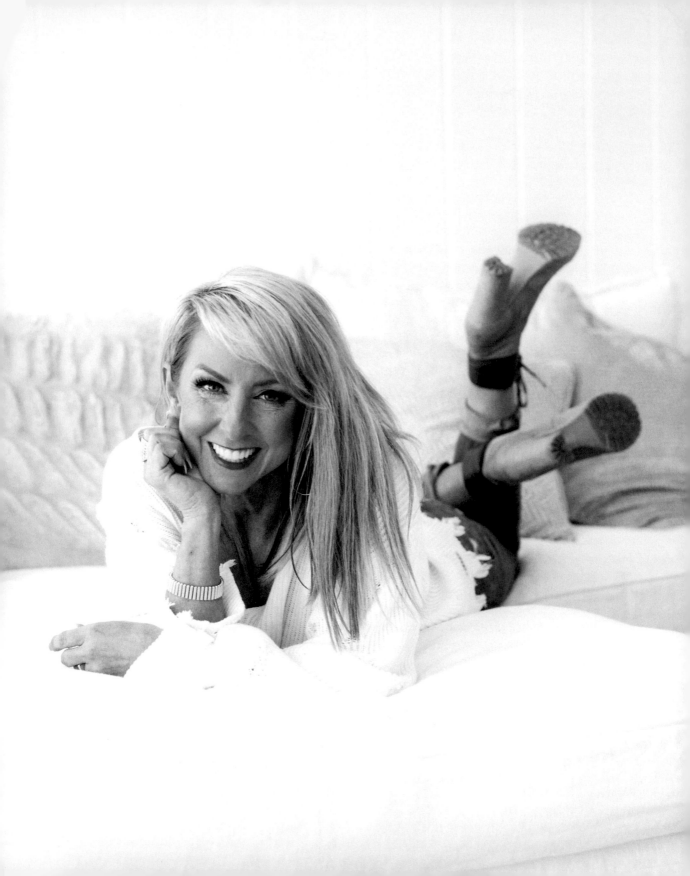

CHAPTER 1

MY STORY IS YOUR STORY

I'm a wife and mother of two, and I pride myself on being a mom first—all else comes second. Next to family, my life pretty much revolves around helping people live happier, healthier lives. I've created and starred in more than 200 exercise videos; written a *New York Times* best-selling book about productivity, *Push*; and hosted a top-ranked podcast on health and wellness, *The Chalene Show*. Yet even with my own 30 years of experience in health and wellness, I, just like you, fell into the "diet trap"—constantly trying to eat less, or following one person's arbitrary set of food rules, only to lose weight, gain it back, and slow my metabolism in the process.

Growing up in the Midwest (I'm a Michigan girl), I thought it was normal that most of the adults I knew, including those in my family, were overweight and always either on a diet or talking about when they would start the next one. I remember how unhappy they all seemed and how, no matter what they did, those same people were *still* overweight. As a child, I put one and one together and formed the belief that going on a diet would make you unhappy and overweight. I surely didn't want to diet, so I turned to exercise. I figured that as long as I did long bouts of cardio every day, I wouldn't gain weight and I would be happy. I still needed to watch what I ate, but surely I could out-exercise my "weight gain" genes!

Fear fueled my extreme discipline. I was terrified to miss a workout. I lived in a constant state of low-grade panic. Little did I realize I was creating a vicious cycle. The more

BTW...THIS EXTRA SPACE ISN'T JUST FOR MY NOTES, IT'S FOR YOUR NOTES!

I exercised and the fitter I became, the less effective my workout was as my metabolism and body adapted to it by burning fewer and fewer calories. The harder and longer my workouts, the slower my metabolism worked. The slower my metabolism worked, the more I had to cut back on calories. Cutting back on calories triggered my body to believe I was in a state of famine, which in turn signaled my body to store fat and slow calorie burn even more. Like a hamster in a cage, no matter how fast or how hard I worked, I wasn't moving.

As all of this was going on, my career as a fitness professional continued to take off. I was asked to develop programs for the nation's top health clubs. I became a featured expert in health and fitness publications, speaking at conventions and filming several fitness videos a month.

Even though I was thought of as one of the world's most recognized fitness trainers, I felt like I had no business being there. I never talked about how many hours I had to exercise each week just to maintain my weight. This embarrassed me. Even at my leanest, I never felt fit or strong enough.

WAKING UP TO HOW MESSED UP THE FITNESS WORLD IS

One day, as I was preparing to start shooting a new consumer fitness program, one of the producers scheduled a call with my husband. I thought that was odd. Why would the producer want to discuss preparations for the project with him instead of with me directly? Bret took the call in our home office, and I went about my business. When he finished, I could tell he was disturbed, so I pestered and prodded and poked until he reluctantly opened up.

This producer had suggested that Bret have a conversation with me about getting in tip-top shape for the project. Said producer added, "We think her next program would crush the market if she maybe lost a little weight, tightened up, you know . . . just really got that inspirational physique that all women want."

OR TALL ENOUGH, OR SMART ENOUGH, OR PRETTY ENOUGH, OR YOUNG ENOUGH . . . YOU GET THE PICTURE.

I felt my face flush. I can't even tell you how ashamed and humiliated I felt that someone had called my husband to share this suggestion. In my overactive imagination I pictured a roomful of executives, red pens in their hands, gathered around a high-def blown-up photo of me. I could picture them circling every dimple, wrinkle, roll, and stretch mark. Of course, the call only confirmed what I was saying all along in my own head. Even though the conversation had been private, I felt exposed to the world. This was confirmation of my deepest insecurities; I didn't belong here.

But I wasn't going to go down without a fight. I thought maybe if I lost a few pounds I would actually feel like I deserved to be called a health and fitness expert. (Holy cow, that's hard to type. It's just so crazy to me now to look back and see how unhealthy all of this was!) Whether fueled by the shame or fear of being found out, in that moment I stopped caring about my health. I had been given my orders and I was on a no-fail mission to lose weight via any means necessary.

I wanted desperately to prove myself worthy of an identity I felt I didn't deserve. Although I rarely weighed myself, that day I jumped on the scale. I looked between my toes and through the tears in my eyes to see that I was *already* at the lowest weight I had ever been in my adult life. How was I going to lose weight when I was already eating a clean diet and exercising for hours and hours a day?

OR SO I THOUGHT

I decided to go on a *serious* diet!

I was determined to get a body that people would find inspirational and prove to the producers and the world that I *belonged*. First, I tried a diet created for fitness models to get them ready for competition. That didn't work. Then I tried a low-fat, high-protein crash-meal plan. Nothing changed. I tried going the low-carb route, then gluten-free. I tried only drinking shakes, tracking just my macronutrients, eating like a cavewoman, and following several popular diets you've probably toyed with, too. You name it, I tried it. Over the course of the next 90 days, I did them all, but nothing worked.

There had to be something wrong with me. I decided I had only one thing left to do, and that was diet *harder*, or crash diet. I cut my calories and portion sizes back even further and added even more exercise to my daily grind. I rarely drank water so I wouldn't hold on to extra fluids. (BTW, drinking less to look leaner is one of the *worst* pieces of advice floating around fitness circles!) Sound miserable? It was. But after a few weeks, guess what? I lost a few pounds, enough to please the producers.

When you shoot a consumer video, a team of people have to sign off on every detail, including hair, makeup, and outfit for each cast member. Most fitness folks would think it a dream come true to be in a workout video. I, however, was now feeling very self-conscious. There I was, 45 years old, standing half-naked in my tight shorts and crop top awaiting approval from a table of decision makers. After months of dieting, I had never been so thin or felt so weak.

I carefully followed the eyes and subsequent facial expressions of each person as he or she scanned my body up and down in silence. If someone had a comment, it was often whispered to another member of the production team—presumably so as not to embarrass me. Picture yourself standing half-naked in front of a small group of adults whispering comments about and judging your physique. I know it's their job. I know they were just trying to make sure I looked my best, but I wanted to scream, "Make it stop!"

When they were finished examining me, they said, "You look really good! We're really happy with your body." On our first day of shooting, I posted a few pics to my Instagram. I knew I looked gaunt and that my muscles had lost their volume. A few people commented things like, "You've lost weight and you look horrible!" and "Chalene, are you anorexic?" But 99.9 percent of the comments were alarmingly positive. To this day, people ask me what diet I was following when I shot that workout. Now you know.

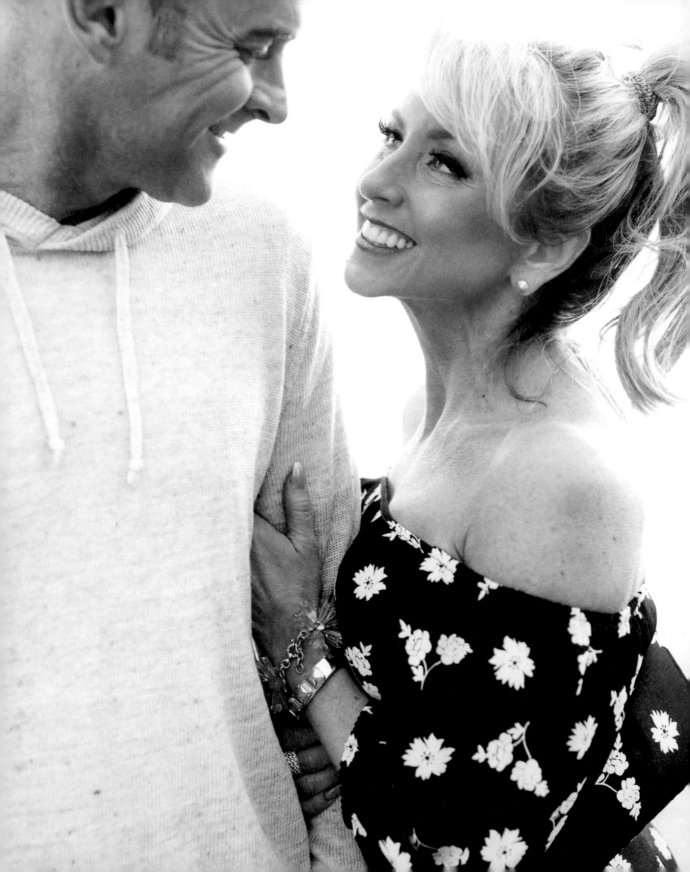

Looking back I realize how messed up it all was. At the time, I was knee deep in an industry that categorizes you as "healthy" based on how low your body fat is. Period. It had nothing to do with health. I was being celebrated for my efforts despite how unhealthy I truly was.

No one made me do it; I did it to myself. I take full responsibility for my decisions and actions. I could have declined the project, but I didn't. I wanted to look the part. My mental and physical states were deteriorating. Between takes I would rush to my dressing room and cry for no reason. My emotions were out of control. My skin, sleep, hair, and hormones were a mess. All I could think about were the foods I could and couldn't eat. I felt like such a fraud. The shoot included several workouts and lasted about a week. Once it was complete, it wasn't like I went crazy. I didn't binge or overindulge. I just returned to my previous (and still very disciplined) eating and exercise habits. Within a month's time so, too, returned the couple of pounds that I had lost—and then some.

I DIDN'T REALIZE UNTIL LATER HOW MUCH HAPPINESS IS IMPACTED BY PROPER NUTRITION.

HOW DID THIS HAPPEN TO US?

Sound familiar? Surely you have your own story of weight gain, weight loss, or just not being able to lose a pound despite your best efforts. Regardless of the details that separate our stories, there are certain things I'm sure they share in common. When we gain weight after a diet, we blame ourselves. We let time pass and then we go on another dumb diet. Each time it becomes harder because now we've trashed and slowed our metabolism, which makes weight gain inevitable. (It sucks!) We wind up miserably disappointed in our bodies, annoyed by everything in our closet, angry about the situation, and desperate to find that magical diet.

Diet Facts

- 95 percent of people who go on a diet gain all the weight back, and then some. (This means 95 percent of dieters feel like failures.)
- Quick fixes often turn into long-term problems.
- Weight loss supplements are a great way to waste your money.
- Diets disrupt gut health and hormone balance.
- Diets increase stress hormones that slow the metabolism and tell the body to store fat.
- Hitting your goal weight doesn't mean you're healthy.
- Diets diminish your confidence.
- Dieting is associated with increased steady weight gain and higher incidences of binge eating.
- Those who regularly diet are five times more likely to develop an eating disorder than those who don't.
- Most diets cause an imbalance of hunger hormones.
- Restricting calories slows the metabolism. Nutritional ketosis, when used sporadically, increases the metabolism.
- Banning any one food group as "bad" results in the tendency to binge and eat those foods.
- There is no one diet or superfood that works for everyone.
- Most diets are deficient in the essential nutrients needed for optimal physical, mental, and cellular health.
- Counting calories is questionable . . . at best.
- Going on a diet is dumb and you're smart!

One-size-fits-all diet and exercise programs leave us feeling like failures. But why did we ever think they would work? From an evolutionary standpoint, our ancestors had to thrive despite seasonal changes to their diet and activity. The idea of a standard, year-round diet is only as old as the Industrial Revolution and the advent of commercialized farming, urban labor, and mass food production. Consumerism moves at a much quicker pace than human evolution.

That's why, with the 131 Method, I will guide you step-by-step through the process of customizing your personal plan. You'll understand what's really going on in *your* body and how to take control of your health; then you'll design a plan that fits your own unique lifestyle. The 131 Method isn't a one-size-fits-all plan with simplified rules or a universal list of what you can and cannot eat. That's called a diet, and diets are dumb, *but you're not.* To date, more than 50,000 individuals have experienced the 131 method through my online program. When you follow the 131 Method, you'll confidently learn why certain foods affect you the way they do. (Even foods that are supposedly "healthy" for others can be terrible for you!) You'll also learn to phase your diet and how to improve your health with simple lifestyle changes. Dieting has a potentially harmful effect on all relationships and ultimately your happiness. Diets impact how you feel about food, yourself, and others. Diets have the power to rob us of our joy, fill us with self-doubt, trigger addiction and self-loathing, and set us up for a lifetime of feeling inadequate. When diets fail, we take to highly edited Instagram posts as if to pour salt in the wound of self-comparison.

PLEASE READ HER STORY!

The first week I lost 6 lbs. My wedding ring fit again. I lost 15 pounds and over 20 inches in the first time through all three phases. I eat when I'm hungry. My brain fog lifted; my energy is steady from the time I get up until the time I go to bed. I sleep better. My bloating went away. The 131 Method has changed me. I never feel deprived. I feel satisfied. I am able to make positive choices. I can actually sit in a room with people eating ice cream or chips and I am not craving that type of food, nor do I feel tempted. It's so amazingly weird to feel this good. I finally feel very comfortable in my own skin.
—DARLENE HIME

REPEAT AFTER ME . . .
DIETS ARE DUMB—I'M NOT!

You know all of this to be true. You know diets don't work, yet it's so common to repeat the cycle over and over. Change can be scary, even when we know it's the right thing to do. Change is good! Your body thrives on change.

THE FOUR S'S: SCIENCE, SELF, SUCCESS, AND SANITY

Before I go into the details of the 131 Method, I'd like to start with a few guiding principles. Naturally, there will be moments when you will question the process, especially when so much of the information in The 131 Method flies in the face of what you've been brainwashed to believe about diets, health, and wellness. When that happens, return to this page and review what I call the Four S's to help you build your confidence and personalize your experience.

Science: When presented with any suggestion that that doesn't sit right with you, check the science. Consider the date of the research and which organization commissioned the study. If the research is several years or even decades old, there are likely newer findings to consider. Keep in mind that big food companies and food marketers, and even prescription drug companies, have a financial interest in finding and paying the right researchers who will come up with results that favor their products and services.

Self: No one knows you like you. When evaluating lifestyle and dietary changes, consider your age, experience, track record, disease risk, personal history, financial situation, and preferences. Then make your choices based on what you know about yourself. This doesn't mean you have permission to make excuses, but it does mean you know what is going to work for you better than anyone. Factor in what you know about how your brain and body respond. The only person who ultimately decides exactly how you do this is you.

Success: How do you define success? I ask you to consider more than just your physical objectives. That goal of looking like an Instagram fitness model might result in a great-looking bikini bod, but at what cost? Consider what it means to be healthy from a whole-person perspective. How you define success will dictate the actions and choices you're willing to make. You have to know how you define success because your plan and approach must be geared toward that objective. Success to you may be to have no more headaches, lose weight, or resolve knee pain.

Sanity: You get to decide what to eat, when to eat, and how you need to customize the 131 Method. Should you struggle with a decision, ask yourself, "What is best for me? Will this new habit make me unhappy, or is it just part of the process of becoming a healthier version of me?" The journey to a happier, healthier you should improve your mental well-being, not make you feel crazy.

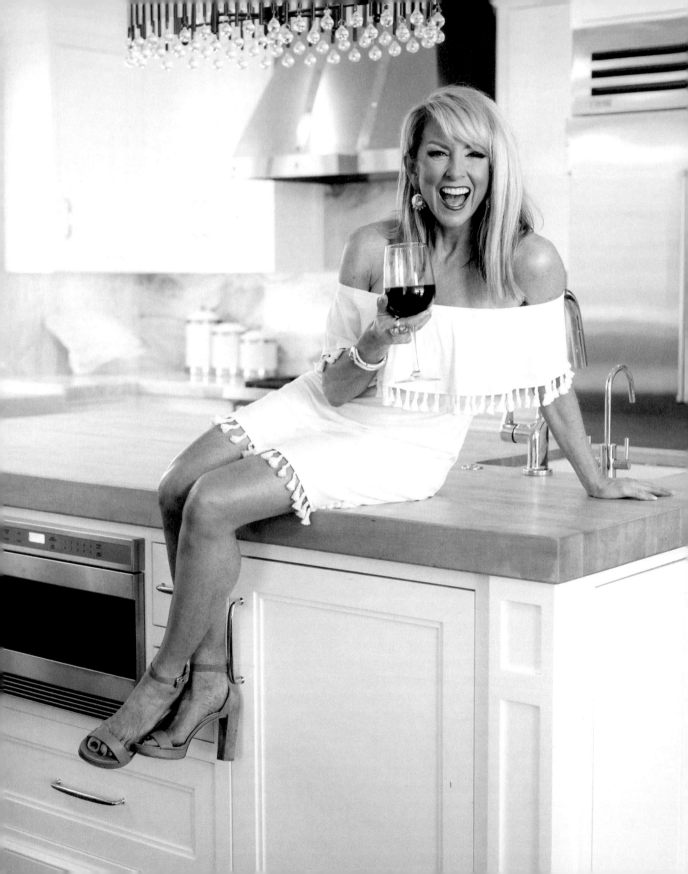

CHAPTER 2
HOW THE 131 METHOD WORKS

WE CAN FIX THIS—HERE'S HOW

We can and *will* fix the dieting trap. I've helped tens of thousands of people just like you end this vicious cycle, find freedom for diet dogma, and transform into happier, healthier people. And you cannot mess this up. Just please remember that I ask you to follow each chapter in the order I've laid out (no skipping ahead). I promise this method will work for you because it will be co-designed by you (a soon-to-be highly informed version of you!).

I suspect the biggest difference between this approach and anything else you've tried is that *you* will be in charge. My role is to be your guide. This book is a condensed, high-level summary of the very intricate system that makes up your metabolism. I will simplify the science, sort through myths and misconceptions, and offer a framework for you to make this work on your terms. You won't need me to tell you what to do. You've been down that road before. Instead, I'm going to give you all the information and options you need to make the right choices for the next 12 weeks. You can apply none, some, or all of the suggestions I make. What you put in is what you will get out. (You need to own it!) I'm going to offer my suggestions based on peer-reviewed research, but they will be just that: *suggestions*. It's your body and your health, and ultimately you have to decide what is important.

GET EXCITED! YOUR WHOLE LIFE IS ABOUT TO GET BETTER

← WINE? YUP. WE'LL TALK ABOUT ALCOHOL SOON.

HERE'S HOW THIS BOOK WORKS:

There are 7.7 billion people on the planet and no two of us are exactly the same. Unlike a typical diet, when you follow the 131 Method you'll customize the approach to work for you. To do that, you need a strong understanding of how your metabolism works. In the first chapters I will simplify the latest research and findings on metabolism, plus energy use and storage. You will understand how your food impacts your hormones, what it takes to speed up your metabolism, and how to improve gut health and use stored body fat as fuel. Fear not! You're going to master this stuff, including the latest research on how your body was meant to heal.

I PROMISE TO KEEP THIS STUFF INTERESTING, LIKE A MINI SKIRT: SHORT ENOUGH TO KEEP YOUR ATTENTION AND LONG ENOUGH TO COVER THE IMPORTANT PARTS! YOU'LL BEGIN TO FEEL LIKE AN EXPERT BEFORE YOU'RE EVEN HALFWAY THROUGH THE BOOK.

Now before we start talking meal plans and recipes, we're going to dig into the stuff that matters—mind-set. I'll help you understand what it takes to shift your thinking, drop the dieter's mentality, and create the habits that fortify your success.

I know that some readers will want to skip the why of the 131 Method and jump to the "What do I eat and when?" section. Those are the people still searching for a diet, a quick fix. Not you. You're not interested in wasting time. You understand that in order to end the cycle of dieting and become the healthiest version of yourself, you need to commit to understanding how your body works. The mystery of your metabolism and the secret to true health come together when you understand a few key principles: homeostasis, the role of inflammation, inflammatory foods, how your gut microbiome impacts hormones, your weight, and overall immunity. By understanding these things first you'll know why your body responds and reacts the way it does. This foundation will give you the information you need to customize every part of the 131 Method.

Next we'll set aside the science to help you get prepared to start! We'll dig into mind-set and uncover subconscious and often habitual thinking that may be holding you hostage. I'll share with you how minor adjustments you make today can help ensure your success, including establishing accountability, creating measures, increasing water intake, getting better sleep, choosing the right type of exercise, supplements, and more. I'll also teach you how to customize your meal plan using your personal favorites or selecting from the more than 100 simple and delicious recipes you'll find in Part III. And throughout the book you'll find inspirational stories from people just like you who have changed their lives and turned their health around by adopting the 131 Method.

It's in Part II of the book that I'll break down the three different cycles, or dietary phases. The 131 Method consists of three different phases: Ignite, Nourish, and Renew. Each phase lasts four weeks. Because each phase has been designed to tackle a primary health objective, you'll cycle or change up how and what you eat. In each phase you spend three weeks following a specific dietary approach. After the first three weeks, you can continue to follow the meal plan for one more week, or you can choose to fast and refuel. (Chapter 5 goes into the whys, how-tos, and ins and outs of fasting, but don't worry! It's not mandatory and there are plenty of options for me to share with you.)

Finally, I'll help you to understand how to maintain your healthy lifestyle long after 12 weeks and apply the principles of the 131 Method to your life.

Let's break down the phase framework:

- **1** health objective for each phase
- **3** weeks of diet phasing
- **1** week to fast and refuel

DIET PHASING = FREEDOM!

PHASE 1: IGNITE

KETO-ISH

The first phase is Ignite. Ignite cranks up your metabolism and sets it on fire! Your body will go from sugar-burning to fat-burning mode, or ketosis, and learn to use stored body fat as fuel. On Ignite you'll enjoy satisfying, delicious meals high in healthy fats and low in carbohydrates. You'll also learn how to use intermittent fasting to supercharge your fat-burning results and stabilize your appetite. You'll eat foods that reduce inflammation, balance hormones, and promote gut healing.

Depending on your goals, on the final week of Ignite you'll follow an optional plan to fast and refuel. Should you choose to fast, you'll spend the first few days on a custom-designed and supported fast to rest the gut, correct your appetite, and emotionally detach from food. You'll finish out the final Ignite week with a personalized refueling plan to help you reengineer your newly rebuilt immune system.

PHASE 2: NOURISH

EAT MORE GREENS

Nourish builds on the fat-burning foundation of Ignite while increasing your body's ability to metabolize micronutrients found in whole foods and plants. Over the course of these three weeks, you'll gradually cut back on animal proteins and increase consumption of vegetables and plant-based healthy fats.

As in Ignite, the fourth and final week of Nourish ends with fasting and refueling. During the first few days of that week, you'll start with one of four fasting options to rest your gut. You'll finish out the week with a personalized refueling plan to boost immunity and increase gut microbiome diversity.

MAKING PEACE
WITH CARBS

PHASE 3: RENEW

Renew is the last four-week phase. By the time you reach Renew, you will have mastered fat burning and intermittent fasting and dramatically improved your insulin sensitivity. You will have figured out which foods are personally problematic and, as a result, will see reduced inflammation

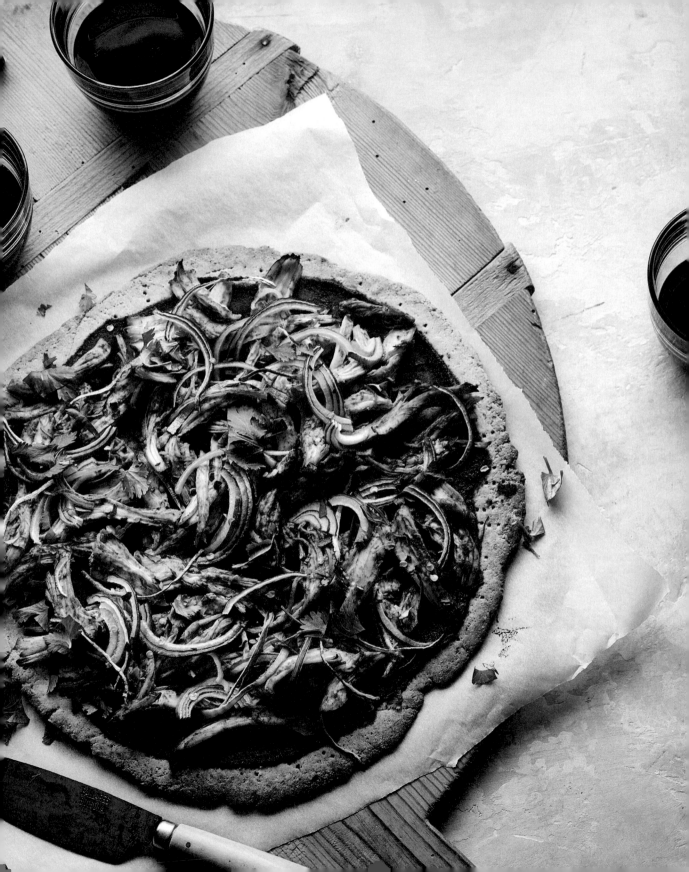

and water retention. Most of all, you will feel amazing! Renew will teach you how to use fats, proteins, and yes, even carbs, for energy! It's in Renew that your body will effectively use all macronutrients for energy, which is called macrophasing.

Macrophasing, which is explained in detail in Chapter 8, provides the ultimate approach to metabolic flexibility by changing or "phasing" your macronutrient ratio of carbohydrates, protein, and fats every two to three days. With guidelines and my recipes, you'll design a meal plan to best suit your lifestyle. You'll enjoy carbs, fats, and proteins and experience the joy of a metabolism that works with you, not against you.

Just as in previous phases, the fourth week of Nourish ends with an optional personalized fast and refueling plan. By that point you'll be a 131 Method pro!

CHOOSE YOUR HARD

I'm a realist. I'm not going to sugarcoat the fact that changing our beliefs and challenging much of what we've been force-fed for decades is going to take some work.

The struggle is real.

One of my closest friends recently started the 131 Method. I texted her to see how it was going. She replied, "Great! But it's really hard to pay attention to what I'm putting in my body." To which I texted back, "True! But it's also really hard to be unhealthy and look and feel older than your age . . . not that you do, because you're gorgeous and hot, but you know what I'm saying." We have to choose our hard.

To no avail I embarked on an exhaustive Google search to figure out who originally coined the phrase "Choose your hard." The first time I heard it, I was at a Tony Robbins motivational event. It stuck. I've considered having it tattooed next to the tiny palm tree on my right ankle that I got on spring break at age 18. (Dumb idea.) The fact is, we do have choices, and sometimes all options involve some difficulty.

There are going to be setbacks. Expect them and press forward. There are going to be days when you find your progress unsatisfying. You may be tempted to drown your frustrations in a box of doughnuts, but instead you'll choose your hard. You'll choose the *right* hard.

Oh, and good news: the most difficult choices almost always come with the greatest reward! It's hard to study. But it's rewarding to earn your degree. It's hard to grow a big baby in a tiny body. But it's pretty darn rewarding to give a child life. I promise to simplify this process for you. It would be disingenuous to suggest it will be easy, but the rewards that await you are immeasurable. Choose your hard. I know you'll choose wisely.

PERMISSION TO DISAGREE IF YOU HAVE TEENS!

The fact that you probably bypassed 10 popular diet books before landing on this gem, coupled with the fact you're actually taking the time to read and absorb *131 Method*, means you're not just smart, you're badass. You're a truth seeker. You don't mind rolling up your sleeves to do the work. I ask you to make a vow not to give up, not to see this as an all-or-nothing kind of thing, but a process, a journey we'll take together. We are better together. Everything is easier when you have the support of others, which is why I want to encourage you to be a part of our 131 community by going to www.131method.com.

You are the smartest and the coolest! I'm already in love with your determination. I wrote this book *for you*, and I'll be with you all the way.

Let's do this . . .

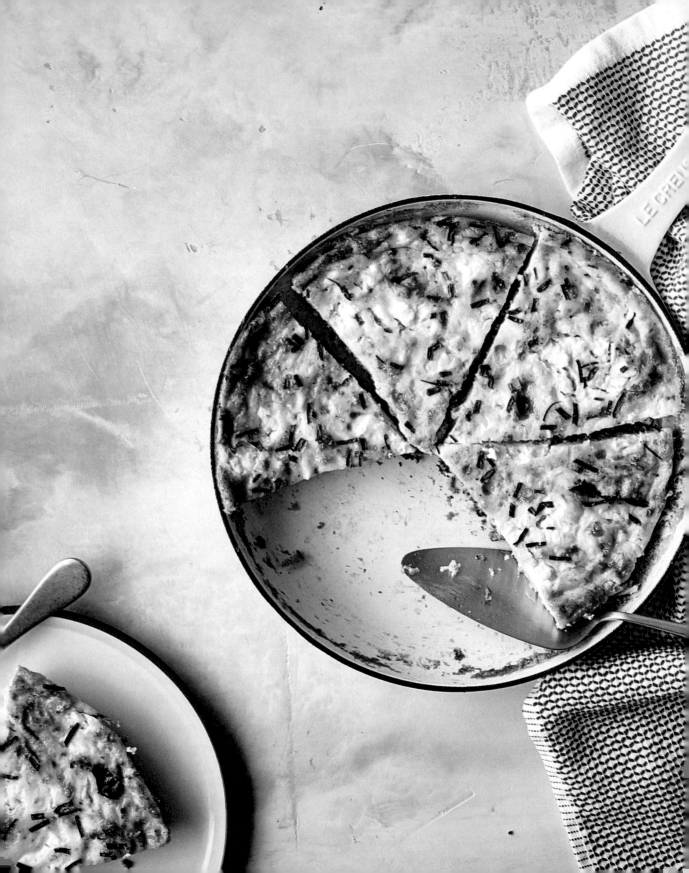

CHAPTER 3
THE DRIVER'S MANUAL YOU NEED TO READ

The universe runs on rhythm. Rhythms gives us patterns that create predictable order. Whether it's the phases of the moon, seasons of reproduction, or our sleep pattern, nature works in cycles, seasons, or phases to bring order to the otherwise unpredictable.

The physical body experiences a multitude of these cycles or phases, such as sleep and awake time, and breathing and ovulation, just to name a few. These produce patterns that are evident in even the smallest cellular level.

The 131 Method starts by working with this very primal design as it relates to our diet. Our ancestors' diets changed or phased due to natural changes or seasonal availability of resources. Diet phasing is a key component of what makes the 131 Method work. You'll learn more about the how-tos in Chapter 4. First, let's get into *why* this works: homeostasis.

Every function and every system of the body is meant to keep us alive. The body tunes in and accommodates subtle shifts in our nutrition, movement, sleep, stress levels, and more to maintain internal stability, or *homeostasis*. It's sensing and predicting patterns and then adapting to them to ensure survival. Homeostasis is sometimes referred to as the body's "set point," the status (including weight) at which your body stubbornly wants to remain.

WHY THIS WORKS

While adaptation is our primitive brain's way of keeping us alive, homeostasis can also keep us feeling fluffy, fat, and frustrated! Regardless of what you eat, your body is programmed to figure out how to adjust energy expenditure and maintain the status quo. This is also why, regardless of the diet, many people experience initial weight loss. Homeostasis simply has not yet had a chance to take hold. You think, *Whaaahoo! Yes! Finally!* You're excited to buy smaller jeans and ready to become a card-carrying lifetime member of whatever diet tribe you've just discovered.

But when you stay on that diet for an extended period, what results is the natural and frustrating process of homeostasis. You gain back all that weight—and probably more—as your body does what it was designed to do. Welcome back the 10 pounds you once lost.

To figure out how to hack this process, I turned to the work of scientists who have studied how to avoid physical adaptation and plateaus. Their studies usually focused on changing exercise training protocols at regular intervals in top-performing athletes. This training approach is sometimes referred to as periodization, cross-training, cycle training, or phasing. In recent decades this approach has been widely accepted as the most effective way to obtain optimal physical results. The 131 Method applies this same biological principle in the form of diet phasing.

DIET PHASING

ITS KINDA LIKE CROSS-TRAINING YOUR NUTRITION.

Diet phasing is as old as human evolution. Scientists agree our Paleolithic ancestors thrived on completely different nutrients with each change of season. The changing availability of food and resources necessitated seasonal variation in their diet for basic survival.

Using that knowledge and employing the right sequence of diet phasing helps your body avoid homeostasis. By changing things up, your metabolism doesn't have time to adapt or slow down. The result is increased metabolic flexibility, which is your tool!

Metabolic flexibility is how we get the body "unstuck." It's the process by which we are able to use carbohydrates, fats, and proteins effectively through a complex communication system in which nutrients are used or metabolized as energy rather than stored as fat. A flexible metabolism means that when you eat healthy fats, which I'll explain, the body learns to burn fat as fuel. Eat more carbs, and the body can return to using stored glucose (carbs) for fuel. The body is so smart, but it hasn't evolved much since the days cavemen roamed the neighborhood.

Diet phasing in the right sequence works with your biology to increase metabolic flexibility. Each phase of the 131 Method helps you efficiently improve your metabolism while simultaneously healing the gut. Diet phasing delivers so many cool things:

- Hormone balance
- Freedom from obsessive dieting
- Balanced insulin sensitivities
- Increased metabolic flexibility
- Increased gut microbiome diversity
- Seasonal convenience
- Freedom to eat a wide variety of foods

INFLAMMATION: THE SILENT ENEMY

Inflammation is like fire. It's necessary in some instances, but when left unattended and out of control, the potential effects are deadly. Experts now know inflammation is the root cause of countless preventable diseases. There are two types of inflammation, acute and chronic. Understanding how inflammation works will have a dramatic impact on your ability to reach your long-term health goals.

Acute, or localized, inflammation is the body's way of fighting off foreign invaders, healing damaged tissues, and getting rid of infections. When you cut your finger, the tissue around the cut becomes red, swollen, and painful. Your immune system immediately sends fluids to stabilize the area, stop the inflammation, and start the healing process. Acute inflammation is sudden and often visible, and it doesn't prevent you from continuing on with your life.

But when it's chronic, or systemic, inflammation robs us of our ability to thrive. Chronic inflammation can be triggered by an internal injury or something the body perceives as unwelcome, such as chemicals, metals, environmental toxins, debris, and even certain foods. Chronic inflammation often occurs slowly and silently, sometimes over the course of days, weeks, months, even decades. It is associated with so many preventable diseases and disorders, including diabetes, cancer, asthma, multiple sclerosis, Alzheimer's, arthritis, depression, lupus, gall bladder disease, heart failure, gum disease, anxiety, infertility, dementia, Crohn's disease, irritable bowel syndrome, atherosclerosis, and many more.

Chronic inflammation often begins in the digestive tract. Eating highly processed foods may be a cause, but it's not just these foods that create chronic inflammation. Even so-called healthy, clean, or natural foods can cause severe and silent inflammation when the body identifies a particular food as a threat, for example food allergies and sensitivities. Emotional stress, physical stress, infections, viruses, other illness, certain synthetic fibers, lack of sleep, certain kinds of latex, adhesives, plastics, and lifestyle choices also contribute to chronic inflammation.

Have you ever stepped on the scale only to find that you gained five pounds overnight? Or looked in the mirror and thought, *Why is my face suddenly so puffy?* Are there days when you can't get your rings off? Those are all signs of systemic inflammation, and it is most often the result of something you ate.

Besides unexplained weight gain and puffiness, other signs and symptoms of inflammation include sore joints, headaches, skin disorders, rashes, migraines, bloating, digestive discomfort or other digestive issues, fatigue, puffy eyes, dark circles under the eyes, depression, anxiety, brain fog, stiffness, runny nose, itchy eyes, low energy, and difficulty healing—just to name a few. If you experience one or more of these symptoms, there's a good chance chronic inflammation is to blame. But don't worry—you're going to fix it with the 131 Method.

LET'S BE HUMANS, SHALL WE . . .

HEALTHY HAPPY HUMANS

Bret and I love to entertain. One year we decided to go all out and host a catered dinner to celebrate the New Year with a small group of couples. Considering the guest list and our own food preferences, I decided to splurge and hire a local chef to prepare a delicious menu using natural and whole-food ingredients. Just to be safe, I suggested he have a few vegan options as well. The appetizers alone were mind-blowingly delicious. It was going so well—that is, until someone spoke the words certain to bring any meal among friends to a screeching halt: "Oh, we can't have that; we're on an elimination diet." The chef scrambled in vain to defend the ingredients of every item. The couple maintained their steadfast dedication and declined every appetizer, every entrée, and every beverage, referencing their combined two-week weight loss as if to strengthen their own resolve. "I've never been so lean!" announced one of them. I smiled and thought to myself, *or so miserable.* (#truestory.)

I'll just bet you know someone who has done one of those super-strict elimination diets. You know the type—the ones where you're supposed to completely cut out, well, pretty much everything. Good luck with that.

There's no question that cutting out inflammatory ingredients can help to identify food intolerances and minimize symptoms of inflammation. The problem is that most elimination diets ask you to give up everything, cold turkey, for 30 days or more. Fantastic concept, just very unrealistic and frankly unnecessary for most of us. These diets focus around what you can't have. You might spend two weeks, 30 days, or another period practicing white-knuckle deprivation, with no plan for how to live and what to eat once you reach the finish line. And by the way, not all inflammatory foods are problematic for *all people*. Popular elimination diets fail to consider this very real fact.

Add a teaspoon of honey on some of these diets and you've "cheated." Substitute your favorite breakfast pancake with a healthy whole-food version of eggs, pumpkin, and stevia and you're in violation. Stray even once and the remedy is to restart your 30 days (even if the food in question is not at all problematic for you). Deprivation is depressing and demoralizing and often leads to feelings of inadequacy.

BUT WAIT . . . DOESN'T THE 131 METHOD SUGGEST ELIMINATING INFLAMMATORY FOODS?

Yes, but the difference is that *you* decide. This is not a hard-line, strict, all-or-nothing elimination diet. Rather, you decide what to eliminate, what to cut back on, and what food you simply don't want to give up at the moment. Instead of focusing on foods you must avoid, you'll approach your menu from the standpoint of how wholesome abundance makes you feel.

Knowing that inflammation results when we consume things our body identifies as foreign allows us to make empowered, personalized decisions rather than relying on a list of foods deemed "approved" or "forbidden."

Let's say you realize alcohol and you just don't get along. But it's your birthday, so you throw back a cupcake and chase it with a margarita. That doesn't make you a cheater. (Please drop that word from your vocabulary. *Cheater* is a word we should use for those who break their vows, not cupcake eaters.) It also doesn't mean you start over or you've failed. It means you made an informed decision, and you'll become keenly aware of how that decision made you feel and move forward.

Let that sink in. You are in charge of every decision.

. . . AND IT MAKES YOU VERY HARD TO BE AROUND!

For the experienced dieter, sitting in the driver's seat is going to require a shift in mind-set. Hard-line diet rules may feel safe, but they only perpetuate the cycle. As with a 16-year-old whose mommy lays out her clothes and writes her English paper, blind dependence stunts confidence and self-sufficiency.

You're very bright. A smart cookie like you doesn't need to see sugarcoated, neon-green puffed rice cereal on a "not allowed" list to know it's not a healthy choice. If you can't live without it, who am I to stop you? It's your life, and only you are responsible for the way you look and feel.

BUT WAIT . . . HOW WILL I KNOW WHAT I SHOULD ELIMINATE?

Don't worry! I'll make the process painless. I'll give you all the information you need to make informed decisions. You'll decide, line item by line item, which ingredients you want to cut out, which you're more comfortable cutting back, and which foods you simply would like to keep in your diet for now, with the option to reevaluate them in the next phase. Life is too short to give up everything just because someone says so.

You're simply too smart to not have a voice in this process. I will teach you how to personalize the decision of which inflammatory foods to remove. We'll do that together in Chapter 6.

Hey, I'm human. So of course I indulge from time to time— but when I do, I pay attention to the price I pay. The result is a changing palate. I don't crave junk the way I once did, and it's not because someone told me I couldn't eat those foods. It's because those foods make me feel bad. We don't look forward to things that make us feel bad. I promise you'll find that the more natural your food, the less you'll crave the fake, hyperpalatable processed foods you once loved.

SHE LOST 80 POUNDS!

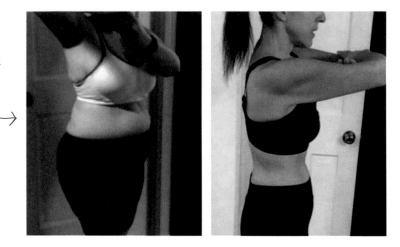

I've lost 80lbs! Before the 131 Method I had been on a diet for as long as I can remember. I was put on a diet by a doctor in elementary school. My initial motivation was of course weight loss. What I didn't know was that my mind-set was about to change significantly!

Within the first two weeks my bloat was gone. I noticed soon after that my skin and eczema had cleared up. I was no longer waking up with horrible back pain from IBS. Then my joint pain was GONE! I wasn't hungry anymore. I was SATISFIED! I wasn't obsessing over what my next meal would be or how many points or calories I had left for the day. This has given me a second chance at life. Freedom from the food/diet prison I have been in for so long! I now actually live and am present and enjoy life.
—MARIA M.

HEALING YOUR GUT: MEET A FEW TRILLION OF YOUR MOST IMPORTANT ALLIES

The *microbiome* is the term used to describe all the good and bad organisms in and on the body—and there are a lot of them, including bacteria, yeasts, viruses, and fungi. Without a doubt, microbes matter. The greatest population of these microbes reside in the digestive tract and make up your gut microbiome. We now know your gut microbiome has a greater effect on your weight and overall health than your genetic makeup!

The microbiome is considered an endocrine organ, responsible for the balancing and production of your major hormones. By improving the health and diversity of your gut microbiome, you can minimize symptoms often caused by hormonal imbalance, symptoms related to such conditions as polycystic ovarian syndrome (PCOS), perimenopause, menopause, anxiety, depression, osteoporosis, Hashimoto's disease, and more. You can't change your genes, but the good news is that you can change and improve your gut microbiome by developing better habits regarding nutrition and sleep and minimizing exposure to toxins.

The tiny microorganisms that inhabit your gut are responsible for the digestion, absorption, and activation of key nutrients that are vital to hormone production and regulation. The gut microbiome influences mood through the production of key neurotransmitters and plays a major role in immune function. It's the first line of defense in our gastrointestinal tract, skin, and mucous membranes, deciding what is a body's friend or foe.

Later we will talk in depth about increasing the diversity of the microbes that live in your gut. For now, know that on the 131 Method, you'll be doing some of the most important things you need to do to heal your gut. You will:

- Reduce inflammation.
- Generate autophagy via fasting (see Chapter 5).
- Rest and reset the gut by resting your digestive system via a variety of fasting options.
- Avoid overuse of antibiotics as well as over-the-counter and prescription medications.
- Increase water intake.
- Diversify your diet and increase foods that feed good microbes: fibrous plant foods (organic when possible), healthy fats, and high-quality proteins.
- Increase gut microbiome diversity with fermented foods and/or high-quality probiotics.

- Minimize intake of sugar, refined carbohydrates, and processed oils, which feed unhealthy microbes.
- Minimize exposure to environmental toxins by avoiding lead, mold, mercury, parabens, fluoride, glyphosate, and phthalates.
- Be active for at least 30 minutes a day, five days a week—but avoid over-exercising!
- Reduce stress.
- Get seven to eight hours of sleep each night.

Gut health is way more important than you might think. If your gut isn't quite right, it impacts every function of your mind and body. Healing the gut is the foundational step when it comes to sustained, healthy weight loss.

IT KINDA IS ALL ABOUT THE GUT

There is a growing body of evidence to support the connection between gut health, hormone dysfunction, autoimmune disease, and—you guessed it—your weight.

The digestive tract is where primary nutrient breakdown and absorption occur. Your gut lining, when functioning properly, serves as a barrier between what you consume and what's absorbed into your body. Your gut and gut microbiome make up approximately 80 percent of your immune system. In case I haven't made it abundantly clear, gut health is a really, really big deal.

What Is Leaky Gut?

Your gut lining is a highly sensitive and intricate system. You might be surprised to learn your gut lining is less than one cell in thickness, thinner than tissue paper. It's also far more sensitive than most of the skin on your body.

Compare for a moment the thicker skin on your fingertips to the one-cell thickness of your gut lining. Now think back on a time when you got a sliver in the tip of your finger. Most likely your finger and the area around the sliver became red, painful, and inflamed. If you were lucky you got some relief from a pair of tweezers. But if not, eventually the swelling created by the inflammation forced the foreign body out.

Imagine that same foreign object working its way into your much thinner, much more sensitive digestive tract. When this happens, the gut lining becomes inflamed, but you might not experience any symptoms. In fact, most of us have no idea when this occurs. But over time that gut inflammation creates systemic inflammation, resulting in damage to the intestinal walls. This damage creates a thinning of the already very thin gut lining. This condition is commonly known as leaky gut.

Leaky Gut in Plain English

A healthy gut lining is composed of teeny, tiny, tight connective junctions (think basket weave). These tight junctions are supposed to act as a filter or strainer, keeping waste products out of your system. When those connective junctions are damaged, it's like trying to strain your pasta with a colander that has large holes in it. Those holes (or loose connections) allow particles that were not meant to enter the body to make their way in before proper digestion or absorption has occurred. Unfortunately, even if you're eating a super-balanced diet, proper absorption becomes more difficult when the gut can't do its job as designed.

I hate to be the bearer of bad news, but there's a very good chance you have leaky gut. In fact, eight out of ten people have leaky gut and don't even know it! Welcome to the club!

MAYBE WE SHOULD HAVE BEDAZZLED JACKETS MADE?

NEARLY EVERY PREVENTABLE DISEASE CAN BE TRACED BACK TO GUT HEALTH

It is believed leaky gut can lead to chronic fatigue, Parkinson's, Alzheimer's, weight gain, hormone disruption, skin disorders, yeast infections, IBS, candida, constipation, malnutrition, chronic joint pain, osteoporosis, brain fog, ADHD, infertility, irregular menstrual cycles, hair loss, anxiety, depression, and just about every autoimmune disease you can think of. Leaky gut or intestinal permeability as you'll find it referenced in the scientific literature, is very likely robbing you of your true health potential. And it's not just fake or inflammatory food that is to blame. Many factors have an impact on our gut health. They include:

- Elevated stress
- Highly processed foods
- Infections
- Food toxins
- Personal food sensitivities
- Poor sleep habits
- Toxic exposure, including to metals like mercury and lead, glyphosate (aka Roundup), and environmental pollutants
- Elevated blood sugar levels
- Inadequate nutrients, antioxidants like vitamin C, selenium, and zinc
- Physical stress, like intense or long workouts and/or injuries
- Oxidative stress

The first step to healing leaky gut is to minimize inflammation. And we're going to learn how to do that using the 131 Method. When I think about the relief you're going to experience doing this I get pretty hyped. The more people who experience the 131 Method, the more convinced I am that inflammation is the thief of vitality. When I spot someone with swollen ankles and a bloated belly struggling just to get out of their car, I imagine a red neon sign flashing above their head that reads,

"INFLAMMATION." I want so desperately to rush over to them and tell them they could have total relief. But that would be awkward. So instead I'm counting on you to inspire those around you with your personal transformation! One by one we'll change the world together.

SHIFT YOUR BODY INTO FAT-BURNING MODE BY UNDERSTANDING KETOSIS AND THE KREBS CYCLE

Whether you have a Toyota Prius parked in your driveway or not, the fact is, you're driving a hybrid. To understand the fascinating biological system of metabolism, let's start with the engine, aka the Krebs cycle. The Krebs cycle is a chemical process that occurs within the mitochondria, taking fuel and converting it into energy.

If you've been following standard American dietary guidelines, you've likely been avoiding fats and have become accustomed to eating far more carbs than our bodies were ever designed to process. The body converts these carbohydrates into sugar and ultimately glucose. In this state, your body becomes conditioned to run on sugar for energy. You're a *sugar burner*.

What most people don't realize is that our bodies have the ability to run efficiently on alternate fuels. The Krebs cycle can use sugar *or* fat to make that energy. With the 131 Method, you're going to learn how to switch between fuel sources and effectively become a *fat burner*.

Think of your body as a hybrid car that can run on either gasoline or electricity. Both work efficiently, but the driver has the ability to determine which fuel source to use based on their nutritional choices.

When we eat carbohydrates our bodies take those fuels and break them down into sugar, or glucose. Oh, and P.S., "carbs" doesn't just implicate bread, ice cream, cake, potatoes, and rice. Carbohydrates are found in many healthy foods, including grains, beans, fruits, vegetables, and even nuts. Carbs are great when we eat the right kinds in the right amounts for our bodies. How much to eat is different for each one of us, and that's what we'll be figuring out on the 131 Method!

It's important to know that even protein can be converted into sugar through a process of gluconeogenesis. When we consume excess protein, find ourselves under considerable stress, or when carbohydrate intake is low and protein consumption is readily available, the body can break down protein (amino acids) and convert those compounds into sugar. This is why when you're first starting out, it's so helpful to track your macronutrients (we'll discuss this more when we get to the Ignite phase).

If consistently provided glucose and/or high amounts of protein, the body will use glucose for energy because it's abundant and easy. It also stores any excess glucose in the liver and muscles as glycogen. When the body runs out of quick glucose to use for energy, it looks for glycogen. Once we burn through all of the glucose and glycogen, the body searches for an alternative fuel.

THERE'S MORE THAN ONE WAY TO DO THIS!

The next most readily available fuel, for most people, is fat. The body has the ability to break down fat and fatty acids to produce ketones (sometimes called ketone bodies) for energy. Those ketones provide ample physical and mental energy! Shifting the body into a state in which glucose and glycogen stores are diminished and it's burning ketones for fuel is known as ketosis, or *fat-burning mode*.

With enough available body fat, a person could potentially live for 60 days without food (obviously not advised or optimal). This is *precisely* because our body has the ability to convert existing fat into ketones and convert ketones into energy.

Once in a state of ketosis, you will likely experience increased focus, greater energy, better sleep, and reduced hunger or cravings. The brain actually prefers to function on the energy of ketones. Ketones have more energy per gram than glucose. Ketones can provide the same energy, or more, and can provide you greater brain clarity. It's worth noting there's also emerging research that suggests a diet low in carbohydrates and high in healthy fat can be used therapeutically for treating type 2 diabetes, weight-loss resistance, neurological disorders like Alzheimer's and Parkinson's disease, epilepsy, chronic headaches, sleep disorders, autism, and even some brain cancers.

There are many ways to get into ketosis. We'll focus on two. The first is by shifting your macronutrient ratio by increasing your healthy fat intake and dramatically decreasing your carbohydrate and protein intake. To do this, 70 to 80 percent of the calories in your diet will need come from healthy fats, while your intake of carbohydrates will be between 5 and 10 percent. (We'll be diving into macronutrient ratios in the next section!)

The second way of achieving ketosis is by depleting your body's glucose stores by allowing more time to pass between meals, a process known as intermittent fasting (see Chapter 5). If you can stretch the amount of time from your dinner to your first meal of the next day, you will most likely be able to shift your body to a point where it's using ketones for energy during the time that you're not eating. As you gradually extend the time between those meals, you'll cut down on the number of hours you're eating food each day, reducing your "eating hours" to about an 8-hour window. In other words, you'll be eating all your meals and snacks within 8 hours of the day and fasting in the other 16 hours. (You'll be getting your beauty rest most of that time anyway!)

After the birth of my two children, I was suffering from severe postpartum depression and struggling to lose weight. I decided to give the 131 Method a try . . . In the first month I noticed amazing changes. I had more energy, I wasn't feeling as depressed, my stomach issues were less frequent, I lost more than 5 inches and 10 pounds, and my clothes were literally loose! **—MAGGIE R.**

LONG-TERM KETO PITFALLS

You probably know someone who has planted their "Keto For Life" flag firmly in the sand. It's hard to miss the ketogenic diet's recent popularity. It seems every magazine cover and cookbook has been quick to capitalize on the "keto" craze. I myself wondered what would be the harm in following a strict ketogenic diet indefinitely when the benefits seem so abundant. The temptations are there.

There are a few things to consider. First, unfortunately many desperate dieters take in some of the details with little or no understanding of why or how long to follow such a program. The worst assumption people make is to assume that becoming a fat burner can be achieved simply by eating more fats, and grossly underestimating carb and protein intake. Off to the market they head for butter, bacon, burgers, cheese, and mayo. This long-term approach usually leads to disastrous results such as weight gain, skyrocketing cholesterol, constipation, un-balanced hormones, thyroid disruption, and increased inflammation, leading to pain and further confusion. The truth is, becoming a fat burner (getting into a state of mild ketosis) requires more than just increasing fat intake. Most people miss the significance of first depleting glucose and glycogen stores, replenishing with micronutrients found in fruits and vegetables, understanding why precise macronutrient tracking is essential, and learning that not all fats are equal in dietary value.

UNDERSTAND MACRONUTRIENT RATIOS TO MASTER KETOSIS

When thinking *macronutrients*, think *macro*, as in big. There are three types of macronutrients: protein, carbohydrates, and fat. All foods are made up of macronutrients and contain calories. Micronutrients are the opposite. They don't contain calories. Micronutrients are tiny, as in *micro*, and they're contained within macros. You'll understand both, but let's start with the big guys, macronutrients.

We need to eat all three types of macronutrients—fat, carbs, and protein—for optimal health.

FAT

Outdated research linked foods high in saturated fat, such as eggs and meat, to high LDL cholesterol, the "bad"

I CAN'T TELL YOU HOW MANY DOCTORS STILL REFERENCE THIS OUTDATED SCIENCE WHEN TALKING WITH THEIR PATIENTS.

cholesterol. Research also correlated heart disease with elevated LDL cholesterol. Recent science finds that people over the age of 60 who have high LDL cholesterol actually live longer than people with low LDL.[1] Because of this study and countless others, many in the scientific and medical community are lobbying their colleagues to drop the cholesterol-heart health myth. At a minimum we need to reevaluate the cholesterol guidelines, healthy fat consumption, and heart disease. Eating healthy fat doesn't make you fat. There are countless benefits to incorporating foods containing quality fats, including plant-based fat as well as healthy animal fats contained in fish and high-quality meat, into your diet. Consider these benefits:

- Fats are the building blocks of hormones.
- Fat lubricates joints.
- Fats help us and our skin look good.
- Fats help us feel better.
- The brain is nearly 70 percent fat, so we think our best when we're getting enough fat in our diets.
- Fats reduce inflammation.
- Fats help with nutrient absorption.

NOT ALL FATS ARE
HEALTHY FATS

There are two main types of fat: saturated and unsaturated. Saturated fats, like coconut oil, palm oil, animal fats, and the fat in cheese, are solid at room temperature There are healthy and unhealthy saturated fats. If you're eating poor-quality saturated fats, you're not going to feel good. Once you learn which saturated fats are healthy and how to balance how much of them you eat, you're going to see and feel an amazing difference in your health almost immediately.

Unsaturated fats are typically liquid at room temperature. The two main types of unsaturated fats are polyunsaturated fats (the fats in nuts and seeds, vegetable oil, corn oil, and sunflower oil), and monounsaturated fats (olive oil, nuts, certain seeds, canola oil, avocado). Polyunsaturated fats are called the essential fats; because our bodies cannot make them, we have to consume them. They are composed of omega-3 and omega-6 fatty acids. The challenge is to eat the rightly balanced amounts of them. Most of the food we eat is overloaded with omega-6s. This imbalance of omega-6s to omega-3s contributes to inflammation. Things like processed foods, conventionally raised and or processed animal meat, lunch meats, and vegetable oils are loaded with inflammatory properties including omega-6s. Omega-3s are found in foods like chia seeds, flaxseed, walnuts, avocados, fatty fish, and grass-finished meat.

Ideally, for every gram of omega-3s you consume, you should have one to four grams of omega-6s. Both are important and necessary, but there's plenty of omega-6s in the American diet. It's not that omega-6s are bad; we just need to limit our consumption to healthier omega-6s and work to increase consumption of omega-3s, found in both plant-based fats and *quality* animal fats, to keep inflammation in check. (You'll learn more on page 153 about the nutritional difference between conventionally farmed meat and grass-fed, grass-finished meat.)

PROTEIN

When people hear the word *protein*, they often think of animal proteins like chicken, beef, seafood, and eggs. But if you don't eat animal products, you can get protein from vegetarian sources such as tempeh, beans, nuts, seeds, and a variety of vegetables.

Our digestive enzymes break down proteins into amino acids. The body distributes these as needed for hair and nail growth, muscle and tissue development, immune system wellness, building healthy cell membranes, and more.

CARBOHYDRATES

Listen, carbs aren't bad. Carbohydrate consumption provides us with valuable nutrients. The problem isn't the carbs, the problem is our overconsumption of carbs. Carbs provide a much-needed balance of fuel for the body. Research today shows a clear correlation between increased consumption of simple carbohydrates and an increase in all disease risk factors. The amounts and types of carbs that we need to thrive are very different from what we've been taught in the past. There are three main types of carbohydrates:

- **Simple carbohydrates** have the greatest effect on your blood sugar levels. They include sugar, honey, and fruit juices. These carbohydrates are quickly and easily absorbed by the body, then converted into glucose, the sugar that's used by your body for energy.
- **Complex carbohydrates** are found in vegetables, whole grains, oatmeal, brown rice, quinoa, and most fruits and beans. These are great sources of fiber and include important vitamins and minerals.
- **Fibrous foods** travel through the large intestine and feed the "good" bacteria in your gut microbiome, helping support the immune system. Fiber aids in digestion, gives you the sensation of being full, and regulates blood sugar levels. (It's excreted as waste at the end of the digestive process.) On nutritional labels, the grams of dietary fiber are usually included in the total carbohydrate count. Because fiber is the type of carbohydrate your body can't digest, many people calculate "net carbs" by subtracting the fiber from the total amount of carbs.

Many factors impact your sensitivity to carbs, including your DNA, the health of and variety within your microbiome, your dietary history, and what you're eating as well as the ratio of fiber, fat, protein, and more. Each of us can expect a unique response. (Doesn't that fact alone just solidify how pointless one-size-fits-all diets are?)

CARBS ARE GOOD FOR YOU... OVERCONSUMING THEM IS NOT.

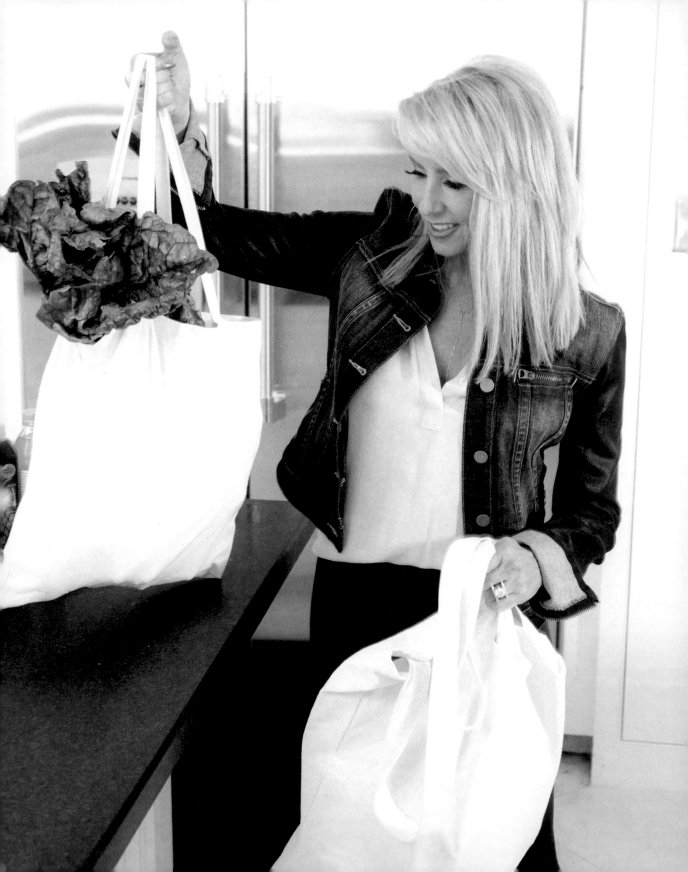

Carbs break down to glucose. Glucose signals insulin to increase. Insulin, a hormone, acts as your gatekeeper, the one who lets glucose into your cells. (It also regulates fat storage.) When we consume more carbs than we were biologically designed to consume, glucose levels rise, and our insulin gatekeeper, the guy who holds the keys, gets lazy. Glucose then stays in the blood, because insulin either isn't showing up or isn't working. This condition is known as insulin resistance.

INSULIN IS THE FAT STORAGE HORMONE!

While your gene expression, lifestyle, aging, and ethnicity affect insulin sensitivity, the most powerful factor is lifestyle and diet. As insulin begins to become less effective at messaging the body, the pancreas begins to produce even more insulin. Eventually, over months and years, this leads to chronically high insulin levels, which leads to weight loss resistance, hormone disruption, and potentially prediabetes or even type 2 diabetes. A growing population now faces nonalcoholic fatty liver disease from this faulty insulin response, not to mention an increased risk of liver damage and even heart disease.

In order to improve gut health, diminish inflammation, and balance hormones, it's important to keep insulin in check. Balancing insulin helps regulate hunger, cravings, energy, and fat storage. Balancing insulin helps you to effortlessly manage your weight and improve your overall health!

As I mentioned previously, one way you can move or shift your body from burning sugar to burning fat (ketosis) is by changing the ratio of nutrients you eat. To do this over the course of one day, your food intake should consist of macronutrient ratios in the neighborhood of 70 to 80 percent of all calories from fat, 5 to 10 percent from carbs, and 10 to 20 percent from protein.

I KNOW THIS SOUNDS CRAZY! DON'T WORRY! I'LL WALK YOU THROUGH IT.

Remember that these are just general numbers. There are many variables to take into account when determining the right ratio for you. Some people burn through carbs faster and more efficiently than others. I explain later how to know which carbs work best for you.

Vegetarian Protein Sources

These are great sources of plant-based proteins:

FLAXSEEDS

OLIVES

MACADAMIA NUTS

LENTILS

TEMPEH

CHICKPEAS

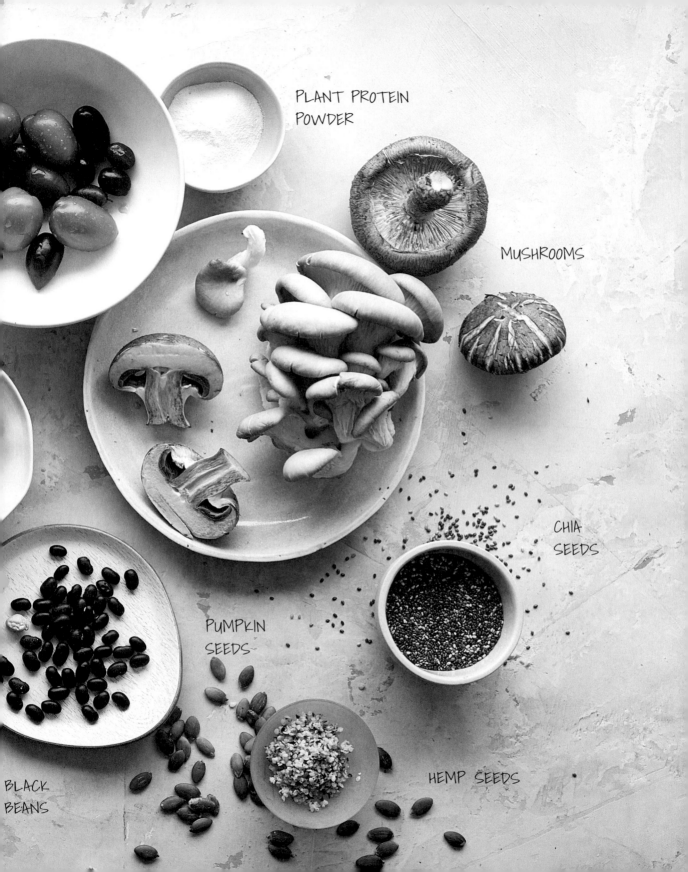

PLANT PROTEIN
POWDER

MUSHROOMS

CHIA
SEEDS

PUMPKIN
SEEDS

HEMP SEEDS

BLACK
BEANS

Healthy Fats

To help your body get in fat-burning mode, consume adequate healthy, anti-inflammatory fats. Here are the top sources:

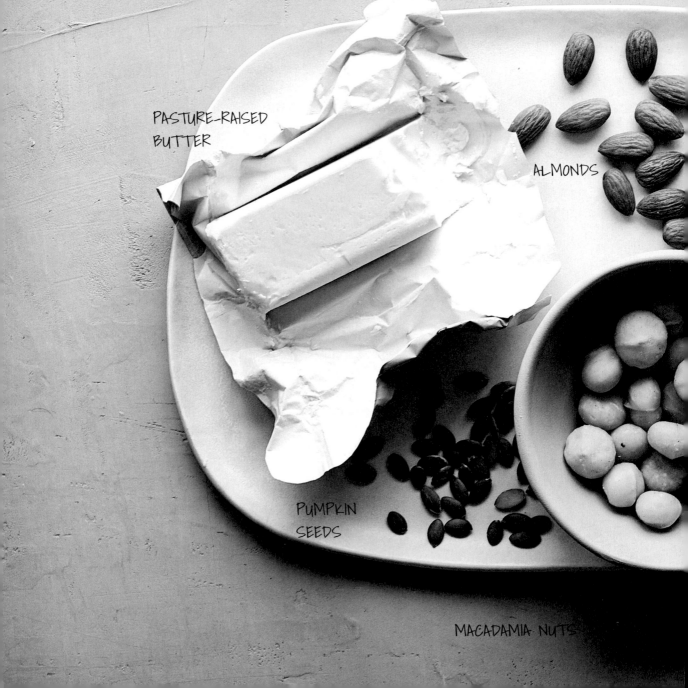

PASTURE-RAISED BUTTER

ALMONDS

PUMPKIN SEEDS

MACADAMIA NUTS

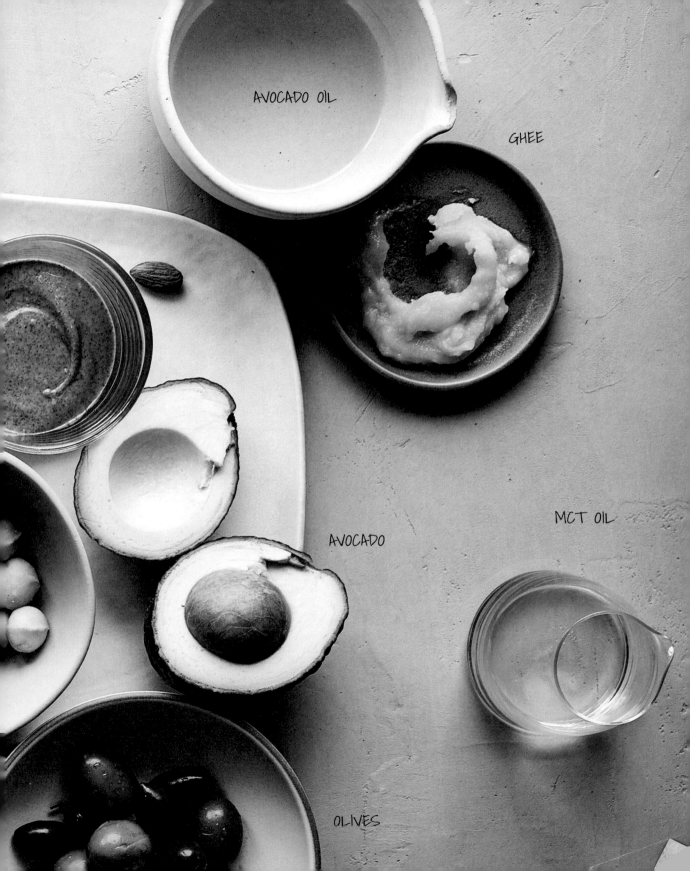

AVOCADO OIL

GHEE

AVOCADO

MCT OIL

OLIVES

Low-Carb Veggies

To maximize nutrition and get your vegetables in while eating low carb, these are the best vegetable choices:

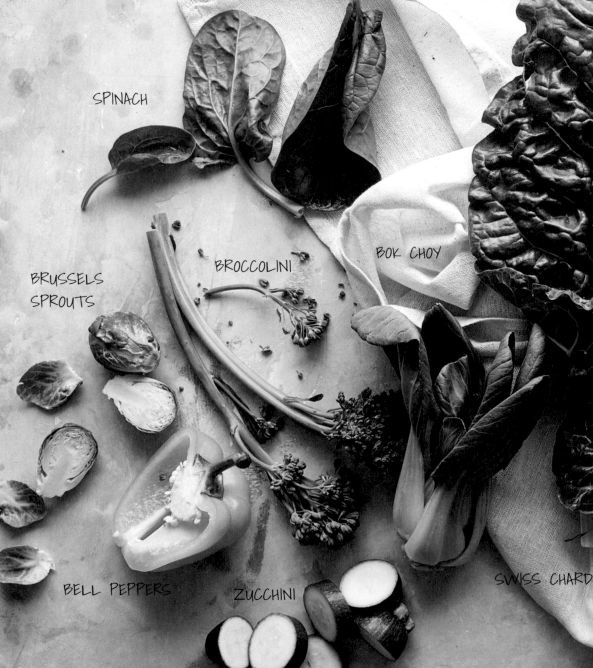

SPINACH

BRUSSELS
SPROUTS

BROCCOLINI

BOK CHOY

BELL PEPPERS

ZUCCHINI

SWISS CHARD

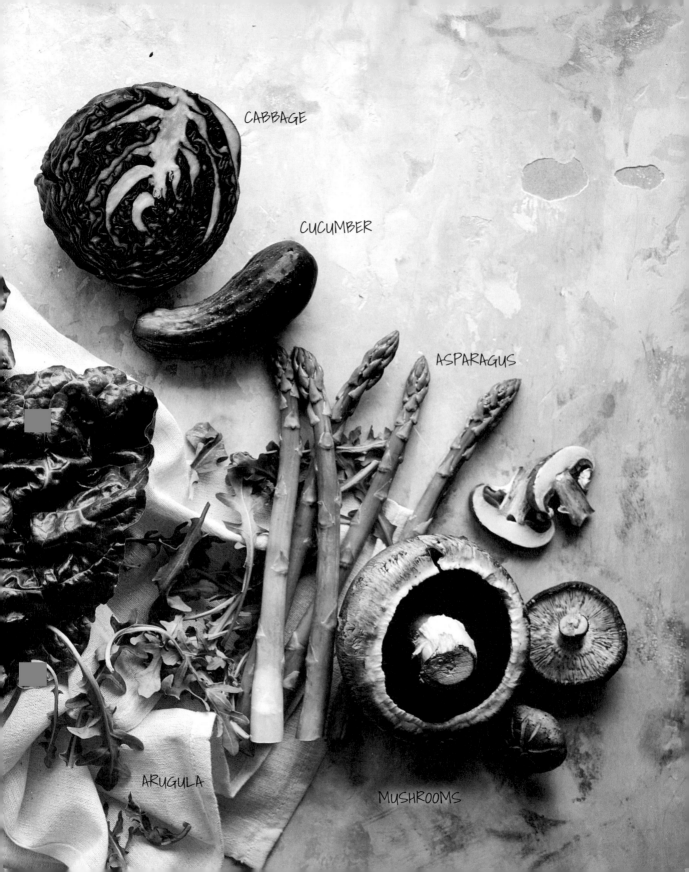

CABBAGE

CUCUMBER

ASPARAGUS

ARUGULA

MUSHROOMS

THE ROLE OF INSULIN IN KETOSIS AND HUNGER CUES

It takes each of us a different amount of time to get into ketosis. Most people are able to shift into ketosis in around two weeks with appropriate dietary changes. Some people can reach ketosis in as little as five days. I'm not proud to admit that for me and my husband, Bret, the speed at which we can transition into ketosis has morphed into a marital competition. And I may or may not have slipped sugar into his morning coffee to maintain my status as Fat Burning Queen. Be patient and do not compare your process to that of anyone else. And for heaven's sake, don't compete! If you are insulin resistant, not exercising, dealing with hormone imbalances, used to eating a diet high in carbs, or under more stress than usual, this transition can take longer for you.

The key to shifting your body into fat-burning mode is that there's very limited sugar storage in your body. Once you've shifted from burning carbs and are instead burning ketones, if you eat something that spikes your insulin levels, well then, your body jumps out of ketosis and you're back into just restricting calories—which you now know doesn't work on its own. That's why, as with all of these things, you have to understand *how* it works. I enjoy delving into the science of everything, not just so you can be a smarty-pants and explain things to others, but so you can make intelligent decisions. So when you do make exceptions to guidelines in the program, you know what the consequences might include and make the right decision for you.

YOU HAVE SO MANY OPTIONS!

You can experiment with macronutrient ratios and intermittent fasting, together or separately, if you want. You might be thinking, *There is no way I am going to eat a diet that's 70 to 80 percent healthy fats. I don't care if they're healthy. I'm going to feel terrible.* Or you might think, *I've tried that before and it didn't sit well with me.* Maybe your body doesn't digest fats well. Maybe you've had really great success eating a diet that's low in fat, high in protein, and moderate in carbs, and you're just trying to fine-tune things and figure out if you've got leaky gut going on. You can continue with whatever feels right for your body.

You'll see that I encourage you to try to get into fat-burning mode for as many days as possible; ideally you'd want to spend a minimum of two weeks in fat-burning mode prior to fasting to reduce your insulin levels. Insulin levels create inflammation and throw our hunger hormones out of whack.

High levels of insulin can contribute to joint pain and swelling, cause us to hold on to abdominal fat, crave sweets, increase blood pressure, and make us feel fatigued around the clock. Pay a visit to your family doctor and she's likely to check for high blood pressure and high cholesterol, yet high levels of insulin are one of the most pervasive and often ignored health risks. When insulin is not regulated it's nearly impossible to lose weight, a condition known as metabolic syndrome. Long before someone is diagnosed as pre-diabetic, insulin levels are likely in the upper ranges as they try to balance blood sugars. Worst of all, high blood sugars (high insulin) aggravate the system. The body knows this excess sugar doesn't belong, and you guessed it . . . it works overtime to fight it by creating inflammation. That inflammation makes the body ache, joints swell, and hands, feet, and eyes puffy. Not only is insulin responsible for the regulation of fat storage, it is also one of the three most powerful hunger hormones.

When hunger hormones are out of balance, no amount of discipline is enough. Only by regulating our hunger hormones can we truly get a grip on the emotional reasons and non-hunger-related triggers that make us want to keep eating.

MEASURING LEVELS OF KETOSIS

Now that you understand how ketosis aids in fat loss, brain function, hormone regulation, and more, you're probably pretty excited to put this to the test. You may be wondering how long it will take you to get into ketosis and how to know if, in fact, you've flipped that switch. The answer to both questions depends on a few factors, including how strictly you limit your carb intake and reduce stress, and of course your personal energy requirements.

One of the easiest ways to know you're in ketosis is simply to recognize the physical signs, keeping in mind that these will vary depending on your history of high blood sugar:

- Diminished hunger
- Feeling satiated for longer periods between meals
- Decreased cravings
- Increased thirst
- Decreased bloating and water retention (ketones are natural diuretics)
- Increased mental clarity, focus, and energy, but no jittery feelings
- Fruity or metallic taste in the mouth
- Increased energy
- Decreased energy (most notably experienced by those newly transitioning)

Ketosis is a sliding scale. Technically speaking, even trace amounts of ketones in your blood and urine means you've made the switch, metabolically speaking, and you are in ketosis. Congrats! To achieve the fat burning, hunger regulation, and mental benefits of ketosis, you need only produce trace amounts of ketones. The higher your ketone levels, the more profound the effects. Having a good sense you're in ketosis is a start, but it's motivating to know with certainty. Achieving higher ketone levels requires crazy-strict dietary adherence and patience—and frankly, barring certain medical conditions, most individuals do not need to reach high levels as the sacrifices are difficult to maintain.

Do you have to test ketone levels to be successful? You do not. However, it's helpful. Knowing you're in ketosis and specifically how high your ketone levels are will help you tailor-fit your macronutrient ratios and understand what degree of ketosis makes you feel the best!

There are several affordable ways to measure your ketone levels, listed below from least to most effective at the time of this writing.

COMPARISON OF URINE AND BLOOD KETONE LEVELS

Level of Ketones	Urine Ketones	Blood Ketones
Negative Amount	<0.5 mmol/L	<0.5 mmol/L
Trace Amounts	0.5 mmol/L	0.6–0.9 mmol/L
Low	1.5 mmol/L	1.0–1.4 mmol/L
Moderate	4.0 mmol/L	1.5–2.4 mmol/L
High	8.0 mmol/L	2.5–2.9 mmol/L
Very High	16 mmol/L	>3.0 mmol/L

Urine: Ketone levels can be measured using disposable strips that can be found online or in most pharmacies. Simply dip one of these strips into a sample of your urine and wait 30 seconds for the strip to change color as an indication of ketones present in the urine. Urine strips are an inexpensive and convenient way to test for ketones. They may be effective when you are first starting, but as your body becomes fat adapted, the urine test becomes less and less effective.

Breath: Portable breathalyzers, also found online, provide a real-time indicator of ketone bodies present in the breath. Once you're over the hurdle of initial setup, these devices are fairly simple to use by plugging into the USB port of your computer. While considered more accurate than urine strips, be sure to read reviews, as device price does not always reflect accuracy.

Blood: The ketones measured by blood tests are different from those detected by urine strips. Blood tests measure beta hydroxybutyrate, or BHB, which is considered the gold

REMEMBER, YOU DO
NOT HAVE TO DO
THE TEST . . .
BUT IT HELPS.

standard method for testing ketones. With a simple finger prick and drop of blood, this type of testing provides more accurate readings for elevated ketones. Low-cost ketone monitors (many of which measure glucose as well) are available online or at most pharmacies.

AUTOPHAGY: TAPPING INTO YOUR BODY'S MIRACULOUS ABILITY TO HEAL NATURALLY

To age in reverse seems to be the stuff of movies, such as *The Curious Case of Benjamin Button*. Yet slowing the aging process is the nonfiction story of autophagy. When you activate autophagy within your body, you slow down aging, minimize inflammation, and boost your body's natural ability to fight off disease. In the 131 Method, we'll be activating autophagy through fasting!

Autophagy (meaning "self-cleaning" or "self-eating") is a naturally induced process whereby dead or damaged cells are killed off in order to generate new cells. "Think of it as our body's innate recycling program," says Colin Champ, M.D., a board-certified radiation oncologist and assistant professor at the University of Pittsburgh Medical Center. Autophagy is a powerful, all-natural healing process you have the ability to induce through specific practices around sleep, exercise, and nutrition.

Your body is a miraculous machine with self-healing mechanisms that in many cases you can activate simply through your nutrition. Autophagy is one of the most potent healing devices you have. You can reap the benefits of autophagy naturally and safely; there's no need to take pills, and it doesn't cost a dime. Your body was designed to do this for you. Autophagy is one of the many fascinating ways in which your body heals.

*****

The more I've come to understand our biology, the more I geek out on this stuff—and that's coming from a girl who once despised science class. I hope you're beginning to make that shift and finding yourself fascinated by what your body has the ability to do for you. Now, don't let this science-y stuff intimidate you. There won't be a pop quiz later in this book. But I want you to soak this stuff up! The more you understand about your body, the more control and confidence you will have. That's one of the core principles of the 131 Method. Now get excited—in the next chapter I'm going to walk you through exactly how to apply these things and truly experience what it looks and feels like to be healthy from the inside out.

MARK MY WORDS—YOU'LL BE HEARING ABOUT THIS A LOT IN THE NEXT FEW YEARS!

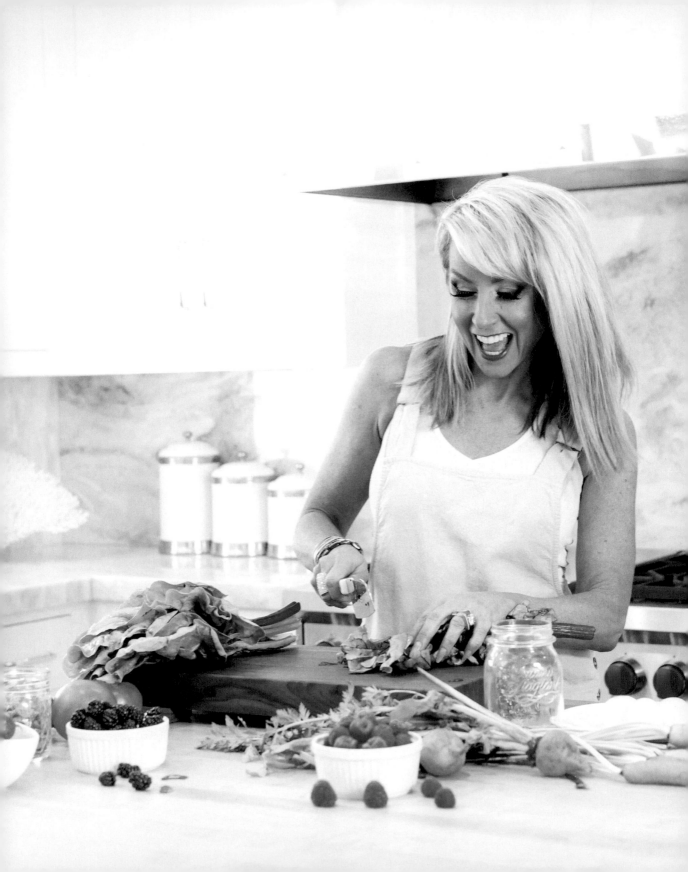

CHAPTER 4

PREP FOR SUCCESS

After reviewing the results of my brain scan and nutritional panel, I was advised that my brain was much older than my chronological age. In no uncertain terms, my treating neurologist, Dr. Daniel Amen, let me know the cognitive decline and brain fog I had been experiencing weren't my imagination. I was on the fast track to early-onset Alzheimer's and autoimmune diseases.

When I got this news, my first thought wasn't about me but about my kids. I couldn't bear the thought of them having to care for me. I don't even like it when they see me without lipstick, so the idea of them looking after my personal hygiene was enough to light a fire under my butt. They became my "why."

Your "why" is what will motivate you to develop the discipline you need to start making changes and turn them into consistent daily habits. In the 131 Method, we'll find your "why" so you have something to lean on as you work to replace old ways of thinking and bad habits with good ones to help you to live a younger and healthier life. But desire, or your "why," isn't enough on its own. To truly succeed, you will need to be prepared mentally and physically.

Preparation is the act of getting something ready. Think of the steps you find in this chapter as getting ready for the healthiest version of yourself. Could you skip ahead a few chapters and just wing it? Sure, but your success would be short-lived.

WHY ARE YOU MOTIVATED TO MAKE A CHANGE?

WARNING: DUCK
AND COVER. I'M
ABOUT TO LAUNCH
A TRUTH BOMB.

Lasting success requires preparation. To prepare for the success you deserve, let's talk about the following: hydration, sleep, exercise, your hunger meter, accountability, and establishing your starting point.

YOUR BELIEF DETERMINES YOUR OUTCOME

It starts with mind-set. We all deserve to live up to our true potential, to live our best possible lives. We also know to do this we have to change some things. Change can be uncomfortable and change takes persistence. So we try, and we stumble. We try again and we slip and finally we give ourselves permission to quit.

There's no point in blaming your genes, vacation plans, or the sabotaging ways of your passive-aggressive roommate. There's only one person responsible for your greatness and it's you. The only thing standing between tolerable meritocracy and you crushing it is your mind-set. We give too much power to external circumstances but the fact is, if you want to make a change, you must take radical responsibility for your optimistic outlook.

I know you want this time to be different. The good news is you are 100 percent in control of the outcome. Your beliefs are the single most powerful influence over the outcome you desire. As outcomes go . . . if you believe you will fail, you probably will. If you believe you will succeed, you're right!

Wait. Don't move a muscle. Let that sink in.

I've been teaching people how to take control and turn every area of their lives around for more than 25 years. Whether I'm coaching someone to be more organized, start a home business, or lose weight, before we start I always ask:

Do you believe it's possible for you?

I tell those who answer, "I hope so" or "I just don't know" not to waste their time. Only once you believe it is possible are you ready to make it happen.

QUITTING ALL-OR-NOTHING THINKING

When it comes to mind-set, one of the hardest habits to break is thinking in terms of all or nothing.

Holding yourself to a standard of perfection destroys confidence and virtually halts progress. If you have perfectionist tendencies, you've likely found yourself reasoning, "Well, if I can't do it perfectly, what's the point? I'm done." Nowhere is this more pervasive than when it comes to diet. I like to call this way of thinking the dieter's mentality.

Dieter's mentality follows a cycle of strict adherence, which leads to feelings of deprivation, then overindulgence, followed by guilt and shame! The all-or-nothing way of thinking triggers a fight-or-flight reaction. To quit makes us feel as though we've escaped danger. Even fleeting thoughts of failure or "blowing it" or "falling off the wagon" subconsciously give power to perceived obstacles. Mess up or lose your determination, no problem! Just quit.

DROP THIS OLD WAY OF THINKING

But this mentality doesn't jibe with the 131 Method, because it's not something you're on or off. This is a knowledge-based program designed to inspire lasting change. Everything you learn and every change you make moves you closer to the healthiest version of yourself.

Unless you're part unicorn, it's normal to doubt yourself. We're hard-wired to search for potential danger. So, learn to be acutely aware when negativity pops in your head. Acknowledge and replace self-doubt with thoughts consistent with your desired outcome.

You're a human, so you're going to mess up. You're going to have a meal or two you regret. You'll step on the scale after a week of your best effort only to see it hasn't budged an ounce. So what! Expect it and keep going.

Show yourself grace. Be realistic. Be kind. Right your rudder and get back on course.

It's time to deprogram your old way of thinking. Rather than focus on what you wish you could improve, or detailing your missteps, acknowledge your progress and move forward. Start with a clear vision of the healthiest version of yourself. What would that look and feel like? Visualize yourself and know that you can achieve it.

At 49 years old I was 30 lbs. overweight. At the time I was trying every diet to lose weight and on top of that I would work out several hours a day, 7 days a week despite terrible ankle pain. I was literally killing myself to lose weight but not getting anywhere! I began the 131 Method and from the beginning started shedding pounds like crazy. Even when I felt like I was "cheating" I still lost weight. My ankle was finally pain free after 8 years!! I have lost a total of 30 lbs.! My blood work confirms the changes I've made will help me to avoid my family history of heart disease and diabetes.
—VERONICA C.

Oh gosh, how hasn't my life changed? I know what to do. I'm soooooo focused and I did not really expect that. My business is improving as a result. I feel empowered and brave. I'm in control and I did it while making my own rules. I'm smarter, sexier, younger, and in control of my life. I'm free. **—KAREN W.**

STAY HYDRATED

It's estimated that 20 to 30 percent of us are chronically dehydrated. Yet, hydration is essential for every bodily function. Even slight dehydration negatively impacts the digestive process, creating conditions such as constipation, irritable bowel syndrome, bloating, and more. Perhaps one of the more motivating facts about hydration is that increased water intake can increase metabolic rate. In a study of healthy men and women published in *The Journal of Clinical Endocrinology & Metabolism*, drinking as little as 2 liters (approximately 60 ounces) of water daily increased participants' metabolic rate by as much as 30 percent, thereby boosting daily energy expenditure by nearly 200 calories.[1]

For more than 30 years I was a full-blown diet soda junkie. I pounded diet soda all day, every day, 365 days a year, thinking I was properly hydrating myself. While I was aware that the soda that quenched my thirst was nothing more than chemicals, colors, and artificial sweeteners, I knew nothing about the effect it had on my metabolism and overall gut health.

Today I drink water—between 75 and 125 ounces—all day, every day. I drink it because I crave it. I crave it because drinking water has become a habit. Drinking tons of fresh filtered water every day helps me maintain energy, control my weight, and improve my gut health.

I NEVER THOUGHT THIS WAS POSSIBLE

If you want to make sure you're drinking enough water, instead of relying on some mathematical equation, let me make this super simple: Try to drink at least 75 ounces of water every day. I promise that will suffice, and if you can get yourself to drink more, even better. The color of your urine also says a lot about your state of hydration. When we are dehydrated, our kidneys, which filter waste, tell the body to hold on to water. This results in less water in our urine, which causes it to become more concentrated and darker in color. Make it your goal to have pale yellow, almost clear urine.

The likelihood of drinking too much water is rare, because the body can process more than 30 ounces of water per hour. Of course, no one wants to wake up several times a night to go to the bathroom, so minimize water intake after sunset. This one habit is a game changer. Decide today to stop hydrating with sodas, juices, artificially sweetened diet drinks, syrup-sweetened coffees, sweet teas, and sports drinks. They may offer minimal hydration, but at the cost of gut health. Bottom line—just drink water.

I encourage you to make a serious effort to increase your water intake now by simply being more conscious of your habits.

INCREASE DAILY WATER INTAKE TO 75 OUNCES OR MORE

Obviously, hydration needs vary from person to person. Activity level, climate, age, height, weight, sodium intake, diet, and exercise all impact how much water you should be drinking. Rather than overcomplicate the matter with formulas or mathematical equations, let's keep this simple: Set a goal to drink a minimum of 75 ounces every day. Hitting this one goal often creates a snowball effect, leading to more healthy habits.

When you want to transform a behavior into a habit, you have to simplify the process and make the action as "mindless" as possible. The easier the action, the more likely the habit will stick! Also, remember when your mom took you back-to-school shopping? You couldn't wait to wear your new outfit or show off your supercool lunch box on the first day. New gadgets get us excited about things that might otherwise feel commonplace. Apply this principle to your goal to drink more water.

When I wanted to hit my personal goal of drinking 75 ounces of water daily, I found myself struggling to remember how many times I had refilled my water bottle. I decided to purchase three super cute 25-ounce insulated water bottles, the kind that stays cold for up to 24 hours. I filled all three bottles each night with my Lemon-Ginger Cayenne Water (see recipe on the next page), ready to drink the next day.

I saved time and no longer had to track how much water I had consumed. When all three bottles were empty, I'd hit my mark. Eventually I designed three coordinating water bottles to represent early morning, midmorning, and late afternoon. My next task was to figure out an easy way to carry the three full water bottles to the office without weighing down my purse or clanking back and forth on the floorboards of my car. In an evening with my sewing machine, I designed a simple carrying tote to transport three 25-ounce water bottles to and from the office. Eventually my social media family persuaded me to make them available for everyone. You can check them out at www.131bottles.com.

TIPS TO HELP YOU DRINK MORE WATER:

- Buy a new water bottle! To be specific, look for BPA-free plastics, stainless steel, or glass water bottles.

- Infuse your water with herbs, fruits, or cucumber. Some flavor ideas: basil, strawberry, lemon, mint, cantaloupe, ginger, or cucumber.

- Try my favorite Lemon–Ginger Cayenne Water recipe: Set aside 1 gallon distilled water. Next, squeeze 2 large lemons into a large blender. Add 3 cups of the water, as well as 4 peeled knobs of ginger, a dash of cayenne pepper, and 5 to 10 drops of liquid stevia (to your taste). Blend on high for 30 seconds, and then strain the mixture. Add this strained concentrate to the remaining water and store in the refrigerator.

- Get half your water in before lunch and the other half before dinner, so you don't get up as much during the night.

- Think of your water bottle as your lifeline. Have one with you at all times! Seeing it will remind you to drink throughout the day.

- Treat your water bottle like you do your smartphone. You know that "something is missing" feeling you get when you've left your cell phone in another room? Create that same relationship with your water bottle.

- If you love bubbles, drink natural sparkling water. You can add citrus fruit and herbs.

- Avoid artificial sweeteners. If you must add sweetness, use natural products such as stevia, but in limited amounts.

- Think of your bathroom breaks as a good reason to get up and move!

YOU SHOULD FEEL NAKED WITHOUT A WATER BOTTLE IN YOUR HAND

WATER AND ELECTROLYTES

Stay hydrated! We often confuse hunger with thirst. Never is this more important than during fasting. Make it a goal to consume a minimum of 75 ounces of water daily, or enough so that your urine is nearly clear. Electrolytes include sodium, calcium, potassium, chloride, phosphate, and magnesium, which are normally found in our food. Electrolytes allow us to sustain hydration on a cellular level. These nutrients also help us to transmit nerve impulses, regulate blood pressure, contract muscles, sleep, and so much more!

Symptoms of electrolyte imbalance:

- Muscle spasms/cramps
- Headaches
- Dizziness/weakness
- Irregular heartbeat, higher blood pressure
- Numbness
- Confusion/mental fatigue
- Muscle fatigue
- Insomnia
- Brain fog

ELECTROLYTE SUPPLEMENTATION

If you feel like you're drinking a ton of water but are still dehydrated and experiencing any of the symptoms above, please consider using a supplement. Some of these supplements contain carbs. Not a big deal. The benefits of proper electrolyte balance far outweigh the risks. Here are some suggestions:

- Himalayan sea salt or Celtic sea salt with lemon juice
- Epsom salt baths (for magnesium)
- Trace mineral liquid supplements or electrolyte powders
- Bone broth (with extra pinches of salt or a squeeze of lemon for more electrolytes)

Quick Tip: Try adding a quarter to a half teaspoon of Himalayan sea salt to my favorite Lemon–Ginger Cayenne Water (page 59).

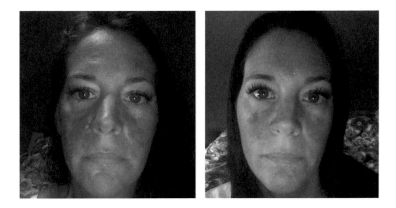

Before starting the 131 Method I struggled with several health issues like migraines, rosacea, PCOS hormone imbalance, plus anxiety and depression. Following the 131 Method changed my life. I lost 30 pounds in two months and gained my health back. I no longer take antibiotics or over-the-counter meds, my depression and anxiety have lifted, and by healing my gut I was able to clear up my face. Getting healthy has improved my focus and energy. Overall I feel like a different person. **—KARA M.**

Magnesium

Magnesium is important for over 300 reactions in the body including hydration, bone health, and more. Too little magnesium could cause muscle cramps, weakness, insomnia, depression, anxiety, and hypertension. Here are top sources of magnesium.

BRAZIL NUTS

ALMONDS

MOLASSES

SEAWEED

PUMPKIN SEEDS

BEANS

BUCKWHEAT

AMARANTH

COCOA

DARK LEAFY GREENS
(SPINACH, BROCCOLI/-
BROCCOLINI, BRUSSELS
SPROUTS, ARUGULA,
SWISS CHARD, KALE)

Potassium

Potassium is an important electrolyte. It helps keep your body hydrated and is important for nerve and muscle contraction. Too little potassium cause could side effects such as muscle weakness, fatigue, and hypertension.

Top sources of potassium include:

RAISINS

POTATO WITH
SKINS

AVOCADO

SQUASH

SUNFLOWER SEEDS

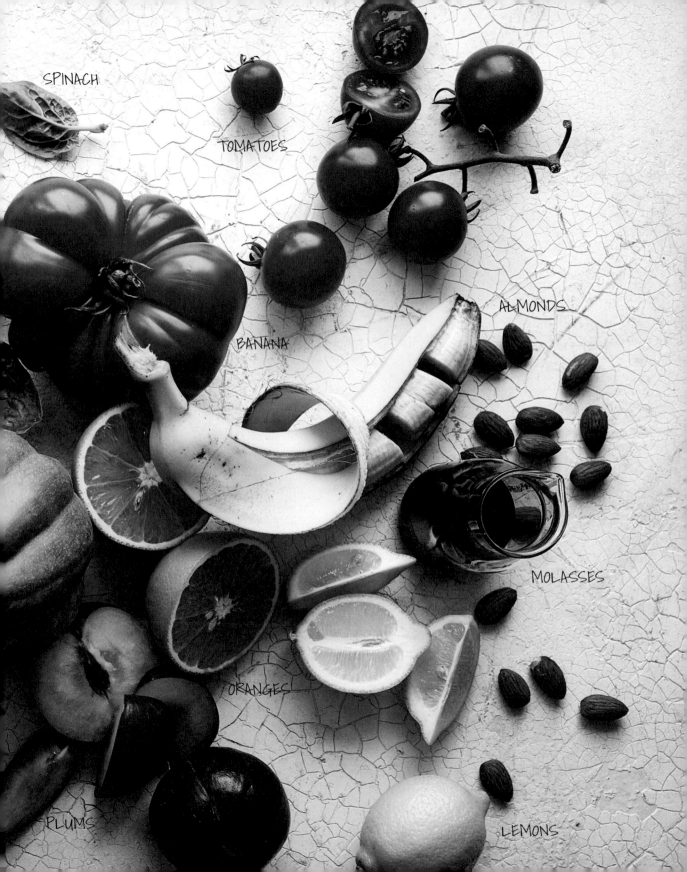

SPINACH

TOMATOES

ALMONDS

BANANA

MOLASSES

ORANGES

PLUMS

LEMONS

Calcium

Calcium is vital for your heart health, muscle contractions, nerve functioning, and blood pressure as well as bone and teeth formation. Here are top sources of calcium:

TAHINI

ORGANIC FULL-FAT DAIRY FROM PASTURE-RAISED COWS (BUTTER, YOGURT, MILK)

BONE BROTH

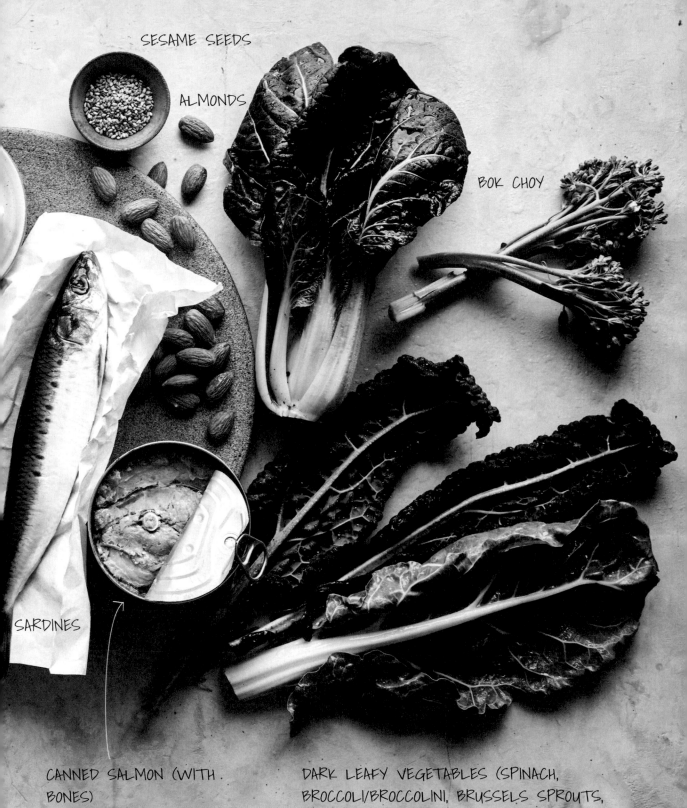

SESAME SEEDS

ALMONDS

BOK CHOY

SARDINES

CANNED SALMON (WITH BONES)

DARK LEAFY VEGETABLES (SPINACH, BROCCOLI/BROCCOLINI, BRUSSELS SPROUTS, ARUGULA, SWISS CHARD, KALE)

GET SOME SLEEP

When I met with experts about the damage to my brain and the seriousness of my leaky gut, the first order of business was to fix my sleep. For more than 20 years, I wore my sleep deprivation like a badge of honor. I rarely felt tired, so long as I was in a constant state of stress and pounding a steady stream of diet soda. I proudly proclaimed, "I'll sleep when I'm dead" or "Sleep is for the weak!" Wrong.

Sleep is for the *smart*. We cannot be sleep deprived and have optimal health. When we are low on sleep we experience multiple changes to our bodies that lead to what I call a slow system shutdown. Our stress hormones rise, blood glucose levels increase, hunger hormones kick into overdrive, and cognitive function is diminished.

Ever wonder why, when you're short on sleep, nothing sounds better than carbs? That's because sleep deprivation changes our cravings, turning on an intense desire for carbohydrates and sugar-laden foods. When we don't get enough sleep, the brain struggles to make healthy decisions about how much and what type of food to eat.

Adequate sleep is essential to regulate insulin and blood sugar, making weight management and a speedy metabolism much easier to attain. Two hormones that play huge roles in appetite suppression and hunger, leptin and ghrelin, depend on sleep for proper regulation. Leptin is made by fat cells and signals the brain when we're full. Leptin's counterpart, ghrelin, is a hormone manufactured in the gastrointestinal tract that stimulates hunger, even though you may have just had a meal.

A study from researchers at the University of Colorado, Boulder, found that by simply restricting sleep to about five hours a night for as little as one week, participants gained an average of two pounds.[2] The impact of sleep on inflammation, brain health, and weight cannot be underestimated. One of the best ways to improve your

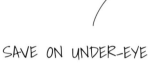

SAVE ON UNDER-EYE CONCEALER . . . GET MORE SLEEP!

sleep quality is by regulating the hormones that help us sleep. And as luck would have it, the better your sleep, the more balanced your hormones become.

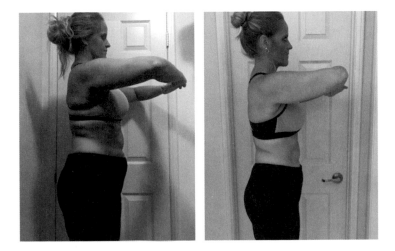

I feel smarter, I'm not falling asleep in my car, I'm sleeping at night! I have more energy. I'm excited every day to learn something new. It's about me, no one else. I have more energy and enthusiasm and I lost 35 pounds overall. —DUSTYN F.

SLEEP SUPPLEMENTS

In an ideal world, our bodies would be able to produce nearly all the vitamins and minerals they need for proper function and restorative sleep. The reality is, most of us are grossly deficient in some very key areas. While the 131 Method takes a "start with food" approach, you may want to consider supplementing where you are deficient.

Knowing where you might be deficient and determining appropriate dosages can be tricky. When in doubt, it's always best to work with an integrative care provider.

You can start by asking your doctor to order blood work to identify your specific nutritional deficiencies. If that is not an option, there are many direct-consumer-access labs that allow you to request blood work without having to make an appointment and trudge over to your usual doctor's office. Start by researching at spectracell.com and nutritionallyyourstestkits.com.

In the absence of lab work, tune in to your own body and consider the standard guidelines that follow:

Magnesium: Dr. Michael Breus, "The Sleep Doctor," praises the sleep-promoting, stress-reducing, disease-protecting power of this essential mineral. Magnesium is also important for energy, metabolism, blood pressure regulation, blood sugar control, and central nervous system function. Magnesium isn't just good for sleep; it's good for your gut! Magnesium deficiency is associated with poor gut health plus heightened stress and anxiety. Magnesium is the fourth most abundant mineral in the human body.[3]

Magnesium plays an important role in the functioning of your body and helps reduce the risk of impaired insulin response. Magnesium also aids in the regulation of sleep. Even if you eat a healthy diet it's possible you're not getting enough of the foods known to be high in magnesium such as dark leafy greens, seeds, nuts, squash, broccoli, meat, dark chocolate, and even high-quality, toxin-free coffee.

Melatonin: Melatonin is a hormone made in the brain by the pineal gland; it also helps to regulate mood, sleep, and wakefulness. Here are some natural ways to increase melatonin production in the body:

- Avoid artificial lighting at least an hour before bed.
- During the day, make sure you get full sun exposure.
- Eat foods rich in tryptophan, which is a precursor to melatonin; these include red meat, turkey, nuts, and eggs.

TIPS FOR BETTER SLEEP

1. Avoid caffeine after noon.

2. Tap into circadian rhythms by avoiding screen time one to two hours before bed.

3. Put your phone in another room or on airplane mode while you sleep.

4. Avoid eating two to three hours before bed. Allow the body to rest, not digest, at night.

5. Drink decaffeinated teas like chamomile, peppermint, or ginger in the evening.

6. In bed, use an eye mask and/or earplugs to shut out light and noise.

7. Lower room temperature while sleeping to mid 60s Fahrenheit.

8. Dim lights of electronics with removable blackout stickers.

9. Increase magnesium and/or melatonin via diet or supplement from a reputable brand.

10. Avoid alcohol.

11. Avoid sedatives.

I was in a dark, unhealthy place after having a miscarriage. I blamed myself for the poor lifestyle choices. After the miscarriage I put on weight, stopped ovulating and I had very irregular cycles. I began to research and came across Chalene and the 131 Method. It has truly changed my life for the better. The 131 Method taught me the importance of a healthy and happy lifestyle. I have discovered the power of eliminating inflammatory foods and fasting and I have lost 35 lbs. I am now ovulating and my cycles are finally regular. The 131 Method has truly changed my life. —**TALLARA A.**

MOVE THAT BODY, BABY!

> YOU ONLY NEED TO EXERCISE ON THE DAYS YOU WANT TO BE IN A GOOD MOOD.

The 131 Method isn't just about a getting a flat stomach or losing inches and pounds. You're on this journey to optimize your health, and exercise is just one aspect of getting there. Exercise helps us live longer, manage our mood, regulate digestion, improve sex drive, reduce blood sugar, increase productivity, regulate insulin, diminish risk of disease, and improve sleep. According to the PURE Study, the largest study of physical activity tracking 130,000 people in 17 countries by the Population Health Research Institute, doing just 30 minutes of physical activity five days a week was associated with a reduced risk of death and cardiovascular disease.[4] If your goal is to live longer and be healthier, then these 30 minutes of exercise at least five days a week are non-negotiable. Period.

Each day someone writes me to say how much they want to exercise but that they just "don't have the energy." (Gosh I hope this doesn't sound unsympathetic. That's not my intention. But you need to hear the truth.)

If you don't have the energy to exercise, it's because you don't exercise.

Energy begets energy. Just stop dwelling on your lack of energy (which only diminishes your energy) and start moving. Make a deal with yourself. Commit to 5 minutes of exercise with a good attitude. After 5 minutes I guarantee you'll start to feel some energy. If you're starting from scratch, don't try to begin with a 30-minute run at track star pace. As a matter of fact, don't start with something you know you're going to hate. Pick something that sounds fun, like a bike ride, yoga, ballroom dancing, Pilates, or strength training, and do it for 5 minutes. Add a few minutes every day until you reach your goal.

Hey, I have an idea! Download any podcast app and search for *The Chalene Show* (that's my health and lifestyle podcast). I have over 300 hours of free content designed to boost your mojo and improve your mind-set. Most episodes average 30 minutes! Perfect! And I would be honored to keep you company on your next power walk.

And as if all of that wasn't awesome enough, exercise can help you lose weight, improve body composition, and boost your body image!

Our bodies were designed to move. Movement improves every aspect of the body: memory, heart health, cognitive function, skeletal strength, bone density, muscle development, libido, confidence, and more. All forms of exercise create some type of oxidative stress. Oxidative stress in small doses can be beneficial; in excess it deteriorates systems like internal rust. Research has shown that it actually prompts our cells to become stronger and younger as they increase production of antioxidants. Your body has a limited capacity to do this to control free radicals, which is why too much stress is detrimental, even if it's in the form of exercise.

How much exercise is too much? As with all recommendations, it depends on many individual factors. However, signs of overtraining include fatigue, loss of appetite, increased appetite, difficulty sleeping, difficulty recovering from workouts, low energy, lack of libido, hair loss, lack of motivation, irritability, anxiety, and depression. Pay attention to the way you feel before and after workouts.

The bottom line is this: You need to move your body every day for at least 30 minutes. This doesn't mean you need to train for a marathon or practice CrossFit every day, but you should work to get your heart rate elevated and keep your muscles strong. You've been given a gift—your body. Honor it. But when you do "go for it," listen to the way your body responds. Vary workouts. Mix up days of high intensity with days of low intensity. Remember that things like a walk, gentle swim, steady bike ride, or yoga are also great activities. Whatever your taste in activity, you can find plenty of free or low-cost programs online. So watch some online videos, follow fitness people on social media, download an app, or join a Meetup group in your city. No excuses!

HEY . . . YOU SHOULD TRY ONE OF MY WORKOUT VIDEOS!

UNDERSTAND AND RECALIBRATE YOUR BROKEN HUNGER METER

I want to help you prepare for this journey. If you were planning to drive across country and suddenly discovered your fuel gauge was broken, you'd prioritize getting it repaired before you set off on your way.

So let's calibrate your hunger meter before we start.

First, *hunger* and *appetite* though often used interchangeably, are very different things.

Hunger is a physical sensation that drives us to eat food. It is created and regulated by hormones. True hunger happens when energy stored in the body is in short supply. When you transition from being a sugar burner to becoming a fat burner, you won't feel as hungry because you'll be using stored body fat as fuel. Therefore, unless your body fat is too low, there's plenty of available fuel on board, and it's unlikely you'll feel true hunger.

Appetite, on the other hand, is primarily psychological. Appetite is having the desire to eat. It can be influenced by true physical hunger, but our hormones do not necessarily regulate it. Consider the last time you may have gone hours with no food, felt the physical pangs of hunger, and then had a thought or image or even a scent kill your appetite.

When we eat for reasons other than physical hunger, it is typically identified as "emotional eating." This doesn't imply you're truly emotional in a crying-in-your-hands kind of way. Emotional hunger or emotional eating are coping behaviors related to food that are triggered by emotion or feelings. This can happen when you feel something and your brain wants to make you comfortable and keep you safe, so it kicks into "protector" mode and tells your body to fix it or soothe it with food.

AWARENESS AND UNDERSTANDING MOTIVATE BIG CHANGES

There is another kind of eating that has nothing to do with hunger. As a society, we've formed habits and cultural routines that have disrupted and even damaged our ability to regulate our hunger. These routines and habits tend to trigger appetite. Think about the last time you gathered with friends, woke to the smell of bacon, or joined the office staff for a potluck. The automatic response is to eat. It's commonplace to enjoy a movie with a large bucket of popcorn and a supersized soda. But are we eating because we're hungry or because it's a habit, an accepted norm?

Maybe you are feeling boredom, fear, sadness, confusion, or anxiety. Or maybe you worked at a job you don't love for eight hours, then came home to unclog the toilet, make dinner for six, finish five loads of laundry, help out with a science project, and put four kids to bed—and now your husband is giving you bedroom eyes. You respond by rolling *your* eyes. You're exhausted and can't help but think, "I want a loaf of bread! And a bottle of wine!" Food (and beverage) becomes a simple way to soothe that has nothing to do with true hunger.

The good news is that you have the ability to correct both appetite and hunger with the 131 Method. Ultimately, you want to maintain a healthy weight and have a relaxed, positive relationship with food. No one wants to obsess about food or be forced to rely on willpower. All of this can and will be repaired as your hormones become more balanced.

When your hunger hormones are balanced, which you will begin to experience in the Ignite phase, you will feel satisfied for longer periods between meals. Balancing your hunger hormones, however, does not impact the other reasons you might feel the urge to eat, like emotional eating. It's important to identify the difference between true hunger and appetite that is triggered by some type of feeling.

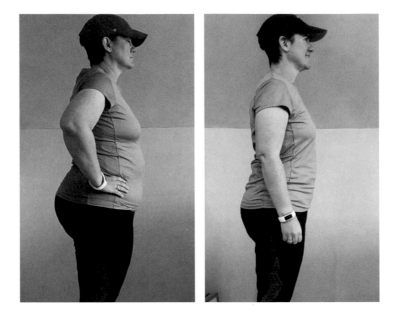

I was a fast-food junkie and hated to cook. I am no longer constantly hungry. I've lost 39 pounds so far. I went from a size 22 pants to a size 12. No starting over, no feeling like I failed. This is a marathon, not a sprint. And I'M winning! —**KRISTIN A**.

TRUE HUNGER VS. EMOTIONAL EATING

For the next week, each time you have a desire to eat—whether triggered by emotion or true hunger—use a diary (or the 131 Method Workbook at www.131method.com) to record your answers to the following questions:

1. What physical sensation am I experiencing, such as stomach pain, headache, etc.?

2. What about my situation may have triggered my desire to eat?

3. What time of day is it?

4. When was the last time I ate?

5. What was the macronutrient makeup of my last meal?

6. What emotions or feelings do I have in this moment, such as boredom, frustration, or exhaustion?

7. Am I craving a particular food?

8. Am I thirsty?

9. Am I experiencing true hunger or an emotional desire to eat?

If you ate a snack or a meal:

10. If I ate, what did I eat?

11. How did I feel after I ate? (describe both your emotional and physical feelings)

12. Was I multitasking while eating?

13. Did I eat slowly?

14. Was I satisfied after eating?

15. Did I choose to eat something that improved my health or was my choice based on convenience?

PULL OUT YOUR CELL PHONE AND SNAP A PHOTO OF THESE QUESTIONS SO YOU HAVE QUICK ACCESS THE NEXT TIME HUNGER STRIKES.

SYSTEMS OF ACCOUNTABILITY

You are not a robot. There are going to be days when everyone and everything is on your last nerve. On those days it can be challenging to flex your discipline muscles and do what you know you need to do. Don't go at it alone! By building systems of accountability, you dramatically increase your chances of success. Here are some of my favorites:

Identify Your "Why." What is it that inspires you to make these changes? What is it you want so badly that you're willing to develop new habits and change beliefs? Identify your motivation. Put words and emotion to it. I don't mean to get sappy on you, but I really do want you to put this book down for a moment, close your eyes, and feel the emotions that are attached to your WHY!

The Important Person Promise. Think of somebody who means the world to you, someone who cares about your health and well-being. I want you to make that person a promise. Let them know what you're doing and how much they mean to you. Be specific in communicating your goals. Rather than ambiguities such as "I'm trying to get healthier," be specific, saying something like "I am going to lose 20 pounds, get eight hours of sleep a night, and do yoga at least three times a week!" Make them a promise and then keep it!

Do This with a Buddy. People who take on a health goal with a friend or family member have nearly double the success of those who go it alone. Pick an accountability partner who will do the program with you and won't let you off the hook.

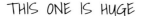

THIS ONE IS HUGE

Keep a Daily Journal. The act of writing or journaling by its very nature keeps us accountable and present. Use a daily journal to write about what you're experiencing and to track your exercise, meal times, hydration, and what you ate each day. (Consider using the 131 Method Workbook to organize your notes and progress.)

Make a Public Proclamation. When you go public with your health objectives, the world becomes your cheering section. You'll be much more likely to follow through when people are rooting for you. So tell the world what you're doing! Announce it on social media, tell the gals at the office, and let your BFF in on the news! When you include others in your quest, they're less likely to expose you to unhealthy temptations. You'll probably inspire others to join you! We're often quick to let ourselves down, but rarely do we want to disappoint others.

Join the Community. If you're having difficulty finding a good accountability partner, join an online support community like the one featured inside our online program, www.131method.com.

Post Your Progress. Nothing is more authentic or inspirational to others than sharing your journey. Keep your tribe posted. Share your progress with us by using the hashtag #131Results on Instagram and Twitter.

A PHOTO WILL TELL YOU SO MUCH MORE THAN THE SCALE.

Just halfway through and I have already lost 21 pounds! My golfer's elbow completely disappeared within two weeks. My hot flashes are gone! But I think the biggest benefit is that I'm healing my gut and getting healthy from the inside out. I don't feel hungry, and eating this way has been simple . . . even with two kids, a full-time job, and volunteering at church! **—CALA O.**

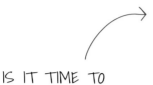

IS IT TIME TO BREAK UP WITH YOURS?

SCALES CAN BE RUDE

When you set out to accomplish a goal, it's important that goal has specificity. If weight loss or any type of physical transformation is your objective, having a measure by which to gauge your progress is imperative. It's hard to hit a mark you never identified.

To be honest, I'm not a fan of traditional scales. Scales can be cruel pathological liars. Despite what you feel when you step on to that cold square, your weight does not define who you are. We all know people who are at their ideal weight, and they're just as miserable thin as they were when they were overweight. Instead of obsessing over a number on the scale, consider tracking a healthy range of pounds.

Hey, I have an idea! If normal weight fluctuations ruin your day, *skip the traditional scale*!

Obsessing over a number is a waste of your crazy cool life. We've been misled to believe that a low body weight somehow represents health when in reality it only represents one small faction of your overall health.

The number on a scale, even for the healthiest of individuals, will naturally fluctuate due to things such as exercise, muscle soreness (which are just inflamed muscles postworkout), what you ate last, digestion, elimination, time of day, hormones, pre- or postworkout, water intake, inflammation, the accuracy of your scale, and so much more.

Yes, you want to track your progress, but there are lots of ways to do that like using scales that factor in your body composition or having your body fat tested. Just remember that you are a freaking amazing person regardless of what that stupid scale says. I want you to focus on your non-scale victories! The following are some things you can monitor to track your progress. I'll bet you can add a few to the list!

- body fat
- confidence
- clothing fit
- digestion
- fewer medications
- flexibility
- hair
- inches lost
- energy
- mental clarity
- mobility
- nails
- patience
- sex drive
- skin
- sleep quality
- sleep duration
- cognitive function
- easier periods
- stamina
- strength

PREPARING TO PHASE YOUR DIET

As a reminder, the 131 Method consists of three phases—Ignite, Renew, and Nourish—and each phase lasts four weeks. For the first three weeks of each phase, I'll give you specific dietary and lifestyle suggestions. During the fourth week of each phase, you can continue doing what you're doing (following the dietary recommendations of the previous week) or optimize your results with a customized fasting and refueling plan.

Remember, there is:

1 Objective for each phase

3 Weeks of dietary phasing

1 Week to fast and refuel

When developing the 131 Method, I started by prioritizing the most critical components of healthy weight loss. I then tested the ordering of each phase on thousands of people in my online program at www.131Method.com to determine which approach would not only give you quick results but provide you with lasting weight loss, improved gut health, and balanced hormones. While all three phases address a specific objective, every phase will progressively improve both your metabolic flexibility and your gut health.

It is of the utmost importance that you follow the phases in the order outlined, as each one tackles a sequential objective necessary for long-term weight loss and overall health. Each phase is a natural progression from the previous phase. Following the phases in this order builds the foundation for your long-term success.

After you've finished 12 weeks of the 131 Method, you will have the knowledge and experience to practice phasing your diet as a way of life. I explain how to do that in Chapter 9.

Before starting the 131 Method, I'd tried every diet known to man and always fell short. I was always doing it for weight loss. At 48 years old, I had to go on high blood pressure medication, and with my cholesterol climbing, my doctor told me I needed to start eating differently! That's when I discovered the 131 Method. The 131 Method helped me to lose weight, and for the first time in over 25 years I was changing my diet for health reasons. It gave me a completely different mind-set! I was able to go off my blood pressure medication and shocked my doctor with my results! My hands and feet arthritic pain has disappeared! I can't believe the changes, and my skeptical husband is thrilled that I feel so much better. I love that I now know how food makes me feel, off meds and in control of my health. **—MARTHA S.**

MEAL PLANNING FOR THE THREE PHASES

To create the meal plan for each phase of the 131 Method, I consulted with leading experts in integrative medicine as well as a select team of registered dieticians with master's degrees as a minimum qualification. With their guidance and the help of our 131 Method–trained chefs, I've created delicious recipes and doable meal plans.

Here are some tips for success:

- Plan your meals in advance. While many diets tell you what to eat at every meal, I find that's like your mom insisting on what clothes you should wear every day even though you're now a big girl. Armed with the right information, you will be able to make the right decisions for you. You have what it takes to get results without someone else holding the steering wheel. Don't worry! I'm right here in the passenger's seat to help you out. Together we will design a meal plan that works for you and gets you excited!

- Fill out the 131 Method Meal Planning Template found on page 86, before the start of each week. Populate your meal template with your favorite foods, recipes, and meals, provided they meet the suggested guidelines of the specific phases you are on. (Review Part III for recipe ideas!)

- Create a shopping list. Scan every recipe you've selected, and place an asterisk by any ingredient that you don't have (or for which you'd like to find a healthier or more appropriate alternative for yourself). Then add it to your list, and go shopping!

HOW DO I KNOW WHAT I CAN EAT?

The number one question I am asked in our online forum is "Is it okay for me to eat ice cream/sweet potatoes/kale/oranges/tacos/every other food imaginable?" Even the most intelligent and confident of us allow self-doubt to take over when it comes to what to eat. And it's no wonder, considering the quantity of conflicting advice we are constantly bombarded with.

You, however, do not need my or anyone else's permission to eat something. Children ask their parents' permission because they haven't yet developed the wisdom to make informed decisions. If parents never allow their children to develop this skill, what results are teenagers or young adults who don't know how to figure things out for

EVERY MINUTE YOU INVEST IN PLANNING MAKES REACHING YOUR GOAL THAT MUCH EASIER!

themselves. These kids become adults who don't trust their own judgment. Adults who can't make decisions end up living a pretty tortured existence.

Good decision making is a skill. You gather information, think about potential outcomes, and then make a decision. Sometimes it works out. Sometimes it doesn't. But the only way to master anything is by trusting that you're smart enough to make a well-informed decision for yourself.

CAN I GET AN AMEN?

I know you crave a definitive, black-and-white answer to the question "Can I eat this?" I also know you're ready to do things differently, and you want the truth. The honest answer is "It depends!" First, we're all so different with unique DNA, dieting history, and personal goals. Second, it's our decision to make. If we continually look to others for permission or to tell us what we can and cannot eat, doesn't that undermine our ability to take control and accept personal responsibility for our weight and our health? I'm asking you to approach this with your newfound bad-ass beliefs! You are smart enough not just to learn this stuff, but to remember it, own it, and make the right decisions for yourself.

Ask yourself the following questions: Does this particular food I'm thinking of eating fit within the guidelines for the phase I'm on? Does it include ingredients that are likely to be inflammatory? Is this food processed or unprocessed? What do I know about the ingredients? What impact will this have on my overall macronutrient intake? Will this food fuel me or weigh me down? How do I think I will I feel after I eat it (or drink it)?

Once you know the answers to these questions and make the decisions that are right for you, nothing is off-limits. You are a human, not a robot. Instead of restricting or shaming yourself, make wise decisions and informed choices. Indulge when you need to, but make note of how it made you feel physically and emotionally. Bring me a pink-frosted sugar cookie with sprinkles for my birthday and I will eat it! Oh, sure, I'll have a bloated stomach and digestive issues 30 minutes later, but that's why it's a rare occasion—and why I don't keep this kind of thing in my home. That's called balance. Find yours. #beahuman

TRACKING: UNDERSTAND HOW FOOD MAKES YOU FEEL

An important factor in your long-term health and weight management is learning which foods work for you. Most diets create a one-size-fits-all list of "good" and "bad" foods. As I said in Chapter 3, know which foods help *you* thrive and which ones make you feel lousy, and be sure to track them all. While it may seem unnecessary to note how a particular food makes you feel, doing so will give you tremendous insight as to how to customize your diet to meet your needs. Some find that even so-called healthy foods like quinoa, tomatoes, or avocados cause symptoms. Any and all reactions are your body's way of telling you, "Hey, something isn't right here!"

YOU'RE THE BOSS.

Know thine ingredients. If you know which ingredients affect the way you feel, and how they impact your gut and your metabolism, and you're okay with paying a price for a little moderation . . . then go for it! You're too smart to rely on strangers to tell you what's good for you and what's not. Trust yourself.

The more specifically you can identify foods that cause unpleasant symptoms like gas, bloating, lethargy, brain fog, acne, constipation, etc., the more successfully you will be able to personalize a meal plan that allows you to reach your goals. Write down each meal and note which foods, if any, caused symptoms.

The following template provides you with an example of a simple one week menu using the 131 Recipes found in Part III of this book. Copy this form or download your own at www.131method.com. Create 12 copies for the 12 weeks of this program. Use this template to plan your meals in advance for each phase. You'll note that this form is more than just a tool for planning your menus. By using the symptom tracker section of this form, you'll gain valuable insight about the role food plays in how you feel.

MEAL PLANNING TEMPLATE AND SYMPTOM TRACKER

	MEAL #1	MEAL #2	MEAL #3	FOOD SYMPTOMS
MONDAY	Granola Bites	Avocado–Basil Deviled Eggs	Spaghetti Squash Bowl	None Joint Pain Gas Bloat Diarrhea Constipation Reflux Headache—started after eating eggs Anxiety Runny Nose Other
TUESDAY	Granola Bites	Mini Bell Peppers with Goat Cheese	Low-Carb BBQ Chicken Pizza	None Joint Pain Gas Bloat Diarrhea Constipation Reflux Headache Anxiety Runny Nose Other
WEDNESDAY	Bacon Quiche	BLT Pinwheels	Turkey Meatloaf with Buffalo Sauce and Chili–Lime Brussels Sprouts	None Joint Pain Gas Bloat—after brussels sprouts Diarrhea Constipation Reflux Headache—after breakfast Anxiety Runny Nose Other

ALL THESE RECIPES ARE IN THE BACK, BUT PERMISSION GRATED TO CUSTOMIZE AS YOU WISH!

	MEAL #1	MEAL #2	MEAL #3	FOOD SYMPTOMS
THURSDAY	Flaxseed–Cinnamon Muffin	Avocado–Basil Deviled Eggs	Shrimp with Zucchini Noodles	None Joint Pain Gas Bloat Diarrhea Constipation Reflux Headache–again after eggs Anxiety Runny Nose Other
FRIDAY	Bacon Quiche (leftovers)	Spicy Avocado Salad with Pumpkin and Hemp Seeds	Pizza Muffins	None Joint Pain Gas Bloat—after breakfast Diarrhea Constipation Reflux Headache—after breakfast Anxiety Runny Nose Other
SATURDAY	Chocolate Chip "Granola" Squares	Pizza Muffins (leftovers)	Spaghetti Squash Bowls	None Joint Pain Gas Bloat Diarrhea Constipation Reflux Headache Anxiety Runny Nose Other
SUNDAY	Flaxseed–Cinnamon Muffins	Cauliflower Fried Rice	Sea Bass with Mango Salsa	None Joint Pain Gas Bloat Diarrhea Constipation Reflux Headache Anxiety Runny Nose Other

Before I started the 131 Method, I was suffering from anxiety and depression. I had no motivation to play with my two-year-old and couldn't even find the energy to complete simple tasks such as the dishes or cooking. I am now on my third round and in the Nourish phase with a weight loss of 15 pounds, seemingly endless energy, and enjoying life like I never have before! My adult acne is gone! I have a mental clarity that I can't even explain; words just come out so clear and I feel so much wittier. **—JENNIFER F.**

RECORD YOUR STARTING POINT

The 131 Method is the beginning of an amazing journey to improve your health. To do so, you need to develop a system to measure your progress. After all, as the saying goes, "What you can't measure, you can't improve." I recommend you record your physical starting point as detailed below.

You'll need:

- A smartphone to take your pics
- A tape measure
- A scale
- A light-colored, solid background or wall

As much as you may dread the thought of taking photos in a revealing outfit, these pics will be priceless to you later! Progress doesn't always show up on the scale. I promise you'll want to reference these pics, especially if you tend to doubt your results. Use a notebook to track your physical, emotional, and mental progress.

HOW TO MEASURE YOURSELF

- Waist: Find the smallest part of your torso between your belly button and the bottom of your breastbone to measure your waist circumference. Breathe as normal and take your measurement in the middle of an exhalation.

- Hips: Find the widest point of your hips and booty.
- Chest: Measure directly across the widest part of your chest.
- Biceps: With your arm relaxed and at your side, measure both biceps above your elbow around the fullest part of the arm.
- Thigh: Measure the circumference of your upper thigh, approximately six inches down from the top of your leg Be sure to stand with your legs apart and weight evenly distributed. Measure both legs.
- Calves: Measure the largest part of both calves.

HOW TO TAKE PROGRESS PICTURES

DON'T ROLL YOUR EYES! YOU'LL THANK ME LATER!

- Take photos vertically or in portrait mode.
- Use a tripod, set a timer, and/or ask a friend or family member to take them for you.
- Wear something revealing like a sports bra, bathing suit, shorts, or form-fitting clothes. (Save this outfit to wear again in later progress photos.) Avoid taking photos in your underwear or in the nude, even if you plan to never share these. Trust me, you'll thank me later when you *do* want to show off the contrast!
- Stand in front of a plain, light (preferably white) background. (For example, you might stand against an empty wall, a white door, etc.) Try to use the same background each time you take a progress photo.
- Place the camera the same distance away when taking the progress photos, and use the same lighting (or, if using daylight, at the same time of day).

These are for you. And I understand if you feel like you're documenting images that later you could be blackmailed with. I promise you're going to see more in your photos than you will on the scale, and there will be days you'll find yourself grateful for the photographic motivation. Listen, you might even want to share them with me! Of course you're not required to, but please know that doing so provides so many people with the motivation they need to make a change!

131 METHOD INITIAL ASSESSMENT

Date _____

Weight _____

Optional

Body Fat Percentage _____

Resting Heart Rate _____

Bloating (scale of 1–10) _____

CIRCUMFERENCE MEASUREMENTS:

Waist: _____ Hips: _____ Chest: _____

Biceps: R _____ L _____ Thighs: R _____ L _____ Calves: _____

Rate each area below on a scale of 1 to 10, with 10 being the best:

How do you rate your overall health? _____

Rate the comfort of your clothing fit: _____

Does it change day to day from swelling, bloating, or water retention?

Explain: _____

For women, rate how regular your cycle is: _____

How heavy are your periods? Do you have cyclical cramping, acne, breast tenderness, or headaches?

Explain: _____

How regular is your digestion? _____

If necessary, be more specific about bowel frequency/quality, belching, gas, bloating, pain, etc.

Explain: _____

How well are you able to focus or maintain mental clarity? _____

Do you forget things easily, have brain fog or trouble concentrating, or generally feel anxious and restless?

Explain: _____

Rate your overall energy level: _____

How consistent and sound is your sleep? _____

Include here how many hours of sleep you get each night: _____

Do you wake up several times or sleep straight throughout the night? _____

How is the quality of your skin? _____

Do you have rashes, acne, bumps, reactions, dry or scaly skin?

Explain: _____

Rate any pain: _____

Headaches, joint pain, muscle aches? _____ _____

Explain: _____

Rate the frequency of any food cravings (for example, I crave sweets after dinner every single night, 10): _____

Indicate the type, frequency, and when they most often occur: _____

Explain: _____

Rate the intensity of your cravings (example, I cannot go without having chocolate every night, 10): _____

How easy is it for you to identify true hunger versus cravings? _____

Explain (throughout the day, between meals, etc.):
_____

Rate the depth of your relationship with food: _____

Do you view food as a friend, a crutch, or fuel?

Explain: _____

HOLD UP!

Before you flip the page, be sure to complete the assessment on page 90. When you compare your before and after numbers and feelings, you'll be astounded at the changes and results. Remember, who you are is much more than a number staring up at you from a scale. All too often we assign too much significance to that number when we're making improvements in other areas. Recognizing this progress can give you just the mojo boost you need!

It's so easy to forget where we started. I cannot wait to have you look back at your answers just 12 weeks from now! It would make my day if you would share your progress with me! Put this email address, results@131method.com, in your contacts, and set a little reminder on your calendar to send me updates!

WHAT'S NEXT?

There's been a lot of talk about fasting, and maybe you're not exactly convinced yet you can do it or want any part of it. After all, "not eating" probably sounds more like torture than a health strategy. I get it. In the next chapter you'll understand how to tap into an abundant fuel source. I'll take you through the ins and outs of fasting. You'll understand how it can revitalize your health, how to know whether it's right for you, and exactly when and how to implement it in your day-to-day life.

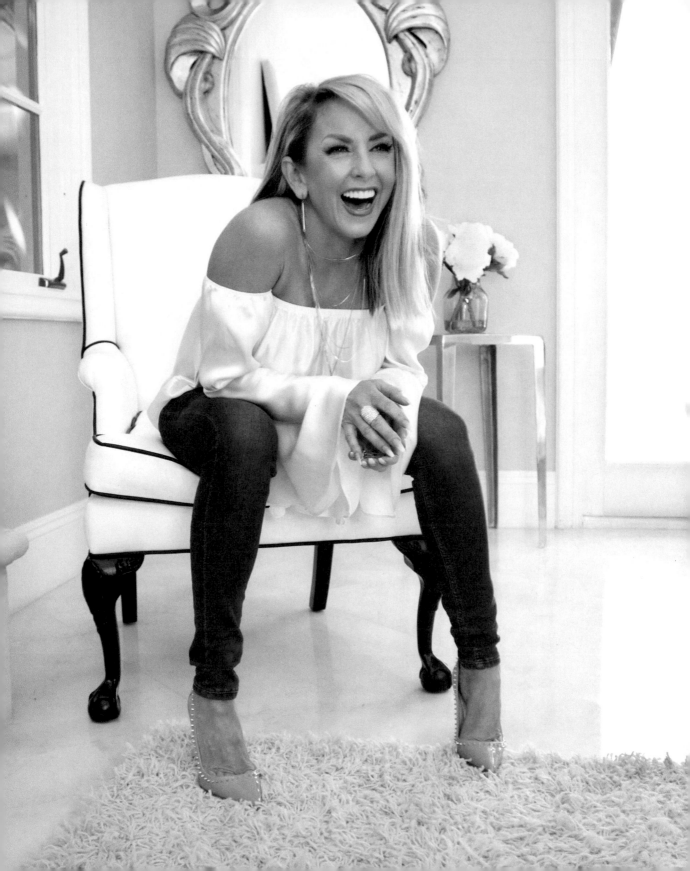

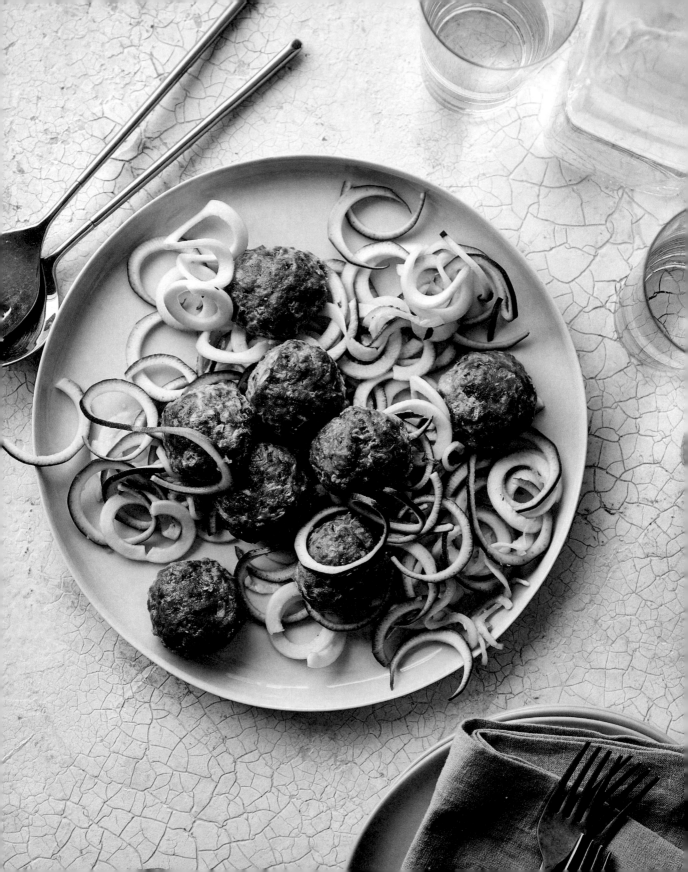

CHAPTER 5

GIVE YOUR GUT A FRESH START: FASTING AND REFUELING

For years I followed and promoted a plan calling for six small meals a day, every two to three hours. Even though I spent much of my time preparing and eating these small meals, I never felt satisfied. Each meal made me hungry for more. This left me feeling deprived and thinking there must be something wrong with me. Not only did eating small meals ramp up my hunger, it was also impossible for me to lose body fat unless I dramatically and dangerously restricted calories. Understanding the difference between calorie restriction and fasting helped me understand why the small-meals approach was never going to work for me.

Technically we all fast at some point each day. (That's why the first meal of the day is called *breakfast*. You *break* the *fast* you were on while you slept.) In this chapter I will share with you the remarkable benefits of extended fasting. However, I want to be abundantly clear that longer fasts are not for everyone.

Bottom line: When in doubt, consult with your physician before fasting. Period. The four types of fasting in the 131 Method are intended to improve your overall health. They are not recommended for quick weight loss. However, once you understand the science behind fasting and you follow the 131 Method to *prepare* your body to fast, you'll see precisely how fasting can support long-term weight loss.

THIS STUFF IS MIND BLOWING!

PINKY PROMISE ME THAT YOU'LL DOUBLE-CHECK THE FASTING CHECKLISTS FOUND ON PAGES 122, 143, AND 160 BEFORE YOU START ANY FAST!

FASTING KICK-STARTS AMAZING BENEFITS

Ironically, it wasn't too many years ago that I warned my loyal fitness followers that fasting was just about the worst thing you could do for your metabolism. I, like many other health experts, believed that if you skipped meals, your body would undoubtedly break down muscle and your metabolism would slow down. Today, I stand corrected. Countless scientific studies have proved those beliefs to be false. As a matter of fact, fasting may just hold the key to improving gut health, rebuilding the immune system, and boosting your metabolic rate.

One of the reasons for fasting's many benefits is that it can kick-start the process of autophagy in your body. In 2016, cell biologist Yoshinori Ohsumi was awarded the Nobel Prize in Physiology and Medicine for his work on autophagy—his discoveries on how cells recycle their content during fasting. Your cells create encoded proteins that seek out dead, broken, diseased, or nonfunctioning cells and break them down to use the resulting molecules to make new cell parts.

Autophagy is awesome because it:

AUTOPHAGY IS AWESOME!

- Naturally increases human growth hormone
- Increases stem cell production
- Lowers insulin levels
- Clears damaged mitochondria and generates new mitochondria
- Prevents growth of precancerous cells
- Reduces some cancerous growths
- Increases fat mobilization
- Improves inflammatory markers
- Increases brain-derived neurotrophic factor (BDNF)
- Decreases risk of metabolic disease
- Improves immune function
- Promotes gut healing

Biogerontologist Valter Longo of the University of Southern California and his team found that fasting increased human growth hormone, increased muscle development post fasting, reduced glucose, lowered blood pressure, reduced IGF-1, normalized C-reactive proteins (which are related to risk for cardiovascular disease), and increased autophagy (soon to be your favorite word). As Dr. Longo and countless other experts, including nephrologist Jason Fung and neuroscientist Mark Mattson, have confirmed, informed fasting, done for the right reasons and with the right preparation, is not only safe for most people, it can help you to live a longer, fuller, healthier life!

Researchers in the Department of Medical and Health Services at Linköping University in Sweden found that consuming one large meal rather than five small meals actually decreases the hunger hormone ghrelin. In addition, their study found that larger meals eaten less often increased energy expenditure.[1] Another study, on morning fasting and obesity, conducted in the department of health at the University of Bath in the United Kingdom, showed that obese adults who were able to delay their first meal of the day experienced a decrease in appetite, a decrease in ghrelin production, and an increase in satiety.[2]

Fasting is an integral part of the 131 Method and offers a variety of scientifically based benefits, including starting and maintaining ketosis and autophagy, regulating hunger hormones, starving down bad gut bacteria to balance your microbiome, regulating your blood pressure, giving the digestive system an opportunity to heal, and helping you identify and break the habit of emotional eating.

FASTING BENEFITS YOUR BRAIN

Fasting does the coolest things ever to your brain! When you fast, you significantly increase production of brain-derived neurotrophic factor (BDNF)—say that five times fast. BDNF is a chemical produced in the brain and blood that is active in the areas of the brain that affect decision making, memory, and clarity of thought. BDNF is also key in

INCREASING BDNF IS LIKE FUELING YOUR BRAIN WITH SUPERPOWERS!

the signaling of the hippocampus to suppress appetite, as well as messaging that tells the body to use stored brown fat (the unhealthiest fat) for energy. BDNF has also been shown to increase the rate at which your body burns energy, increase quality sleep, and promote daytime wakefulness. Are you sold yet? BDNF is also thought to play a role in the reduction of depression, anxiety, and stress. Several studies have linked low BDNF production to depression, sleep disorders, and weight gain.

BYE-BYE, FATTY FAT CELLS

The relationship between weight loss and fasting isn't as obvious as it might seem, so let me break it down. First, while it's likely you'll experience rapid short-term weight loss on a fast, that shouldn't be your primary objective. Sure, stepping on the scale after your first fast can be exciting and motivating, but keep in mind that the number on the scale does not necessarily represent permanent weight loss. Many of the pounds that are gained and lost in quick weight fluctuations are due to water weight.

Remember, when the body is inflamed, it holds water in tissue as a sort of protective mechanism. As you reduce inflammation through fasting, you'll experience less bloating and your body will eliminate unnecessary fluids. Body tissues also hold water based on the sodium content of food. While losing that water can be seen when you step on the scale after fasting, some of that water weight will and should return. Your body requires additional water when you are eating regularly for proper digestion, waste elimination, nutrient absorption, and more.

But here's some good news about those lost pounds: Not all of the weight you lose on a fast will come back. Studies show you can lose up to half a pound of fat per day while fasting! Now we're talking! For example, let's say you complete your first three-day fast, step on the scale, and see that you have lost five pounds. Some of that will be water weight, so you won't have lost five pounds of pure fat—but you may have lost one and a half pounds of fat. I don't know about you, but I would be pretty happy with the ability to lose that much fat in such a short period. And while water weight should be expected to return, you can say bye-bye to the body fat for good!

To help maintain your realistic and healthy expectations for fasting, rather than focus on the scale after your fast, focus on your body's new ability to burn fat and the tremendous long-term health benefits you experience each time you fast. (If you struggle with this concept, you may want to reread the section "Scales Can Be Rude" in Chapter 4.)

FASTING FOR SELF-AWARENESS AND BREAKING THE HABITS OF EMOTIONAL EATING

Many on the 131 Method often remark that the most powerfully transformational piece of the program is the awareness they gain during fasting. We're surrounded by food. It's everywhere. It gets your attention on Instagram. Commercials lure you to the pantry. Family congregates in the kitchen. Coworkers bond over potluck lunches. It's no wonder we end up eating for a million reasons other than hunger. (Don't forget to complete the True Hunger vs. Emotional Eating exercise in Chapter 4.)

Fasting can also be the ultimate reality check, giving you a profound awareness about the amount and frequency of the food you consume each week due to emotional eating, habit, and plain old boredom. Armed with this self-awareness, you can replace these habits with healthier activities. How you prepare for these situations in advance of your fast will help ensure your success.

WANT MORE ENERGY, CLARITY, AND TIME?

I could not believe how good I felt while I was fasting. I can't say I've ever felt that much energy or mental clarity. —**MICHELE P.**

WHAT YOU CAN EXPECT TO FEEL WHILE FASTING

... MOST OF WHICH AREN'T PLEASANT.

If you're like most people, you likely have some preconceived notions about fasting. Maybe you've convinced yourself that fasting requires supernatural willpower or that it'll feel torturous. Most people assume they'll feel sluggish or "hangry." While everyone's experience is a little different, when you prepare for a fast following the 131 Method, you'll be shocked by how good you feel!

Actually, you should expect to look and feel *amazing*. (Remember, our expectations often determine our outcome.) When we fast, human growth hormone production increases nearly fivefold. Human growth hormone is essential for cellular regeneration, tissue repair, and production of collagen for healthy hair, strong nails, and skin that glows. Don't believe it? Take a picture of your skin on day one and again on day three of a fast to document the difference for yourself!

When following the 131 Method fasting protocol, people often report feeling more energy than when they are consuming a normal diet. This is because with greater human growth hormone comes greater energy. Furthermore, ketone molecules produced while fasting deliver a more potent form of energy.

While fasting, you can expect relief from nagging joint aches and pains as inflammation begins to subside. Every system of the body performs more proficiently, and you'll find relief from common discomfort so many of us have just learned to live with. In addition, puffiness disappears!

Before developing the 131 Method, if I had gone so much as five hours without food, it would have been an all-out "Call 911, get out of my way, I don't care what I eat, someone's going to get hurt, I need to eat" kind of emergency. But once I created the 131 Method, giving me choices of how and when to fast, everything changed.

For example, I decided to do a three-day fast in conjunction with a three-day social media conference called Marketing Impact Academy that I host here in Southern California. There were nearly 1,000 participants in attendance, expecting brain-blowing business strategies and social media marketing content to be delivered from the stage by yours truly from 8 A.M. to 6 P.M. Pulling off this event requires that I am fully rested, focused, and mentally sharp.

I distinctly remember each day of the fast waking up and feeling better than the day before. I had spent the two weeks prior to the event preparing my body. Because I was in a mild state of ketosis before I started my fast, day one was breeze. On day two, I recall wanting to eat something for dinner, not because I was hungry, but because I wanted to unwind after a mentally grueling day. I noticed the desire and identified that it wasn't a physical hunger, but rather an appetite triggered by a feeling. Instead of breaking my fast, I downed a cup of bone broth and joined attendees for the event dance party. My energy was very high. I ended up dancing my booty off for three hours! Knowing I probably had overdone it, I expected to wake the next day feeling a bit run down or low on energy. Nope.

By day three, my energy level was through the roof. I felt as if some super-bionic computer had taken over my brain; I was no longer searching for the right word or struggling to remember what I was to present next. I spoke from the stage for hours with laserlike focus. With each hour that passed, I felt better mentally and physically. And not once did I feel hungry. Over the course of the third day, I must have said 20 times to myself, "I cannot believe I'm not hungry."

Over the course of my career, I've led countless multiday events, each of which was stressful and took its toll on me mentally and physically. Not this time. I fell asleep as soon as my head hit the pillow each night and awoke feeling rested, high-energy, and focused.

REMEMBER...THIS WASN'T MY FIRST FAST

I felt comfortable doing this experiment because I did the following to prepare for fasting:

- I developed the metabolic flexibility that comes only after completing all three phases—Ignite, Nourish, and Renew—of the 131 Method.
- I had several successful three- and even four-day fasts under my belt before attempting to do one while simultaneously hosting a seminar.
- I prepared my body in the weeks before starting my fast by getting into fat-burning mode.
- I promised myself that I would end the fast the moment I didn't feel well or it wasn't serving me.

I lost 19 pounds, 3 inches from my waist and hips, and 5 percent of my body fat. I definitely have more energy, a healthier gut (no more daily stomachaches), and fewer aches and pains. I feel younger at 52 than I did in my 40s. My skin looks smoother, and my hair is healthier and has stopped falling out. **—MELISSA H.**

KICK "HANGRY" TO THE CURB: WHY YOU WON'T BE HUNGRY WHEN FASTING

People often worry about fasting for one reason: They're afraid of feeling hungry. When I tell people who follow the 131 Method that they won't be hungry, they think I've lost my mind. But it's true, and here's why.

We experience hunger when there isn't enough of the expected or current fuel source available. That's when the body signals the brain, via our hormones, to tell us to eat. When we are in a sugar-burning state, glucose and glycogen are stored in our system. When we begin to deplete those glucose stores, our hormones signal the brain to create hunger cues such as a growling stomach, headaches, sleepiness, lethargy, anger, confusion, etc. The body perceives a threat—shortage of fuel to keep running—

and the brain screams, "Eat! Eat! Eat or you're going to die!" We answer by eating whatever is in sight, which raises insulin levels, increases hunger hormones, and creates a metabolic cycle of survival. As a result, those hunger hormones are used, confused, and abused and don't know what to do!

Fasting, however, corrects your temper-tantrum hunger hormones. As you transition into the fat-burning mode of ketosis, fat becomes your primary fuel source. Your hunger hormones then signal the brain, "Hey, you can relax, we have plenty of fuel on board." Those hunger cues of the past disappear. Long gone will be the days of starvation-based bad decisions or text messages you shouldn't have sent while you were hangry!

BE PREPARED: NOT EVERYONE WILL BE SUPPORTIVE

Humans have used food to self-soothe and express love since the beginning of time. If we simply thought of food as fuel, healthy weight loss wouldn't be nearly so complicated. The fact is, food is how we express care and concern for ourselves and others. For this reason, you probably shouldn't expect friends and family to be super-excited about your plans to fast. Quite the contrary. However, don't confuse their concern with ill-intended sabotage. Their worries likely stem from a good place. Unlike you, they haven't immersed themselves in the science of metabolism, so their fears arise from a lack of understanding. What we don't fully understand we fear. Here are some ways I suggest handling this:

- Don't talk about it. (That's pretty simple.)
- Share selectively. I'm not suggesting you hide anything or lie, but do you really need to announce to your mom or all your coworkers that you'll be fasting next week? Only if you're prepared to debate your decision. This is your health journey, not theirs.

DON'T TRY TO EXPLAIN FASTING TO PEOPLE WHO AREN'T INTERESTED IN KNOWLEDGE. #FIXEDMINDSET

- Avoid the know-it-all. There are certain people you and I both know who love to tell us what to do, what not to do, and why they know everything. Unless you're looking for a lecture, these folks do not need to know what you're doing.

- Explain your emergency plan. Assure loved ones that you appreciate their concerns and promise to end your fast if at any time you're not feeling well. If you're doing a fast that doesn't include abstaining from food, maybe avoid using the term "fast."

- Exercise good judgment. Avoid discussing your plans with anyone with a known history of eating disorders or with impressionable teens (see parenting tips on page 106).

- Boycott the body shamer. If there's a particular person in your life that triggers negative feelings about your weight or body image, do yourself a favor and stop giving them so much power. What you do and how you do it and why you do it is none of their business.

THE FOUR FASTS OF THE 131 METHOD

At the end of each of the three phases of the 131 Method, you'll have a choice! You can follow the one-week optional fast and refueling plan, or you can continue following the guidelines of the phase you are in. (I know it's going to feel a bit redundant, but at the end of every phase I will remind you that fasting is optional. I will also ask you to take a Fasting Assessment to help determine if it's the right time for you to fast.)

Here's how that will work. Say for example you are on the Ignite phase for three weeks. During the fourth week, you decide that fasting isn't for you this month. No problem! You'll simply extend what you were doing in weeks 1, 2, and 3 and continue it during week 4. This means, if you choose to skip fasting on Ignite, you would continue to practice macro tracking and intermittent fasting for an additional week.

There are four levels of fasting. Each level is more advanced than the previous one. For best results, don't skip ahead to more advanced levels until you have established the metabolic flexibility that comes in later phases of the 131 Method. But you *can* return to a lower-level fast, or choose to skip fasting altogether! The 131 Method allows you to customize every part of the program and still be successful.

When it comes to fasting, it's not uncommon to hear people insist there's only one way to do it. They're wrong. The right way is the way that works for you. The type of fast you select should be determined only after considering your health objectives, current physical condition, how you've prepared in the weeks prior, and what's going on in your life. If fasting might place an undue burden on you or disrupt something important you have planned—like a special dinner or that 5k you've been training for—then skip it for now, but don't dismiss the idea of trying it later.

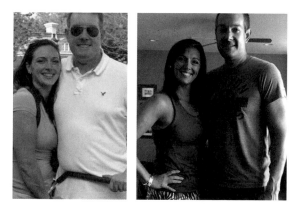

P.S....TONS OF DUDES HAVE SUCCESS WITH THE 131 METHOD

Fasting was intimidating at first. I never thought I could not eat breakfast or work out in a fasted state. Now, I cannot imagine it any different. From working out and following a "diet" to LEARNING what works for me. Living life and enjoying food, and teaching my husband about it, too. Now, we are eating good-quality foods, have less inflammation, balanced workouts of cardio and weights, better sleep, clearer skin without use of expensive products. I used OMAD (One Meal a Day) as my go-to fasting choice and I truly feel that I am aging backward! We've learned to do what works for us. We will never follow a one-size-fits-all diet again. **—BRIDGET I.**

AN IMPORTANT NOTE FOR PARENTS

Parents, when it comes to fasting, we have to be very careful what message we are sending small children and/or impressionable teens. They haven't the maturity or need to understand fasting, and seeing Mom or Dad going without food can create subliminal messaging. In fact, studies have shown that parental role modeling is the single greatest predictor of a child's relationship with food, body image, and dieting. Unfortunately, when parents restrict food, diet, speak negatively about themselves, or obsess over body image or weight loss, the result is an increased likelihood of obesity and diminished self-esteem in their children.

Young children and impressionable teens are likely to interpret fasting as a form of restriction. Kids aren't privy to the knowledge you've consumed in this book, nor is it appropriate for children to fast. For this reason, I always suggest that if you are a parent, consider fasting options that allow you to eat within specified periods of time, such as fasting level 1, 2, or 3. Speak in terms of health, energy, brain function, and longevity around your kids. Instead of foods that are "good" or "bad," refer to foods in terms of how they help you perform or improve the way you feel. Avoid talking about weight, dieting, or your body. Instead of restricting, rewarding, or controlling your child's food intake, role model what it means to be healthy from the inside out. What's more, I also think that shopping, preparing, cooking, and eating healthy food with our family are some of the most important things we do as parents. So, Mom and Dad, keep some food in your fast!

It might seem to you I'm overstepping my boundaries—after all, this isn't a parenting book. You're right, but the fact of the matter is that most of us can trace our issues with food and body image right back to our earliest years of childhood. Those well-meaning yet hurtful comments and unhealthy habits of parents can create a lifetime of struggle for some. The 131 Method gives you the tools you need to change the legacy of health for your family forever.

THIS IS HOW WE CHANGE A FAMILY'S LEGACY OF HEALTH.

LEVEL 1: INTERMITTENT FASTING

Also referred to as time-restricted eating, intermittent fasting will help you correct an appetite on overdrive, burn stored body fat, and give your gut a rest. And to do this, you won't need to count calories, but you will want to watch your macronutrient ratios. When used in combination with a diet high in fat and low in carbs, fasting helps your body deplete glucose and glycogen stores. That's why keeping your carb intake at 5 to 10 percent of your total calorie intake will give you optimal results with intermittent fasting.

Intermittent fasting is considered by many to be the easiest fast to start with. I encourage you to practice several weeks of intermittent fasting before even considering a more advanced fast.

There are countless variations of intermittent fasting. While I suggest you practice it on all three phases of the 131 Method, you'll practice daily intermittent fasting during the Ignite phase using an eating window. This means you will schedule your meals to happen within a particular window of time, such as 12 hours. Technically speaking, if you didn't eat in your sleep last night, you were doing intermittent fasting for however long you slept.

Getting started is a breeze. Begin with the time you want to have your last meal and then count ahead 12 hours to schedule your first meal of the next day. Let's say that you plan to finish dinner by 7 P.M. That means you'd have your first meal (breakfast) no earlier than 7 A.M. the next day.

Start with a 12-hour window for your first few days. Then, every day, delay your first meal by another hour or so, while continuing to have your last meal of the day at the same time. This means breakfast on Monday might be at 7 A.M. On Tuesday you would delay your first meal until 8 A.M. On Wednesday you would postpone breakfast until 9 A.M. and so on until such time that your meals are eaten within an eight-hour window. Using our example, you would eat from 11 A.M. to 7 P.M., then fast from 7 P.M. to 11 A.M.

INTERMITTENT FASTING IS THE PERFECT BEGINNER FAST!

The way you design the timing of your meals should fit seamlessly into your lifestyle with consideration of the time of day you usually have the most robust appetite. Some may prefer an early breakfast and have dinner in the late afternoon. If you tend to be hungrier in the evening, you'll likely have no problem pushing your first meal back to almost lunchtime to accommodate a late dinner.

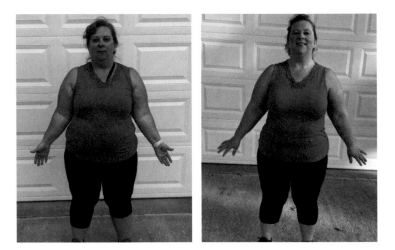

Never thought in a million years that I, Tara, could fast, but I did! Intermittent fasting made it so easy. I've lost 18 lbs. I sleep so much better. Within the first week, I noticed that my feet, knees, and joints didn't hurt like they did. I was taking pain relief medicine almost daily but not anymore. My complexion has improved. I have more energy. I crave real food too! I love the recipes! The recipes help with meal planning ideas! **—TARA Y.**

It's a good idea to track the time of your first and last meal each day using your 131 Method Workbook (available at www.131method.com) or by keeping notes in your smartphone. This will help you progressively and comfortably shorten your eating schedule until you're down to an eight-hour window.

Technically speaking, when fasting for the pure benefits of autophagy, you want to avoid consuming any calories.

Water is of course encouraged, but there's much debate about whether bone broth, your morning coffee with MCT oil, or preworkout supplements break the fast.

Here's the answer: It depends. Strictly speaking, anything you eat could take you out of a ketosis and therefore "break the fast." However, most people have found they can eat a small amount of something high in fat—or mostly pure fat—during their fasting window and still stay in fat-burning mode! So many people during their fasting period still have coffee, coffee with coconut oil, coffee with heavy cream (no sugar), lemon water, MCT oil, or bone broth to help stave off the urge to eat.

If it's any consolation, in all the fasting I've done over the course of the last three years, I have my fat-burning coffee every morning, bone broth in the evening, and small amounts of pure fat when needed. Don't get caught up in the idea that there's only one way to do this. All-or-nothing thinking does not allow for forward progress.

You may be able to eat a handful of nuts in the evening, or even have a preworkout drink in the morning, and not be kicked out of ketosis; others may find that this affects them negatively. It may take some time to build the metabolic flexibility needed to maintain ketosis. You have to trust how you feel during this time.

Honestly, I'm not that nice a person until I have my fat-burning morning coffee. Just typing the words "morning coffee" brings me joy and fills the back of my throat with the smell of that fresh pot! You're in charge here. You get to decide what works best for you! If you're the obsessive rule-following type, then stick with water until your first meal. But if dropping any part of your morning or daily ritual means you'd be putting the greater public at risk, girl go get your coffee!

Intermittent fasting is just one of several simple strategies on the 131 Method that allow you to take control of your hormones, rest the digestive system, and reduce body fat without having to "diet." Each of these strategies, or tools

DON'T GET CAUGHT UP IN OTHER PEOPLE'S RULES. DO WHAT WORKS FOR YOU.

as I like to call them, will help you improve overall health. Using one tool is great but stacking these tools is even better and only works to fortify your long-term success.

While fasting is certainly something humans have done for thousands of years, there have yet to be clinical human studies to assess the long-term effects of intermittent fasting on metabolic adaptation. For that reason, I suggest periodically phasing from intermittent fasting to avoid adaptation. Ideally, this can be done anytime intermittent fasting isn't convenient due to your social schedule, or just because you wake up and really feel like you need to eat. Give yourself some grace. There's a big difference between good habits and obsessive behavior. Avoid making food or the timing of your meals something that interferes with living your life! The 131 Method is all about balance.

I used to use a lot of prepackaged meals and sauces; now I make it all from scratch. I also love intermittent fasting and not eating late at night. **—SARAH J.**

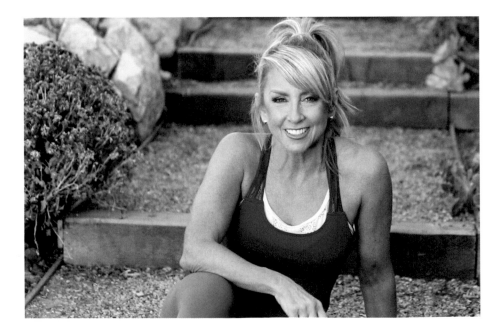

EXERCISE AND INTERMITTENT FASTING

For many years, we have been told to eat before exercising. The idea was that if we exercised in a fasted state, we would be low on energy, have diminished returns, and possibly lose muscle mass in the process. The latest research shows that exercising and intermittent fasting are safe when done together. As with all things, however, you want to listen to your body and give yourself time to become comfortable as you transition from being a sugar burner to a fat burner.

When you are new to intermittent fasting and your body is accustomed to running on the energy provided by glucose and glycogen, you may at first find it challenging to fuel high-intensity workouts. As your body becomes fat-adapted and metabolically flexible, exercise and all physical activity will become much easier. Keep in mind that everyone adapts to ketosis at a different rate. Be patient! Listen to your body. Many people report having more energy during fasted workouts and a diminished postworkout appetite.

Research shows that those practicing intermittent fasting demonstrate no significant difference in physical performance as compared with those consuming food prior to their workout. In one eight-week study, scientists compared maximal strength of those who were fasting and those who were not and found maximal strength was maintained in resistance-trained men when doing intermittent fasting.[3]

Regardless of studies, statistics, and recommendations, what matters is what works for you. Some people feel great exercising in a fasted state. Others take several weeks to make the transition. I want you to learn to listen to your body. If your body is craving rest, rest. If a rigorous workout sounds good, let's do it!

LISTEN TO YOUR BODY, NOT WHAT SOME YOUTUBER TELLS YOU TO DO.

When I first heard that fasting was a part of the 131 Method, I have to admit I was nervous. Like most people, I immediately thought I could never fast beyond 24 hours. I followed the 131 suggestions and got my body into ketosis prior to my fast, and I couldn't believe I sailed through using the shortened window protocol. I was amazed how my body took care of me! I didn't experience any of the discomfort I had anticipated. The shortened window method of fasting was a great stepping stone to extended fasting. I'm now able to complete a three- to four-day fast every month. —DANA M.

LEVEL 2: SHORTENED WINDOW FAST

The shortened window fast (SWF) takes intermittent fasting one step further by reducing the schedule each day during which you consume food. If you've mastered the eight-hour intermittent fasting schedule during Ignite, you'll find the SWF a breeze.

On the SWF, you'll delay your first meal of the day even further, so that you are eating all your meals within a four-hour period each day and finishing your final meal at least two to three hours before bedtime. It doesn't matter exactly when in the day your four-hour eating window occurs—you can have it during the morning, afternoon, or evening if you want. The exact time isn't nearly as important as working to ensure it's at the same time every day for seven days.

The food that you do eat on your SWF should be high in fat and low in carbs to maintain nutritional ketosis. I specifically recommend a range of 70 to 85 percent of your calories from healthy fat and less than 15 percent from carbohydrates.

So how does a four-hour window work? How you customize your four-hour eating window is up to you. You might allow hunger to be your guide. Create quiet, undistracted, peaceful space to enjoy your first meal and then wait until you feel hungry again within your scheduled window. You might also wish to create four smaller meals and eat on the hour for four hours. Or you could play it by ear and do something different each day. Remember, the only rules are the ones you make, and the right way to follow this method is the way that works best for you. (Insert mic drop here!)

Because of the limited number of hours you'll be eating within, it's very likely your intake will be substantially less than what you usually eat each day. That's okay! Remember, this is a fast. Don't worry about calories or try to force down food, as if you'll never make it through the night. Remember, a fat-adapted body can survive on stored body fat for quite some time.

I had wanted to do the three-day fast, but after listening to my body I opted for the shortened window fast. I ate within a four-hour window every day for seven days. The shortened window fast didn't seem like a fast, so I was worried I was doing it wrong until I took some time to listen to my body and notice the results.

My skin has cleared up, the pounds and inches melted off—which is so odd to me because of all the fat I ate. I am one of those people who cut as much fat out of my diet as possible for the last several years, so I definitely had to "trust" the process. I also had dealt with stomach issues in the past when eating fat, so I was very leery to eat any. I was amazed that I had absolutely no stomach issues with the diet and felt satisfied by all of the wonderful recipes I tried. My only disappointment was that I wanted to try more recipes but always found myself feeling so satisfied that I didn't need to eat more! I've got a list of recipes I want to try in the near future. I also found myself naturally drinking more water than ever before.

I also loved the fact that I had time to do more in the day. When only thinking about eating within four hours, I wasn't consumed with meal planning the other times of the day and found myself getting so much done.

I do hope to try the three-day fast the next time I get a chance, but the one thing I have definitely learned to do is to listen to my body. If I don't feel like it's the right time, I know I can do the shortened window fast and still have amazing results! **—LORI F.**

LEVEL 3: ONE MEAL A DAY (OMAD)

The level 3 fast is called OMAD, which stands for One Meal a Day. This one is pretty self-explanatory. OMAD is a practice of fasting an entire day, except for one meal. If you choose OMAD, you'll be testing it for three consecutive days; ideally, you'll want to eat your meal (and any additional calories) within a one- or two-hour window.

IDEAL FOR NEWBIES, STRESS CASES, AND PARENTS.

Which meal you choose is up to you and should be based on your lifestyle and the time of day when your desire to eat is most active. As with all scheduled eating, it's best to choose the same mealtime each day. Parents have often mentioned that they find it most convenient to choose dinner as their meal of the day so they can spend quality time with their children and role-model healthy habits. I love the idea of parents modeling healthy eating for their kids. Our children are always watching. For that reason, instead of talking about diet, use dinner as a time to talk about food as fuel and the power of unprocessed whole ingredients.

AVOID OMAD IF YOU
HAVE A TENDENCY
TOWARD BINGE
EATING

When practicing OMAD, be careful to not to binge or indulge beyond what you would typically eat for a meal. Remember, although fasting comes with many health benefits, it is also a practice in releasing our emotional attachment to food. There's no reason to supersize portions or stuff yourself. Eat to the point of satiety, never discomfort. You're eating only one meal, so the quality of the ingredients is critical. Do your best to create meals with whole, unprocessed foods.

Practice mindful eating. Work to be consciously aware of each bite. To maximize the health benefits of a modified fast such as OMAD, meals should be higher in healthy fats, lower in carbohydrates, and moderate in protein to help you stay in ketosis. The carbs should be complex carbohydrates, and mostly from plants.

Avoid consuming calorie-laden drinks before your one meal. If you're going to eat something before your meal, be mindful of your macronutrients and whether your choice will affect your insulin level and spike your blood sugar. Ultimately, how carefully you follow this recommendation is up to you.

We started the 131 Method at the ages of 59 and 68 to get into better health so that when we are older we will not have to go to many doctors' visits. Needless to say, it was eye-opening, informative, and last but not least, amazing. When we got to the fasting protocols, the OMAD wasn't as hard to try as we thought. We just shortened our eating window more and more so we could have one meal a day . . . We used to think the older you get, the harder it is to lose weight . . . but it's NOT! I'm now 60, and I've lost 55 pounds. I haven't been this size for over 20 years. My husband is 69 and down to his college weight of 175 pounds—a loss of 45 pounds. AMAZING to say the least. :)
—ELIZABETH AND KEN K.

IT'S NEVER TOO LATE TO MAKE A CHANGE!*

LEVEL 4: THREE-DAY MINI-FAST

Level 4 is the most advanced fast, but many consider it the most rewarding. If you have mastered intermittent fasting with an eight-hour eating window and maintained ketosis for several days, you might find your first three-day fast far easier than you've anticipated.

A three-day mini-fast can look like a variety of things as you can customize your experience to meet your needs. Traditionally speaking, a three-day mini-fast might mean you are only drinking water for 72 hours. However, due in large part to the works of Dr. Valter Longo and others, we now know that many of the benefits of fasting can be achieved without fully abstaining from calories or food. This means your three-day mini-fast should be designed to include the support (from a mental, physical, and nutritional standpoint) that you need to be successful.

Regardless of how you design your three-day fast, it is essential you support your efforts with adequate hydration and with special attention given to ensure electrolytes are balanced (as discussed in Chapter 4). I might add the other key component to a successful fast, regardless of type, is that you exercise common sense. If you're not feeling well, end the fast!

A three-day mini-fast probably sounds a bit intimidating. I get it. As a fitness professional, for decades I warned people of the "dangers" of skipping even one meal. Today I am empowered by the research and human studies of great scientists who are helping us to uncover the miraculous healing benefits of fasting. I now have firsthand experiencing preparing my body to fast, and I know that if you follow the 131 Method, fasting will help you rebuild and repair your immune system, improve overall health, manage emotional eating, and help you to keep body fat off for good. By following this plan, you will find the three-day fast to be one of the most healing, powerful, and transforming things you can do for yourself.

NOT GONNA LIE... THIS ONE WILL MAKE YOU FEEL LIKE A ROCKSTAR!

Let's get real. Going without food for three days is going to be much tougher on you mentally than it will be physically. Keep that in mind. Don't set yourself up for disaster. Think about what you have going on, the situations you'll be in, any social engagements you might have planned, your health, and of course your stress at the moment. If you are under considerable stress, level 1 or 2 is likely a better fit.

Your three-day mini-fast starts when you're ready to start it. Select three days during the week that make the most sense for your lifestyle; three days where you simply won't have to rely solely on your willpower. Pick three days during which you can keep yourself quite busy. Try to avoid scheduling your fast to coincide with a big social gathering, or even a close-of-the-soccer-season pizza party. It's not the end of the world if you decide to delay the start of your fast by a day or even a week, if that makes life a little easier. No part of this should be painful or rigid. This whole journey leads to a healthier version of you. This is real life, not a prison sentence.

Once you complete your three-day mini-fast, you will begin refueling and prepare to move on to your next phase feeling lighter, stronger, and more empowered than ever.

Your three-day mini-fast will give your digestive system three full days of rest. Three days is sufficient for most people to burn entirely through their glucose and glycogen stores and truly reap the benefits of fasting ketosis and the process of cellular autophagy.

The benefits of the three-day mini-fast include:

- Extra time. You'll be pleasantly surprised by the amount of money and time saved by eliminating shopping for food, planning meals, preparing food, cooking, and cleaning up after meals.
- Simplicity. The only guidelines are to go without calories for three days. There's no need to calculate or track meals. There's no counting.

- Compliments. Mark my words, you will be glowing and people will notice. As you begin your fast you'll begin to reduce inflammation. Take a few selfies so you yourself can document the reduction in puffiness often present around our eyes, face, hands, and feet.

- Confidence. When you hit that 72-hour mark, you are going to feel like such a badass! There's just no other way to describe it. Many describe the experience as spiritual, and I agree! The removal of distractions and the mental clarity I experience when fasting allow me to feel more connected to God.

SHOUT-OUT TO JESUS!

BEST PRACTICES FOR SUPPORTING YOUR FAST

Support refers to the supplements, liquids, or anything else you might need to take in (including food) in order to make the most of your fasting experience. You may need support because fasting is new or to help you cope, whether physically or mentally.

EXOGENOUS KETONES

I've said it before and I'll say it again, I want you to take a food first approach to your health. However, there are circumstances where you may want to consider supplementation. In part because of the increased interest in the benefits of ketosis, many companies have developed supplements which can aid in the process of entering ketosis.

Exogenous ketones are man-made supplements (*exogenous* describes something made outside the body). As you've learned, your body has the ability to produce ketones naturally. Due in large part to the popularity of the ketogenic diet, the production of exogenous ketones has become big business. There are countless types, manufacturers, and uses to consider. Though your goal should be to produce ketones naturally, there are many individuals who find supplementing with exogenous ketones helps to minimize any discomfort associated with

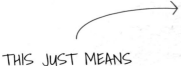

THIS JUST MEANS
YOU'LL FEEL KINDA
"MEH"

the transition into ketosis, which is sometimes referred to as "the keto flu." A quality-ingredient exogenous ketone supplement may be ideal if you have a history of consuming a high-sugar/high-carb diet; if you find it difficult to maintain appropriate macronutrient levels prior to fasting, as may happen with vegans or vegetarians; or if you need to consume more than 10 to 15 percent carbohydrates.

I've experimented with several brands, flavors, and types of exogenous ketones. Without question they are man-made, highly processed ingredients, and I don't endorse their long-term use. Personally, I prefer to get my body to produce them naturally. However, you may find them helpful in getting through a rough day of fasting.

The consumer availability of exogenous ketones is relatively new. There is a lot we don't know yet, so proceed with caution. As with all decisions, you're in charge!

Some things to consider before supplementing with man-made ketones:

- They're an additional cost.
- They are not regulated by the FDA.
- They will not take the place of a fat-burning diet.
- They may produce digestive discomfort.
- To date, there are no studies evaluating the risks or side effects of long-term use.

If you do decide to proceed, look for 10 or more grams of beta-hydroxybutyrate per serving. Be wary of manufacturers that fail to list total grams on their packaging.

FOOD WHILE FASTING

When you're trying to stay in fat-burning mode, carbs will have the most significant impact on your insulin level. Instead of carbs, supplement with foods containing healthy fat, such as avocados, macadamia nuts, pecans, or cashew nuts. Or go for a pure healthy fat like coconut oil, coconut butter, grass-fed or grass-finished ghee, grass-fed butter, or even MCT oil. The oils and even butters can be stirred into your coffee or tea. That might sound strange, but trust me when I say you'll feel surprisingly satisfied. In small quantities, these supplements should allow you to remain in fat-burning mode while continuing to rest your digestive system.

I think it's important to note that many people really miss the act of chewing; others may experience digestive discomfort by consuming pure fat on an empty stomach. So, can you have a handful of nuts or a couple tablespoons of avocado? Sure! In fact, you can have ice cream if you think that's the right decision for you. Just remember that almost everything, even nuts and avocado, contain carbohydrates. The more carbohydrates you consume, the more likely you are to push yourself out of ketosis. For the record, I have yet to do a fast where I didn't have a few nuts. To judge the success of your fast, you need to include your mental state, not just the depth of your ketosis.

KEEP YOURSELF BUSY

In my experience, fasting success is about 10 percent physical and about 90 percent mind-set. My first attempt at fasting was a disaster for three reasons. First, I didn't know the importance of achieving ketosis before fasting. Second, I failed to plan activities to keep me busy and my mind off food. Third, and most significant, was my bad attitude. In the back of my mind I had decided I would quit even before I started. Your beliefs determine your outcome. Start with the right attitude.

WHAT SUCCESS ISN'T 90% MINDSET?!

Today fasting is a breeze for me. I actually love it. I look forward to it because I know how to prepare mentally and physically. Following these tips will help you avoid an unpleasant ride on the struggle bus.

In advance of your fasting days, pull out your calendar and pack it with productivity! Organize your closet, catch up on projects, schedule a garage clean-out, start that book you were going to write. (Most people say fasting is one of their favorite parts of the 131 Method, not just because of the physical benefits but because of the productivity that results.) Or pamper yourself, learn to meditate, take a hike with a friend, or read a great book.

Schedule activities away from food hubs like the lunchroom or the kitchen. During mealtimes and habitual "snacking hours," set a meeting or appointment, or use the time to call your mom. (Legit, call your mom!) If mindless snacking is your nemesis, hang out anywhere other than where temptations can be found.

When all else fails, go to bed early.

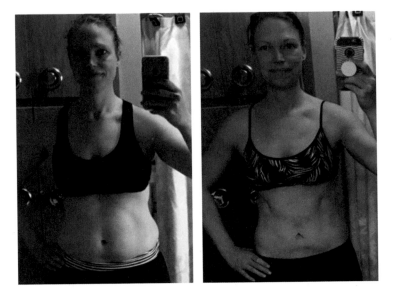

I've lost 20 lbs. and 12 inches and kept it off for almost a year now! I keep cycling through the phases and have fasted four times! I have not had a major sickness in a year! The 131 Method has improved my immune system! I also love my relationship with food now. I'm not hungry or worried about when I'm going to eat next. So freeing!
—RHONDA K.

BEFORE YOU FAST

There are several concepts you'll see I have repeated several times throughout this book. I've done so with the intention of making the message stick. One of those is that fasting is optional.

Fasting is an *option*; it is not mandatory. (As I warned, I'll repeat that message often.) Fasting can be a stressor on the system and should be carefully considered before you begin. Even if you choose not to fast during the entire 12-week process, I promise it will not hinder your success. At the end of each phase, before you begin your fast and refueling, you will find a fasting checklist. I recommend you complete this checklist before deciding if this is the right time and if fasting is right and safe for you. Fasting is not appropriate for all populations.

WHO SHOULD AVOID FASTING

- Infants and children
- People with type 1 diabetes
- Those with low blood sugar (hypoglycemia)
- Those with low blood pressure (hypotension)
- Pregnant and nursing women
- Those recovering from surgery or severe injury
- Those who are underweight or have very low body fat
- People with a history of eating disorders, such as anorexia, bulimia, or compulsive eating ← TAKE THIS SERIOUSLY, EVEN IF UNDIAGNOSED.
- Those on medications that need to be taken with food
- People with heart conditions
- Those suffering from a cold, flu, or other viral infection
- Those suffering from adrenal fatigue
- Anyone suffering from thyroid problems

Remember: *Always* consult your doctor before starting a fast!

PRE-FAST CHECKLIST

Before embarking on a fast, review the following to determine if fasting is appropriate for you at this time:

- ☐ I am not doing this for quick weight loss.
- ☐ I do not have any of the conditions or limitations listed above.
- ☐ I understand that if for any reason I do not feel well, I will end the fast.
- ☐ I have spent at least one week in ketosis (eating exclusively in fat-burning mode).
- ☐ I am fully hydrated.
- ☐ I am not under additional stress.
- ☐ Fasting makes sense for me from a lifestyle standpoint.
- ☐ If at any time I'm not feeling well, I know to end my fast.
- ☐ I have what I need to support or customize my fast, such as bone broth, electrolyte mix, ketone supplements, or anything else I plan to use in support of my fast.
- ☐ I have selected the appropriate level of fast for me at this time.

REFUELING

Refueling isn't just a cute way to describe the fact that you get to eat again! Refueling is intentional and specific and many believe it is perhaps even more important than the fast itself. Refueling gives you the opportunity to rebuild from scratch, to start over and to get it right. Here's what I mean.

When you refuel you learn to listen to your body as you reintroduce and test foods. Done right, refueling will not only give you valuable gut health information, it will also help you to build a stronger gut lining, which in turn means a stronger immune system.

Imagine you had a friend in a relationship with this really rock-solid, awesome guy, the love of her life, her soul mate, the one who wanted to love her, care for her, and buy her cute shoes. Let's pretend this friend didn't realize what a catch she had. In fact, she took Prince Charming for granted, treated him poorly, and never listened. Frankly, she was abusive. You weren't a bit surprised when he said he wanted to "take a break." But now he's decided to give her another chance, an opportunity to start anew.

This, my darling, is the story of your gut!

Fasting and refueling gives you an opportunity to do things differently this time and build something beautiful. This is why refueling is just as critical as the fast itself, if not more so. Refueling is like learning to appreciate and care for one of your most important assets. Think of refueling as a second chance to rebuild a healthy environment in your gut.

During your fast, you gave many systems of the body the opportunity to rest, including your digestive tract. Now you need to slowly and carefully reintroduce solid food. No matter how much you want a big plate of syrup-drenched pancakes, or even something healthy like a kale salad, you must start slowly, or find yourself making a mad dash to the restroom!

Aside from giving you an opportunity to be kinder to your gut, refueling is also an opportunity to create diversity in your gut microbiome and to understand which foods do and don't work with your digestive tract or might be causing inflammation.

When trying to determine which foods cause you digestive distress, it's essential you go about refueling in a way that makes it easy to identify the culprit. That's why I suggest, if at all possible, that you avoid combining foods for at least the first day. If, for example, you develop a pounding headache or painful gas soon after your first refueling meal, you'll want to know which food is to blame. But if that first meal was scrambled eggs, spinach sautéed in olive oil, brown rice, and some sliced avocado, it will be difficult to pinpoint the culprit that's causing your digestive sensitivity.

BE A DETECTIVE!
SOLVE THE CASE

Use your symptom tracker to record what you ate and when. And before you break up officially with dairy, peanuts, tomatoes, or whatever food you suspect of having caused your distress, consider this: The urgency to rush to the bathroom immediately after eating a particular food might have little to do with a potential food sensitivity. Rapid elimination, fast transit, urgent bowel movements, and even diarrhea immediately after a meal can be the result of many gastrointestinal conditions such as irritable bowel syndrome (IBS), candida overgrowth, acid reflux, Crohn's disease, or another illness. If these symptoms persist, repeating each of the three phases of the 131 Method will aid in the healing of your gut. It goes without saying that persistent problems should be addressed by a qualified physician. I would also encourage you to consider working with a qualified integrative medical doctor who specializes in digestive health.

Every time you complete a phase, your immune system will get stronger, your metabolism will get faster, and your digestion better able to tolerate foods that in the past may have been problematic.

REFUELING RECOMMENDATIONS

- Have a plan for reintroduction in advance.
- Eat one food type at a time for the first 24 hours. Combining foods makes it very difficult to isolate which food may be problematic.
- Start with small bites and snack-size portions.
- Allow one hour to pass between eating your first post-fast food and the next.
- Choose easy-to-digest, low-fiber foods such as avocado, bone broth, eggs, nut butters, or cooked vegetables.
- Avoid difficult-to-digest and high-fiber foods with rough or jagged edges, hard nuts such as certain roasted nuts, popcorn, raw kale, red meat, etc.

- Avoid foods high in sugar or carbohydrates for the first 24 hours.
- Avoid reintroducing processed foods, like bread, cereal, or candy. (Trust me when I say you'll regret it.)
- Avoid foods you know (or suspect) to be inflammatory or generally cause digestive discomfort for you.
- Avoid alcohol for at least 48 hours after ending a fast. (Let's just say I learned this one the hard way!)
- Document how foods make you feel using your 131 Method Workbook or the Refueling Tracker (see below).

REFUELING TRACKER

Use the chart below to track your food and symptoms while refueling. Describe your symptoms below each food you list.

Symptom (describe in the space provided)	Food 1	Food 2
Joint/muscle pain, aches, inflammation		
Fatigue, sleepiness, insomnia		
Digestive discomfort: bloating, gas, diarrhea, constipation, reflux, etc.		
Headache, migraine		
Sore throat, stuffy nose, sinus infection, itchy eyes		
Skin rash, redness, acne		
Poor concentration and lack of focus		
Mood disturbance, irritability, depression, anxiety		
Excitability and hyperactivity		
Other: List symptom		
No reaction		

TO DOWNLOAD AND MAKE COPIES OF THIS FORM, GO TO 131METHOD.COM/FORMS

Symptom (describe in the space provided)	Food 3	Food 4
Joint/muscle pain, aches, inflammation		
Fatigue, sleepiness, insomnia		
Digestive discomfort: bloating, gas, diarrhea, constipation, reflux, etc.		
Headache, migraine		
Sore throat, stuffy nose, sinus infection, itchy eyes		
Skin rash, redness, acne		
Poor concentration and lack of focus		
Mood disturbance, irritability, depression, anxiety		
Excitability and hyperactivity		
Other: List symptom		
No reaction		

Using the Refueling Tracker, you'll be able to identify signs and symptoms of foods that are inflammatory for you and foods that should be removed from your diet as you continue to heal your gut.

MOVING ON TO YOUR FIRST PHASE

Congratulations! You're ready to Ignite! Your next step is week 1 of phase 1 of the 131 Method. I encourage you to read through the next three chapters fully before starting the program. And don't forget to share your progress with me at results@131method.com.

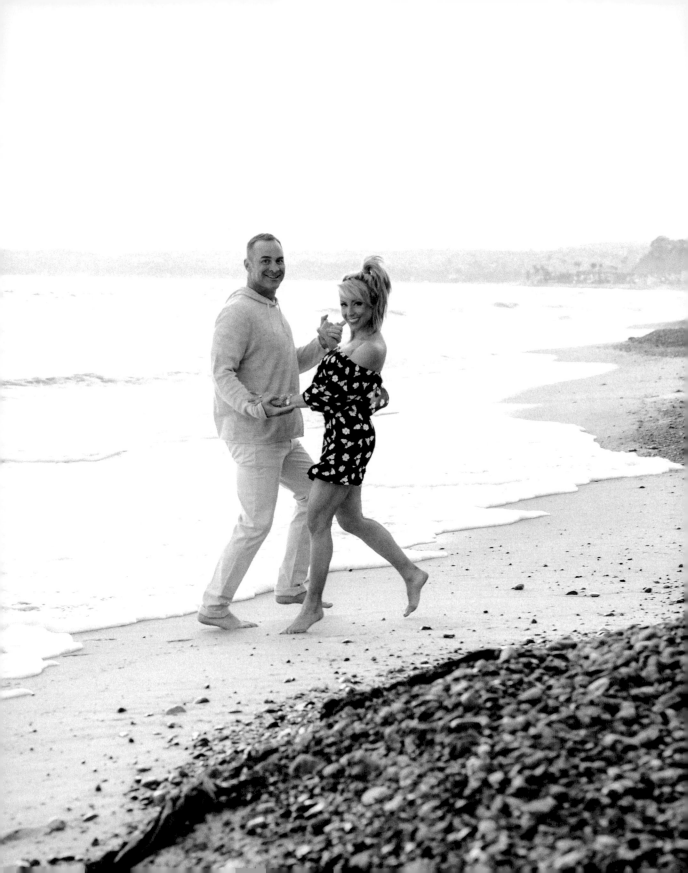

PART II

12 WEEKS TO HEALTHY INSIDE AND OUT

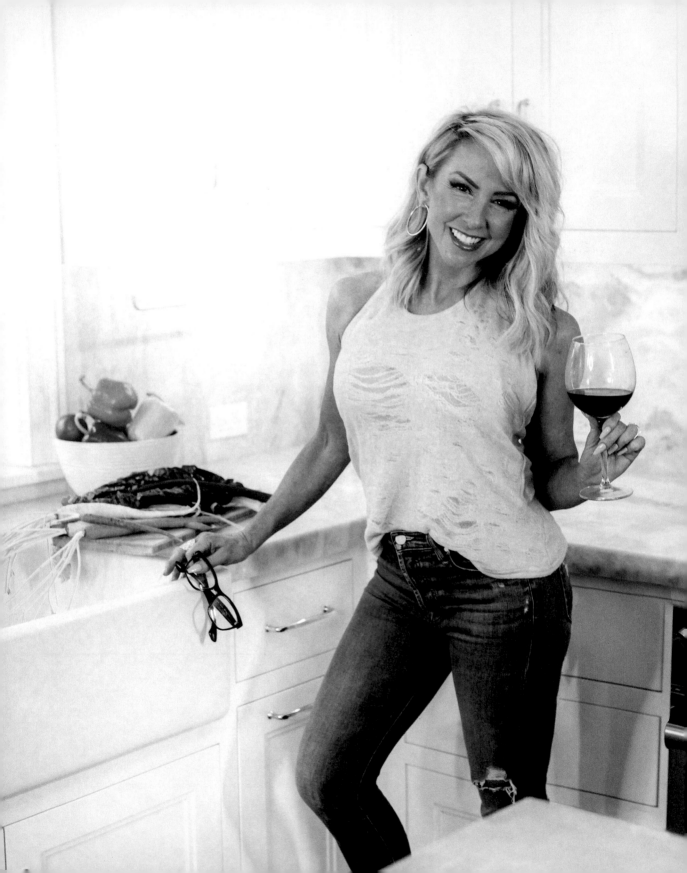

CHAPTER 6

PHASE ONE: IGNITE

WEEKS 1 TO 4

Welcome to your first phase of the 131 Method! Ignite has been designed to set you up for success with the 131 Method. The primary objective of the Ignite phase is to recalibrate your hormones. Over the course of the next four weeks on Ignite, you will build a rock-solid foundation for a healthier, leaner you. By balancing your hormones, you create a domino effect that will result in effortless weight loss, appetite correction, a happier disposition, more energy, better sleep, increased sex drive, clearer skin, stronger hair, and all the good vibes that come with feeling balanced.

I SUGGEST YOU UNDERLINE THIS OBJECTIVE!

When I think about the thousands of people who have benefited from the 131 Method, maintained sustained weight loss, and freed themselves from the diet hamster wheel, they all have one thing in common: they developed a new mind-set. How? By making the distinction between *dieting* and *phasing*. Doing so creates a meaningful shift in how you approach food and your health and gives you confidence that this time can and will be different.

To make permanent change, we have to change more than just our eating habits. We have to change our thinking. To free yourself from the dogma of dieting, you must *stop dieting*. To be in control of your health and your weight, *phasing* should be a way of life. Stop dieting and start phasing. Let that marinate for a minute.

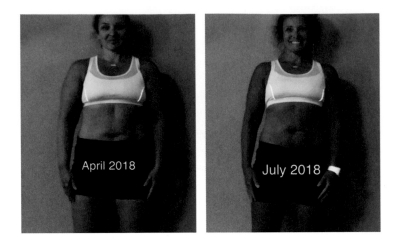

April 2018

July 2018

My endocrinologist told me I needed a thyroidectomy or radiation to remove my thyroid. I had huge reservations and wanted to give my body the chance to heal itself. Since starting the 131 Method I have lost 22.5 pounds, I'm down 3 sizes, and I feel AMAZING. I am excited about life again and my muscle and joint pain is gone! I no longer suffer with bloating. I have incredible energy & my cravings for sweets are gone. I have been able to dramatically cut my thyroid medication and my doctor says I will be off it soon! I am so thankful to have avoided a thyroidectomy and thyroid radiation. **—SUZIE D.**

IGNITE AT A GLANCE

Your goals on the four weeks of Ignite will be to:

- Become a fat burner by tracking your macronutrient ratio. The ideal macronutrient ratio for ketosis is to keep calories in the following ranges: 70 to 80 percent fats, 10 to 20 percent protein, and 5 to 10 percent carbs.

- Practice intermittent fasting; eat meals within an eight-hour window.

- Eliminate or cut back on as many inflammatory foods as possible.

- Increase daily water intake to 75 ounces or more.

After you've completed three weeks following the Ignite guidelines, you'll select a fasting level for week 4 or you can choose to skip the fast and continue on Ignite's guidelines for an additional week.

BECOME A FAT BURNER BY TRACKING YOUR MACRONUTRIENTS

Ignite will teach you how to take control of your metabolism once and for all. You'll be flipping the switch, metabolically speaking, and teaching your body how to be a fat burner rather than a sugar burner. By following the macronutrient ratio outlined in this phase combined with intermittent fasting, you will effortlessly deplete excess glucose and glycogen stores and transition into a mild state of ketosis. This also lowers insulin levels and helps your body access stored body fat for fuel. In turn, this process will begin to correct hormone levels, especially those responsible for hunger and satiety.

Since each one of us is different, it may take more or less time for you to become a fat burner. That's okay. Just stick with it and you'll see results.

Tracking macronutrient ratios, even for the most self-aware eater, is an eye-opening experience. You may be shocked to learn how many of the so-called healthy foods you've been eating convert to glucose, resulting in unwanted stored body fat. But that's all about to change. You are the hero in this story! My job is to be your guide, but let me be frank. You cannot do this without some accountability. Tracking during Ignite gives you accountability and valuable insight.

To be successful, you want to carefully track everything you eat for the next three weeks. Everything! Don't worry, this will become second nature in a matter of days and it's not something you'll have to do forever.

HOW TO TRACK MACRONUTRIENTS

Technology makes tracking your macros a breeze. You can look up the macronutrient makeup of each meal by referring to the nutrition label or via a simple Google search. Next, record the total fat, carbs, and protein for each item. You can do this in a journal, workbook, or your phone's calendar, but I think you'll find using an app far more convenient. I strongly encourage you to use a tracking app!

There are plenty of free smartphone apps that make macronutrient tracking quick and easy, such as MyFitnessPal, Carb Manager, and Lose It! With worldwide nutritional databases that include nearly every category, brand, and restaurant entrée you can think of, all that's left for you to do is to enter what and how much you ate. The more diligent you are about doing this (right down to that bite of pancake you took before putting your toddler's plate in the sink), the more informed and successful you will be. Many apps even allow you to simply scan the bar code to automatically add nutritional facts. Remember, what we don't measure, we can't improve.

THIS IS MY FAVORITE!

Why you should prioritize tracking during Ignite:

- Studies show the average person dramatically underestimates carbohydrate consumption—by as much as 40 percent!
- Tracking gives you a baseline from which to establish customized macronutrient ratios for optimal results in future phases.
- A survey of online 131Method.com participants revealed that those who carefully tracked daily macronutrient ratios had greater weight loss and reported more and better overall health improvements.

Before you start Ignite, schedule 10 to 15 minutes and familiarize yourself with the app of your choice. You'll need to enter some basic information about yourself to get started. Based on height, weight, and goals, it may give you a calorie range. Don't worry about that range for now. Instead enter your desired macronutrient calorie ratios: 70 to 80 percent fats, 10 to 20 percent protein, and 5 to 10 percent carbs. Remember that your goal is for your entire day (not each meal) to match these percentages. Refer to page 134 for more detailed instructions on tracking your macros and using an app.

PRACTICE DAILY INTERMITTENT FASTING

During Ignite, I recommend two powerful tools to help you fast-track your success: intermittent fasting and tracking. You can combine intermittent fasting and macro tracking to quickly and effectively deplete extra glycogen and glucose stores and allow your body to ease into a mild state of ketosis. Intermittent fasting, which is explained in Chapter 5, means that you'll eat your food within a shorter window, or time period, each day. Start with a 12-hour eating window. Then, once you feel comfortable, gradually reduce your eating window down to about eight hours per day. Whereas removing inflammatory foods and tracking your macros are essential, remember that intermittent fasting (like all fasting) is optional, though I highly recommend you experiment with it.

DO THIS FIRST!!!

Intermittent fasting will help to correct your hunger hormones without obsessing over or counting calories. It's also likely you'll be eating one fewer meal than usual. For that reason, Ignite is a phase in which I encourage you to exercise less. Consider shorter, more restorative workouts such as yoga and flexibility training, light weights, walking, and moderate-intensity intervals.

CUT OUT OR CUT BACK ON INFLAMMATORY FOODS

Another thing you'll do on Ignite is eliminate or at least cut back on as many inflammatory foods as possible, which we discussed the importance of in Chapter 3. It's possible some of these foods are things you love and simply cannot give up cold turkey. Maybe you look forward to the occasional pasta dish or enjoying a cocktail on Saturday nights and an absolute ban on these sounds like a punishment. This type of blanket deprivation is one of the many reasons strict elimination diets backfire. When we cut something we're used to eating, the brain triggers our hormones to respond to a perceived scarcity of food. This subconscious reaction is known as the famine response.

GIVE YOURSELF THE GIFT OF GRACE.

Banning food or labeling something "bad," even swearing off carbs, is never a good idea. Instead, give yourself permission to make the right decisions at every meal. No one expects perfection. Do your best, not because you've been told to do so, but because you're learning what your body needs and what makes you feel amazing.

My girlfriend Natalie Jill has celiac disease, which means she has severe reactions to even trace amounts of gluten found in wheat, certain other grains, and other foods. When I asked how she developed the discipline to avoid so many delicious foods containing gluten, Natalie explained that once she's identified a particular food as problematic, the way she feels after eating it becomes part of the food memory. Avoiding a food that makes her feel bad never feels like deprivation.

You can do the same thing. Rather than pulling up the memory of how a food tastes, create a stronger memory around how it makes you feel physically and emotionally. The acute effects of inflammatory foods may include water retention, swelling, bloating, digestive irregularities, nausea, or headaches. They can also cause widespread hormonal disruption. By being aware of how inflammatory foods makes you feel, it's not likely you'll continue to crave them.

WHERE TO START

I'd like you to take a more positive, grace-giving approach than memorizing lists of "good foods" and "bad foods." I'd like you to take a look at the following list of foods that are considered anti-inflammatory, and *add* more of those foods to your diet. Then look at the lists of food that are inflammatory for most people, and make some quick decisions, knowing you can reevaluate later. Using these lists, select either "Cut out," "Cut back," or "Undecided." Consider what foods you are able to eliminate from your diet while still maintaining your happiness; those would be foods you can cut out. If there are foods you are unsure about, ones you simply cannot live without but perhaps you *could* limit your intake, then place a check mark under "Cut back." For foods you're just not sure one way or the other, check "Undecided." This is a journey. You can do this in stages. You hold the reins.

You'll note some of the foods on the inflammatory list are also listed as anti-inflammatory. I know that can be confusing. That's because one person's anti-inflammatory food may cause inflammation in another. While we are all different, you can err on the side of safety by assuming any food that's fake or highly processed is likely to cause low-grade inflammation.

The only way to know with any degree of certainty whether a food is inflammatory or anti-inflammatory *for you* is to conduct your own study. Take notes on how each food makes you feel when you eat it and afterward. Do you truly enjoy the flavors and textures, or does your mind just like that you're indulging in something that's "forbidden"? Does your body feel good after eating something, or do you have inflammatory symptoms like low energy or pain? When you eliminate a food from your diet, do your appearance and energy improve?

Be sure to track what you're eating and how you feel each day, to identify patterns you might not otherwise notice. While you can use a notebook or memo on your phone, you might want to check out the 131 Method Workbook at www.131method.com. Also refer to the Meal Planning Template and Symptom Tracker on page 86.

SHOULD YOU CHOOSE TO BOOZE

While on the subject of what to cut back on, this seems like the perfect opportunity to discuss alcohol. There's a good chance you saw the cover of this book and thought, A personalized plan that involves wine? I'm in!

I'll bet you were a little surprised to see a glass of red wine on the cover of a book about health. I wanted to make the point that nothing is off limits. My role is to help you create an informed decision that supports your current objectives and helps you improve your health in the most comfortable and doable way possible.

Scientific studies routinely find those who drink 1 to 2 glasses of wine per day have a significantly reduced risk of heart disease and greater longevity. Many believe the polyphenols, antioxidants, and anti-inflammatory properties of wine promote longevity, while others suggest a correlation between moderate drinking and a person's ability to manage stress and spend more time relaxing with friends and family.

Truth be told, I've never been much of a drinker. I mean, sure, if we were out with friends I might order a "skinny" cocktail or a glass of wine. I was familiar with the studies suggesting a glass of wine a day was associated with improved health, but the foggy feeling and headache I had the next day made me suspicious of any possible health benefits.

When I decided to track my symptoms, I quickly realized the negative side effects were the worst with "skinny" or "diet" cocktails. To my surprise, the next most problematic (for me) was wine. Curious, I decided to research further. We know alcohol is a toxin (though many would argue it's the dosage that renders it toxic). But I've since learned it's not just the sugar, calories, carbs, or even alcohol content that creates a negative impact. Just as with all food, ingredients, quantity, quality, and country origin make a huge difference.

But here's the kicker—if you're consuming spirits manufactured and bottled in the U.S., there's no reliable way of knowing what you're actually ingesting. Get this . . . (are you sitting down?!) Distilleries in the U.S. are not required to list ingredients on the label, only alcohol content.

Largely in response to the shift in consumers' interest in label accuracy, the European Union now requires nutritional facts, calories, macros, and all ingredients to be listed on alcohol beverage labels.

If you want to know what's in the bottle, and you live in the U.S., you may need to choose European imported spirits. I recently discovered a U.S.-based company that imports zero sugar, organic, all-natural wines from the finest European vineyards. These wines will not spike your insulin level or kick you out of ketosis. To learn more, go to http://www.dryfarmwines.com/chalene.

To be clear, even moderate alcohol consumption increases appetite, disrupts hunger hormones, dehydrates the body, and diminishes sleep quality, all of which can lead to weight gain. As with all things, make an informed decision and always practice moderation. No one looks cuter, sounds smarter, or feels better if they overdo it, even if it is low sugar, organic, and all-natural.

THESE FOODS HAVE BEEN PROVEN TO REDUCE INFLAMMATION.

COMMON ANTI-INFLAMMATORY FOODS

(healing foods that aid in the reduction of inflammation)

- Avocados
- Berries (all), including raspberries, blueberries, and blackberries
- Bone broth made from grass-finished meat*
- Cacao (raw), as well as low-sugar dark chocolate
- Cayenne pepper
- Citrus fruits (all), organic
- Coconut aminos, coconut butter, and unrefined coconut oil
- Eggs from pastured poultry
- Fish, wild caught
- Almond flour
- Cassava flour
- Ghee (clarified butter) made from milk from grass-finished cows

- Gingerroot
- Herbs and spices (all), organic
- MCT (medium-chain triglyceride) oil
- Meat, organic, grass-finished
- Non-starchy organic vegetables:
- Asparagus
- Bok choy
- Broccoli
- Brussels sprouts
- Cabbage
- Carrots
- Cauliflower
- Celery
- Cucumber
- Green beans
- Kale
- Mushrooms
- Onion

- Radishes
- Spaghetti squash
- Spinach
- Swiss chard
- Yellow squash
- Zucchini
- Nuts and seeds, raw (except peanuts)
- Olive oil, cold-pressed, extra-virgin
- Salt, Himalayan or sea
- Starchy organic vegetables:
- Beets
- Butternut squash
- Parsnips
- Sweet potatoes
- Turnips
- Tea, especially green tea
- Vinegar (apple cider vinegar)

YOU CAN FIND SOME WONDERFULLY TASTY SNACKS MADE FROM CASSAVA FLOUR ON AMAZON.COM AND THRIVE.COM, OR AT YOUR LOCAL HEALTH FOOD STORE.

COMMON INFLAMMATORY FOODS

Below is a list of foods most commonly believed to cause inflammation.

Cut out	Cut back	Unde-cided	
			Alcohol
			Artificial colors, dyes, and additives
			Artificial sweeteners (all), including aspartame, sucralose, acesulfame K, saccharin
			Dairy products from conventionally raised cows
			Deli meats containing nitrates or nitrites; processed, smoked, or canned meats from conventionally raised animals
			Fish, farmed
			Flours, refined
			Fried foods
			"Fruit" beverages not made with 100 percent fruit juice
			Grains (even whole grains), including white, wheat and whole wheat breads, rolls, pasta, cereal, wraps, etc.
			Jams, jellies, and syrups (high-sugar, processed fruit products)
			Meat from conventionally raised animals
			Peanuts, peanut butter
			Processed foods, prepackaged goods, most fast foods, and convenience store foods
			Sodas and other sugar-sweetened and artificially sweetened beverages
			Soy products including tofu, soybean oils, soy-based protein powders, soy sauce, edamame
			Sugar and high-fructose corn syrup
			Vegetable oils, including canola and corn, especially hydrogenated oils

* For a discussion of the terms *grass finished*, *grass fed*, and *pasture raised*, please turn to page 153.

POTENTIALLY INFLAMMATORY FOODS

Listed below are foods that may be problematic for some individuals, often due to common processing and/or undiagnosed food intolerances or allergies. Consider removing these foods if signs and symptoms of inflammation or digestive distress persist after removing known inflammatory foods.

Cut out	Cut back	Unde-cided	
			Carbonated waters, low sugar alcoholic beverages
			Milk chocolate, or any chocolate containing artificial colors, preservatives, genetically modified ingredients, or inflammatory oils including corn, soybean, sunflower, canola, and safflower oils
			Citrus fruit
			Some coffee
			Eggs
			Guar gum or xanthan gum (commonly found in protein powders and processed foods)
			Kombucha
			Genetically modified foods
			Nightshade vegetables: bell peppers, eggplant, tomatoes, potatoes (purple, white, and yellow), chile peppers, jalapeños, habaneros, chili-based spices, red pepper, cayenne pepper
			Peanuts and some processed nuts including those with rough edges, such as roasted almonds
			Soy products, fermented, such as tempeh and tamari
			Some stevia products
			Vinegar

I HOPE AT A MINIMUM YOU SELECT "CUT BACK"!

ALL FORMS ARE ALSO AT 131METHOD.COM/FORMS

MAKING SENSE OF LABELS

Far more useful than memorizing a food list is remembering a few important principles:

- Get in the habit of asking yourself if what you're about to eat is real food.
- Read the label.
- Avoid GMO ingredients.
- Avoid foods that have been fortified (meaning the food is nutritionally deficient without added processing).
- See an ingredient not listed in this chapter? Do a quick Google search!
- Watch out for these terms on the nutrition facts and ingredients labels:

  - Artificial ingredients
  - Artificial sweeteners
  - Artificial colors
  - Casein
  - Corn syrup
  - Enhanced
  - Enriched
  - Fructose

  - Genetically modified (GMO), keeping in mind that, at the time of publishing, not all countries are required to label foods that contain GMO ingredients
  - Gluten
  - Monosodium glutamate (MSG)
  - Preservatives
  - Refined
  - Sugar
  - Trans fat

Keep it simple. Ask yourself: "Is this food as close as possible to its original state?"

Prior to finding the 131 Method, I had just received results from a 24-hour urine hormone analysis that showed that my body was overproducing progesterone and making little to no testosterone. My adrenals were high, as well as cortisol levels. When I read that the 131 Method could help balance hormones, I was ready to dive in. This program could not have come at a more perfect time for me. **—TAMMIE W.**

WEEK 4: FASTING AND REFUELING

The 131 Method combines several fat-burning strategies during each phase. One of the strategies offered is a variety of fasting options. However, fasting is just one of many tools and is therefore always optional. If you choose not to move beyond fasting level 1 (intermittent fasting), then you can continue following the rest of the Ignite guidelines during week 4.

Pre-Fast Self-Assessment Checklist

☐ My daily eating window is down to eight hours or less.

☐ I have been following an intermittent fasting protocol for at least seven days (preferably a few weeks).

☐ I feel comfortable and confident with this way of eating.

ARE YOU READY?

☐ I am eating fat-burning foods with 5 to 10 percent of total calories coming from carbs and 70 to 80 percent coming from fat.

☐ I am not sick, pregnant, or nursing; do not have diabetes; and am not on medications that must be taken with food.

☐ I have medical clearance to start a fast.

☐ I am not currently under a high level of stress.

☐ I have reviewed the "Who Should Avoid Fasting" list on page 121 to ensure it's safe for me to fast.

☐ I have on hand some optional items to help support my fast, including tea, coffee, water, coconut oil, MCT oil, bone broth, electrolyte mix, ketone supplements, or anything else I plan to use.

☐ I know that if for any reason I don't feel well during a fast, I should end my fast and consult a physician.

☐ I have selected the appropriate level of fast for me at this time.

If you agree with all the statements in the checklist, then go ahead and select another fasting level from Chapter 5, such as Level 2: Shortened Window Fast, for week 4 of Ignite. Be sure to carefully follow the fasting and refueling guidelines!

***

As you begin to balance your hormones following the Ignite guidelines, don't be surprised if you start to drop the pounds fairly quickly. Excited by your success, and certain you've found the key to your weight loss challenges, you might think, *Hey, this is great! I should just keep doing Ignite forever!*

But don't forget about homeostasis. I can tell you that once your body adapts to what you're doing routinely, weight loss will begin to stall. That's when bad habits and a negative mind-set creep in through the back door. Stay strong. Trust the science. Believe in the process. To reap the rewards of a speedy metabolism, healthy gut, and balanced hormones, you will need to finish all three phases.

THE CURE TO HOMEOSTASIS IS DIET PHASING

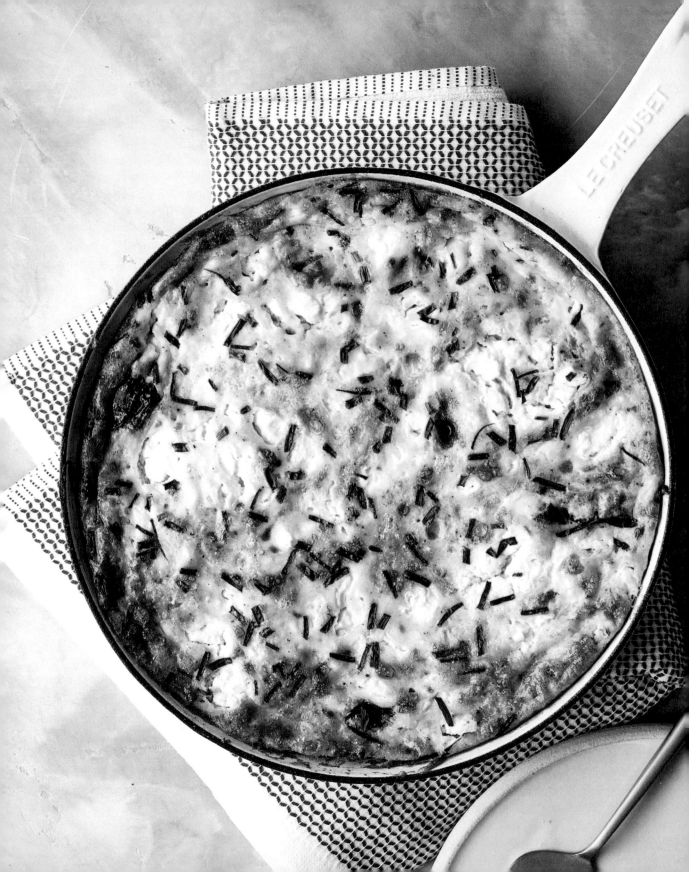

IGNITE MEAL PLAN

This is an example of a daily meal plan for each week of Ignite. Please refer to Part III for your recipes!

IGNITE WEEK 1

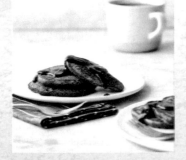

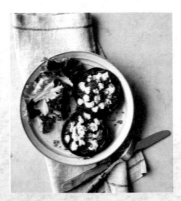

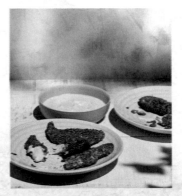

BREAKFAST

Chocolate Peanut Butter Pancakes (page 198)

LUNCH

Stuffed Portobello Mushrooms with Goat Cheese (page 214)

DINNER

Chicken Tenders with Broccolini with Lemon & Garlic (pages 225)

IGNITE WEEK 2

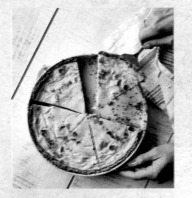

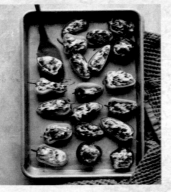

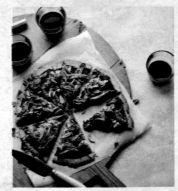

BREAKFAST

Bacon Quiche (page 203)

LUNCH

Mini Bell Peppers with Goat Cheese and Olives (page 212)

DINNER

Low-Carb Barbecued Chicken Pizza (page 222)

REMEMBER, YOU DON'T HAVE TO FAST. INSTEAD YOU COULD REPEAT WEEK 3'S MEAL PLAN. OR FOR MORE OPTIONS CHECK OUT PG 117

IGNITE WEEK 3

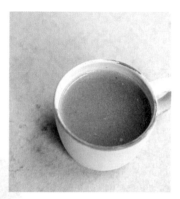

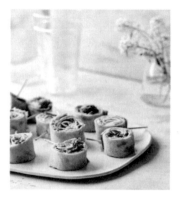

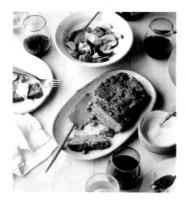

BREAKFAST

Chicken Broth (page 345)

LUNCH

BLT Pinwheels (page 218)

DINNER

Turkey Meatloaf with Buffalo Wing Sauce with Chili Lime Brussels Sprouts (pages 228 and 236)

IGNITE WEEK 4

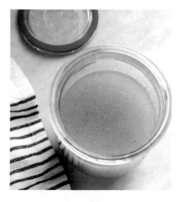

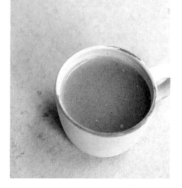

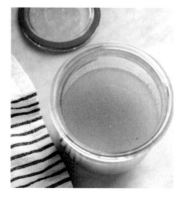

BREAKFAST

Chicken or Vegetable Broth (page 345 and 346)

LUNCH

Chicken or Vegetable Broth (page 345 and 346)

DINNER

Chicken or Vegetable Broth (page 345 and 346)

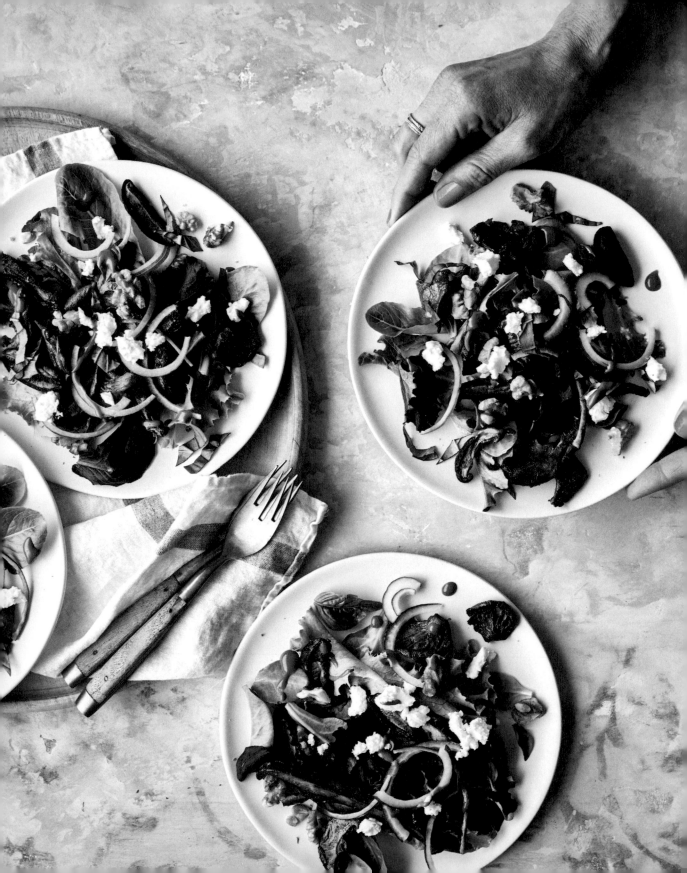

CHAPTER 7

PHASE TWO: NOURISH

WEEKS 5 TO 8

By this point you will have spent four weeks on Ignite, depleting excess glycogen stores, teaching your body to burn fat for energy, balancing hormones, and repairing your digestive health by identifying and eliminating as many inflammatory foods as possible. Nourish builds on the work you've done in the Ignite phase and helps you maximize your results. The primary objective of the Nourish phase is to accelerate gut healing and optimize all functions of the body by increasing the intake of micronutrient-dense superfoods. In other words, we'll focus on quality fuel intake to enhance the performance of your engine!

As you begin Nourish, you will resume intermittent fasting. Just as you did during Ignite, your goal is to achieve an eight-hour eating window daily. Depending on your practices over the past week, you might simply continue as you have been, or you may need to delay your first meal by an hour each day until all meals are eaten within that six- to eight-hour period.

You may be excited to learn that Nourish has been nicknamed the "beauty" phase. You can expect to see marked improvements in your physical appearance, most notably your skin and eyes. Within a matter of days, you will begin to feel like a new person.

MORE PLANTS, LESS JUNK!

As a mom of three, including twins, my body has been through a lot. I started the 131 Method during the holidays and lost over 30 pounds and have kept it off! My journey & results with the 131 Method go way beyond weight loss. I've learned how to identify inflammatory foods for my body AND what healthy habits to adopt, including how to eat to boost my metabolism, balance my hormones, and improve my gut health.
—JESSICA S.

NOURISH AT A GLANCE

Your goals on the four weeks of Nourish will be to:

- Intuitively track macronutrients
- Eat more plant-based foods rich in micronutrients
- Cut back on animal protein
- Prioritize quality ingredients and micronutrients

After you've completed three weeks on the Nourish guidelines, you'll select a fasting level for week 4. As with each phase, the fasting is optional! Not fasting this time? No problem. You'll continue with Nourish's guidelines for one more week instead.

INTUITIVELY TRACK YOUR MACROS

Feel free to put away your app! While every 12 weeks I think it's very important to track your nutrition, it's also useful to learn how to intuitively know what macronutrient ratio your body needs for optimal performance. During the first three weeks of Nourish, instead of *precisely* tracking your macros, you'll begin to practice tracking them intuitively. Intuitive tracking means you will use what you have learned about food and macronutrient ratios to attempt to stay within a range of getting 10 to 30 percent of your calorie intake from carbohydrates. As you approach week 4, you'll want to reduce your carbohydrates to a range of 5 to 15 percent of your total calories to ensure a comfortable transition into your fast. For full macro guidance during Nourish, refer to page 133.

Let's talk about those carbohydrate ranges for a moment. When it comes to an ideal daily carbohydrate intake, the range suggested for you is just that: a range. It's up to you to figure out exactly what percentage helps keep your hunger hormones at bay. Despite what other programs might have you think, there is no one percentage that will work for everyone. Staying in this general range should help most people maintain healthy blood sugar levels and make steady weight loss progress.

What if, shortly after transitioning to Nourish, you just feel stuck or you're not confident in your ability to track macros intuitively? Simple solution: go back to tracking your nutrition with more precision. This is a journey. You'll get better and more confident as you go!

If you're not experiencing the progress you hoped for, you may want to adjust your carb intake to be on the lower side of this range. Each phase is an opportunity for you to do additional testing and tweaking to help you discover the appropriate amount of carbohydrates you need to eat to feel your best and effortlessly manage your weight. We're all different.

IT'S TIME TO THRIVE: EMPHASIZE QUALITY INGREDIENTS

We both know plenty of people who "survive" despite horrible nutrition. I was one of them. My diet was devoid of any real micronutrient density. I believed I was eating a so-called clean diet, which I defined as avoiding fried foods, sweets, treats, and avoiding fat and keeping calories low. That meant a steady stream of diet drinks, processed protein shakes, protein bars, and lean highly processed protein. To make matters worse, due to leaky gut syndrome resulting from my consumption of fake foods and stress,

ALL NATURAL?

When it comes to terms such as *all natural*, the FDA does not have specific rules or regulatory guidelines for the use of this label. This and many other health-related terms are not enforced by the United States Department of Agriculture (USDA). While we assume *all natural* to mean the product doesn't contain anything artificial, the truth is manufacturers can include ingredients that may not be considered natural by most of us. For example, Goldfish crackers and Cheetos are labeled as natural. Oh and by the way, foods containing known GMO ingredients can also be labeled as all natural. While some might argue that high-fructose corn syrup is natural, I doubt many would defend it as healthy. The only way to protect yourself is through knowledge. Keep in mind the more bold the health claims on the packaging, the more likely they're trying to get you to ignore your common sense.

when I did have quality food, my body couldn't absorb the nutrients.

Your body is stubborn enough to survive on just about anything. But low-quality, fake food slowly robs us of our immune system Anyone can survive. You're not about that life. You're here to thrive! To do that, the quality of your food must become a priority.

Quality matters. Whenever possible, eat the highest-quality ingredients available, and that includes your choice of animal meat, poultry, dairy, and fish. Let me keep it real and just agree that this is no easy task, especially when it feels like we're constantly being misled by slick marketing. Food producers bank on our willingness to pay a premium when we believe something is "better" for us, especially when it comes to labels such as "all natural" or even "grass fed," both unregulated terms.

Your best bet when it comes to increasing essential micronutrients in your diet is to look for quality ingredients, and that includes your meats and animal proteins. You'll need to be vigilant. For example, I bet you've been hearing a lot more people using the term *grass fed* or *grass-fed beef*. Most of us would assume if we're paying a premium for meat labeled this way that we are in fact getting meat raised on grass, not on inflammatory GMO-laden grains, (which by the way cattle don't eat in nature). Unfortunately even the term *grass fed* is unregulated.

You see, most cattle, pigs, and other animals, once weaned, are grass fed for a period of months. Some conventional farming operations then move these young animals from grass into over-crowded feedlots to fatten cattle up on a less expensive steady diet of grains to "finish" and fatten them up before slaughter. The more the cow weighs, the more money the producer will receive, and the more affordable meat becomes for the consumer. There's no one stopping these producers from labeling the beef as "grass fed."

That said, when looking for quality meat, it's helpful to look for terms such as *grass fed* and *grass finished*. The quality of an animal's life and the diet of the animal during its lifetime have a significant impact on the micronutrients found in the meat. An animal raised on plants is going to have higher levels of essential vitamins and antioxidants in its food supply. For more than three decades, studies have confirmed the significant nutritional differences found when comparing conventionally farmed animals and pasture-raised animals.[1] Pasture-raised cattle have been shown to have higher levels of omega-3s, antioxidants, vitamin A, vitamin E, and even glutathione (known as the master of antioxidants).[2]

At the moment, your safest bet for high-quality meat, poultry, and even eggs is to look for those labeled "certified organic," "pasture raised," and "certified humanely treated."

KEY INFO!

Look, I understand finding quality ingredients isn't always convenient or affordable. Do your best. Generally speaking, we eat far more animal protein than our ancestors ever did. Biologically speaking we weren't designed to process this much meat. So instead of complaining about the difficulties of finding affordable quality protein, how about you take that same meat budget and invest in quality over quantity. Find a reputable source or local farmers and support them! If you're in the United States, one of my favorite trusted sources is Butcher Box Meats. You can learn more about their amazingly convenient and affordable delivery program and the process for sourcing the quality meats, and even get a discount I've arranged for readers by visiting www.Butcherbox.com/Chalene. My family, extended family, and friends all swear by the difference in taste and quality. Choosing quality may not be most convenient or the cheapest option, but can you really afford to cut corners when it comes to your health?

Quality is equally important for fish and shellfish. Wild-caught fish can provide you with the important balance of omega-3s that help to diminish inflammation and bad cholesterol. Without question, consumer demand for cheap food has led to fish farming and breeding practices that produce fish high in inflammatory contaminates like mercury, lead, fossil fuel, and other environmental toxins, as well as color additives and more. As you might suspect, the most popular varieties of seafood have the greatest likelihood of being genetically modified or farmed in less than desirable conditions. Salmon, tuna, tilapia, and shrimp are some of the most tainted varieties.

Armed with the latest information, you can make healthy choices for yourself and your family. In the United States the USDA requires all retailers to clearly list product origins and method of production (farm-raised or wild-caught) on all fish and shellfish sold. The bad news is, health standards in the fishing industry are not as cut-and-dried as they are with meat and poultry. Plus, many companies purposely mislabel their fish. When buying fish, look for terms such as *wild-caught* and *troll caught*. Alaskan pink or sockeye salmon is always wild-caught, while some Atlantic salmon is farmed. When choosing Atlantic salmon look for wild-caught and troll-caught versions. Troll caught refers to fish that are caught on a hook and line and iced one fish at a time. The careful way that they are handled makes for a premium quality. When in doubt ask questions. Do your best to eat the best, but don't let this stuff make you crazy.

QUALITY OVER QUANTITY

As you begin to feel the effects of your healthy choices, let this motivate you to tighten the reins even further, especially when it comes to sugar, artificial ingredients, and processed foods. Your efforts, combined with your decision to select the highest-quality ingredients available, will result in a substantial decrease in inflammation and hormonal imbalance. Why is this so important? Because when we further reduce inflammation, we get at the root causes of weight loss resistance and nearly all disease markers.

I encourage you to revisit the list of potentially inflammatory foods found in Chapter 6 and consider cutting out additional foods from your diet that simply don't help you to become the kick-ass, super-healthy, super-happy person you deserve to be!

As you increase your consumption of plant-based foods, you will also eat less meat. Now, I didn't say give up beef, pork, eggs, and seafood completely for four weeks (unless, of course, you want to). Instead, just gradually reduce the amount of animal protein you consume to approximately three servings (or less) per week. Not a big deal.

If reading the previous paragraph has you about to close this book, let me remind you who is in charge: *you* are! If this recommendation doesn't sit right with you even after I explain the scientific reasoning behind it, then don't do it. At every turn I want to encourage you not just to tailor and customize this program so it works for you but to make it feel realistic. However, if you've never tried cutting back on animal protein just to see how you feel, what do you have to lose? Attitude is everything! Each phase is just four weeks. You can do this!

MAYBE A FEW POUNDS!?!

When it comes to eating less animal protein, do it in a way that truly works for you and your family. Maybe you're the "cold turkey" kind who is willing to give this a try by not eating animal protein the first day you start Nourish. Or maybe you'd prefer to gradually limit your intake by eating two servings per day the first week, one serving a day the following week, and ultimately cutting back to three servings per week by the end of Nourish.

EAT MORE PLANTS, FEWER ANIMALS

During the Nourish phase, your goal is to improve how your body functions, and the best way to achieve this is to consume more plants. In Nourish, you will enjoy meals that are far more plant dominant.

Many of the compounds naturally occurring in plants help reduce oxidative stress by delivering essential vitamins, minerals, and most notably polyphenols. Polyphenols are natural compounds that act as antioxidants. In plain English, if oxidative stress is like rust on the inside of our cells and tissues, then antioxidants act as rust removers. Antioxidants are nature's way of protecting our cells from unstable molecules created by oxidative stress, which otherwise prematurely break down our cells and tissues.

THAT'S ME, ENJOYING A GLASS OF POLYPHENOLS!

You can think of polyphenols (compounds found in certain plants) as part of the clean-up crew. Polyphenols deliver benefits to your overall health by working to reduce oxidative stress that might otherwise lead to premature aging and system breakdown. One example of a polyphenol common in many fruits and vegetables is resveratrol. Resveratrol is found in the skin of red grapes, hence the purported health benefits of red wine (in moderation of course!).

While polyphenols are essential, they are only one of the many nutritional benefits of increasing your intake of plants. Plant-based nutrients activate autophagy, that powerful cellular recycling process discussed in Chapter 5. By shifting your nutrient intake and eating more fruits and vegetables, as well as higher quality protein, you'll start to feel the difference almost immediately.

FOODS HIGH IN POLYPHENOLS

- arugula
- bell peppers
- buckwheat
- cacao (chocolate)
- capers
- celery
- coffee

- dates
- garlic
- grape skins
- green tea
- hot peppers
- kale
- olive oil

- parsley
- red endive
- red onion
- strawberries
- tempeh
- turmeric
- walnuts

EASING INTO NOURISH

Adding a variety of vegetables to your diet will definitely increase gut diversity and deliver you micronutrient-dense fuel. However, you may find it takes a few days (or sometimes a few weeks) to adjust to the dietary changes. This can be quite common, especially for those unaccustomed to eating a lot of greens. Many vegetables contain insoluble fiber; fiber that can't be digested, only eliminated. Fiber is important, but it can be irrating to the gut lining, especially for those with leaky gut.

By following these tips you can help your digestive system to ease into Nourish: **Transition gradually**. Instead of going suddenly from high-fat foods in Ignite to fibrous vegetables in Nourish, start with easy-to-digest veggies, such as spinach, cucumbers, and lettuce.

THINK CORN. SORRY! TMI!

- **Break 'em down.** Make vegetables easier to digest by finely chopping, shredding, mashing, massaging with olive or coconut oil, or dicing them in advance. Remove the toughest, most fibrous part of the plant, such as the stems found on greens such as kale, spinach, broccoli, cauliflower, and winter greens to minimize digestive stress.

- **Cook vegetables to aid in the digestive process.** Doing so means less work for your digestive system. Insoluble fiber foods are easier to digest when broken down by cooking, steaming, boiling, braising, etc. You can move to raw servings when you feel ready.
- **Chew your food longer.** Take your time.
- **Avoid raw vegetables on an empty stomach.** Start your meal with a protein or fat before eating your greens.
- **Increase digestive enzymes.** You can do so by taking a digestive enzyme supplement or adding a few teaspoons of raw apple cider vinegar to your daily diet.
- **Hydrate between meals.** Drinking too much water at meal time is thought to dilute digestive enzymes, so stay hydrated throughout the day instead.

FODMAPS: THE SNEAKY CAUSE OF BLOATING AND DISCOMFORT WHEN YOU INCREASE PLANT-BASED MEALS

Certain people have a difficult time digesting a class of plant-based carbohydrate known as FODMAPs (fermentable oligosaccharides, disaccharides, monosaccharides, and polyols). If you happen to be one of those people, the more often you eat these foods, the more likely you are to experience unpleasant symptoms such as abdominal bloating, gas pain, and inconsistency of bowel movements. Studies have shown that many digestive conditions like irritable bowel syndrome (IBS) may find relief by reducing consumption of high-FODMAP foods.

Common foods that are high in FODMAPs include:

- Garlic
- Onion
- Wheat, rye, barley

- Some high-fructose fruits such as:
  - Apple
  - Apricot
  - Avocado
  - Blackberry
  - Cherry
  - Dried Fruit
  - Fruit Juice
  - Large Servings of Fruit
  - Mango
  - Peach
  - Pear
  - Plum
  - Prune
  - Watermelon
- Certain vegetables
  - Artichoke
  - Asparagus
  - Beet
  - Broccoli
  - Brussels sprouts
  - Cabbage
  - Cauliflower
  - Eggplant
  - Fennel
  - Garlic
  - Green capsicum/ Pepper
  - Leek
  - Mushroom
  - Okra
  - Onion
  - Shallot
  - Sweet Corn
  - Spices/Herbs: garlic powder, fennel, onion powder
- Honey, agave, and other sweeteners high in fructose
- Dairy products that are high in lactose
  - Cow's milk and products made from cow's milk
  - Custard
  - Ice cream
  - Sheep milk
  - Soft cheese: cottage, mascarpone, ricotta
  - Yogurt
  - Legumes and beans

So what are you supposed to do with this info ? Relax. Assess the situation. I am not telling you to eliminate these foods. What I am suggesting is that if after removing known inflammatory foods you find that you're still suffering from digestive issues and other symptoms that present after a meal, you need to do some further investigating. I like to call this the study of one.

As I started the journey to solve the mystery of my own metabolism, it became abundantly clear I needed to fix my gut. I gradually removed inflammatory foods. I made important changes to key areas of my life as suggested in this book. It was exciting to see and feel results almost immediately. But after almost a year, I still had nagging digestive issues. I started by eliminating a few of the foods on the FODMAP list that I was eating several times per week: beets, beans, and dairy. By eliminating these items for just two weeks my symptoms were gone. Since that time I've been able to gradually add beets and beans back into my diet. (Dairy and I still don't get along.)

Tune in to your body and consider eliminating high FODMAP foods you suspect may be causing your issues. For guidance on an elimination diet, you may want to consult a registered dietitian.

WEEK 4: FASTING AND REFUELING

As a reminder, fasting isn't for everyone. It's also not something you need to do every month. Instead, as you approach the fasting and refueling week of any phase, check in with your body, what's going on in your life, and evaluate if fasting is right for you at this time. If you so choose, you can continue following the rest of the Nourish guidelines during week 4. I can't stress it enough: *you* are in charge of this journey.

PRE-FAST SELF-ASSESSMENT CHECKLIST

☐ I have been able to keep my carbohydrate intake low for at least seven days.

☐ I have been following an intermittent fasting protocol for at least seven days.

☐ My daily eating window is down to eight hours or less.

☐ I feel comfortable and confident with this way of eating.

☐ I do not feel overly hungry or weak prior to my first meal.

☐ I am not doing this for quick weight loss.

☐ For the week before the fast I am following a fat-burning meal plan, with 5 to 15 percent of total calories coming from carbs and 65 to 80 percent total calories coming from fat.

☐ I am not currently under a high level of stress.

☐ I am not sick, pregnant, or nursing; do not have diabetes; and am not on medications that must be taken with food.

☐ I have reviewed the "Who Should Avoid Fasting" list on page 121 to ensure it's safe for me to fast.

☐ I have on hand some optional items to help support my fast, including tea, coffee, water, coconut oil, MCT oil, bone broth, electrolyte mix, ketone supplements, or anything else I plan to use.

☐ I know that if for any reason I don't feel well during a fast, I should end my fast and consult a physician.

☐ I have selected the appropriate level of fast for me at this time.

If you agree with all the statements in the checklist, then go ahead and select another fasting level from Chapter 5, such as Level 3: One Meal a Day (OMAD), for week 4 of Nourish. Be sure to carefully follow the fasting and refueling guidelines!

***

Those who feel they have to follow a set of arbitrary food rules often live life in one of two states: "on my diet" or "off my diet." The latter tends to come with permission to go off the rails until the next diet fad catches their attention. Not good. At all.

MIND-SET MESSAGE RIGHT HERE

As you begin to adopt the 131 Method, I hope it's becoming abundantly clear that progress, not perfection, is the goal. It's easy to slip into despair or self-doubt, to beat yourself up when you make a not-so-healthy choice. Get over it. You didn't mess up—you had an experience. How you deal with that moving forward is what I want you to focus on. We are all a work in progress. We all have room for growth, and your next choice is an opportunity to do better.

Focus on small, bite-size changes you can make every day. Focus on moving forward, taking little baby steps in the right direction. With each day, each week, each phase, your only goal should be just to feel and look a little better than you did before the 131 Method.

NOURISH MEAL PLAN

This is an example of a daily meal plan for each week in Nourish. Please refer to Part III for your recipes!!

NOURISH WEEK 1

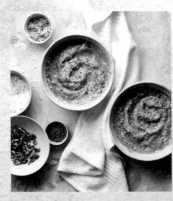

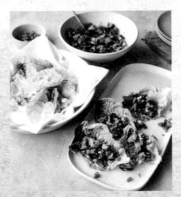

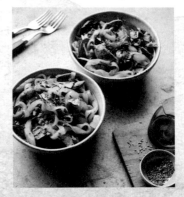

BREAKFAST

Frozen Smoothie Bowl
(page 242)

LUNCH

Vegetable Lettuce Wraps
(page 249)

DINNER

Chicken Lo Mein
(page 262)

NOURISH WEEK 2

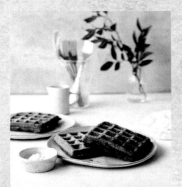

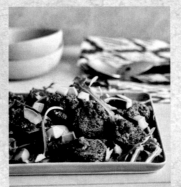

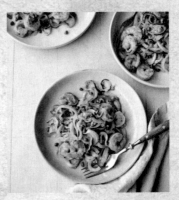

BREAKFAST

Hazelnut Waffles
(page 245)

LUNCH

Lentil Falafel Salad
(page 250)

DINNER

Shrimp with Zucchini
Noodles (page 265)

DON'T PANIC! YOU'RE NOT LIMITED TO BROTH! CHECK OUT PAGE 117 FOR ALL YOUR OPTIONS.

NOURISH WEEK 3

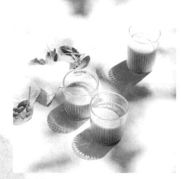

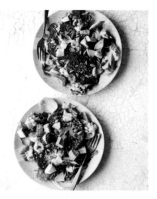

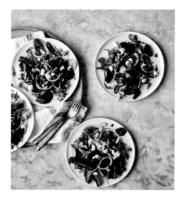

BREAKFAST

Chocolate-Mint Protein Shake (page 254)

LUNCH

Spicy Avocado Salad with Pumpkin and Hemp Seeds (page 253)

DINNER

Warm Mushroom, Goat Cheese, and Walnut Salad (page 257)

NOURISH WEEK 4 (FASTING)

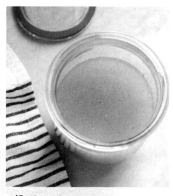

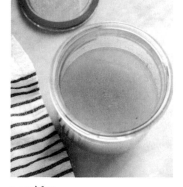

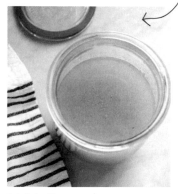

BREAKFAST

Vegetable Broth (page 346)

LUNCH

Vegetable Broth (page 346)

DINNER

Vegetable Broth (page 346)

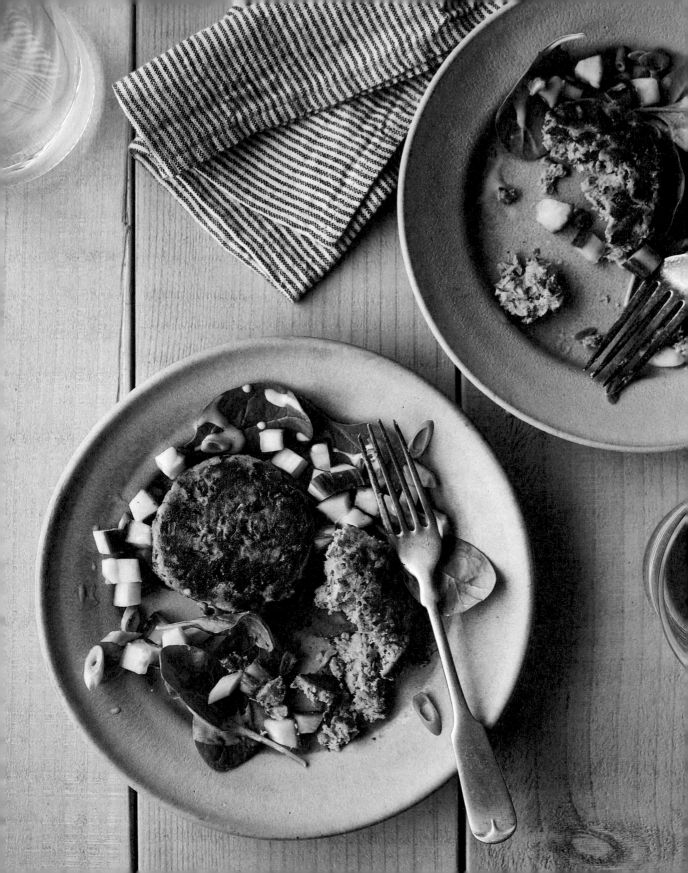

CHAPTER 8

PHASE THREE: RENEW

WEEKS 9 TO 12

Congratulations! You have reached the third phase of the 131 Method. The primary objective of the Renew phase is to reintroduce or refresh your relationship with carbs! The Renew plan further increases the metabolic flexibility you've developed during the Ignite and Nourish phases while simultaneously healing the gut, balancing hormones by reintroducing the right kind of carbs back into your diet. The work you did in the two previous phases will have prepared your body to efficiently use carbs as fuel rather than storing it as fat. By following the very specific weekly design of Renew, you will be able to successfully thrive with carbs, fats, and protein yet continue to make progress!

Have you ever dated or been friends with someone only to realize that for whatever reason you tended to bring out the worst in each other? Most people go their separate ways. But sometimes you realize that by just making a few adjustments you can make it work. If after reading an earlier chapter you cried a little thinking you had to break up with carbs for good, wipe those tears away sister, (or brother)! You are going to love Renew! We're bringing carbs back, baby!

This is another important distinction between the 131 Method and dumb diets. With most diets you commit to eating a certain way, maybe by limiting fat, cutting calories, calculating points, or using special containers. And maybe you experience some success—but as soon as you let yourself be a human again, *bam*, you're right back where you started (plus five pounds). It's not your fault. You're not a computer. You just need a guide.

RENEW AT A GLANCE

Your goals on the four weeks of Renew will be to:

- Master intuitive intermittent fasting
- Increase your metabolic flexibility through macrophasing
- 2 days of Lean Green
- 2 days of Carb Charge
- 3 days of Fat Burning

After you've completed three weeks on the Renew guidelines, you'll have the option to select a fasting level for week 4 or continue with Renew's guidelines for one more week instead.

MACROPHASING =
METABOLIC MAGIC

The meal plans on Renew have been designed to reboot your relationship with carbs By following a precise weekly schedule that cycles fats, protein, and carbs, your metabolism will learn to efficiently switch between each fuel source.

Though this phase does have a bit more structure than the two previous ones, you will still have the freedom to modify the plan to work for you. To do this, you'll need to follow the daily plan for this phase with a bit more precision than Ignite or Nourish. Don't worry, you'll still have the ability to personalize your approach. Renew significantly shifts your macronutrient ratios every two to three days through a process I call macrophasing.

Macrophasing in a nutshell is the alternating of macronutrient ratios every couple of days, which increases metabolic flexibility and promotes efficient use of energy. (I'll explain how this works in a moment.)

We all know that girl who looks great, eats whatever she wants, and effortlessly maintains her weight, while we are in a constant battle to lose those final pounds. Why is it some people have more wiggle room than the rest of us? I used to envy others who could indulge in a slice of pizza or plate of pasta without regret or consequence. Why couldn't it be that easy for me? If I so much as enjoyed the aroma of fresh bread, it showed up the next day on the scale. I was determined to get to the bottom of this mystery. I needed to know what made us different. What is it that enables some people to have more freedom when it comes to food? The answer is *metabolic flexibility*. Get excited!

INTUITIVE INTERMITTENT FASTING

With Renew, you'll learn to apply an intuitive approach to intermittent fasting. During earlier phases, when you began to master the benefits of intermittent fasting, you likely followed a precisely timed meal schedule. Using a schedule to track the timing of your meals helped keep you accountable during the sometimes challenging early weeks of becoming fat adapted. Structure gives us a foundation for success, but inflexible reliance on rules puts us at risk of developing unhealthy obsessive behaviors that can leave us feeling powerless.

Step into your power! Take a moment to honor the fact that you've come this far! Pat yourself on the back for taking the time to better understand what works and what doesn't, and pay attention to what your body is trying to tell you and why.

When deciding how and when to eat during Renew, I really want you to take the training wheels off. It's time to drop rule-based thinking regarding the timing of your first and last meals. Don't get me wrong; while rules provide order and security, rigidity and compulsive thinking can get in the way of your long-term success. Signs you've slipped into a dieter's mentality are clear when diet rules and daily habits are more important than your body's common sense.

My first attempt at intermittent fasting was heavily influenced by my old dieter's mentality. Once I established a schedule for my first and last meal, I stuck to it like a dog

DON'T BE THIS
PERSON

that won't let go of a bone. If I scheduled my first meal for noon, I wouldn't eat it at 11:50 A.M. even if I was starving, weak, and about to pass out. I didn't allow a single bite of food to pass my lips until precisely noon. If I had a dinner date with friends that meant broadening my eating window to 10 hours instead of the usual 8, I considered that day a failure. The diet rule mentality was stronger than my common sense. I ignored what was right for me on any particular day, ignoring even true hunger!

Conversely, there were days when I just wasn't hungry when my first mealtime rolled around, but I ate it anyway. I had yet to learn the power that comes from understanding and trusting my body's ability to know what is best. I believed that to be successful, I had to follow all protocols with exact precision. That, my friends, is dieting. It's not healthy. It's not sustainable.

An intuitive approach to intermittent fasting simply means instead of using your watch or a rule to dictate when to eat, you'll allow hunger and energy to guide you. Ideally, as you approach the fasting and refueling of week 4, you'll want to shorten your eating window to roughly six to eight hours if you plan to do a more advanced-level fast. But again, don't get all caught up in a schedule and overthinking it.

As a result of the 131 Method, I learned that I'm smart enough to figure stuff out. I don't have to wait for someone to tell me what I can and can't eat, what shake or supplement I should take, or that I must do a, b, and c workouts on specific days! I've learned that the "all or nothing" mind-set is a recipe for failure. I feel so much more free. **—JESSICA S.**

MACROPHASING

Maybe you've looked at your previous weight loss attempts or exercise plans as all-in endeavors. This extreme way of thinking results in the broad categorizations of efforts as either "failures" or "successes" with little room for anything in between. That line of thinking stunts metabolic flexibility.

Here's what I mean. Let's say you've got a tight lower back. We can assume part of the problem is lack of flexibility, and that means you need to stretch. But attack the tightness too aggressively by overstretching, and you'll do more harm than good.

Flexibility, whether biomechanical or metabolic, requires planned progression. Each phase of the 131 Method has been designed to create this. Each progression works to develop the metabolic flexibility needed to move to the next phase safely. The next step in your journey, creating healthy metabolic flexibility, is achieved through macrophasing.

From my studies and through the tens of thousands who have adopted the 131 Method as a lifestyle, I know that anyone can increase metabolic flexibility. Macrophasing creates flexibility while maintaining your ability to be fat adapted. You'll do this by enjoying meals that stretch your current macronutrient tolerance.

CROSS-TRAINING FOR YOUR METABOLISM

Macrophasing is a lot like cross-training. To achieve optimal fitness results, top trainers know the importance of changing up routines to keep clients' workouts exciting and push the body to use energy instead of storing it. By cycling different macronutrient ratios in specific amounts over a period of days, you teach your body to use the energy from foods you eat rather than storing it as fat. The result is improved metabolic flexibility. ←

IN PLAIN ENGLISH THIS MEANS YOUR METABOLISM UNDERSTANDS YOU'RE ON THE SAME TEAM!

KETOSIS MAKES
FASTING A BREEZE,
BUT YOU KNEW THAT!

Each week of Renew has three different stages or types of menus: Lean Green for two days, Carb Charge for two days, and then Fat Burning for three days. I'll break down exactly what meals might look like on those days and how to approximate your macros in just a minute. How you organize those days each week is up to you. If it's more convenient to follow Carb Charge days on the weekend, go for it! However, to comfortably transition into ketosis, be sure to finish strong with three consecutive days of Fat Burning ratios before starting a fast in week 4.

You probably have already figured out that it's pretty normal to experience increased hunger on Carb Charge days and sometimes the day after. The increased carbohydrate intake can sometimes create an insulin response even in the most fat-adapted of us. That extra hunger might correlate to a project that's forcing you to expend a lot of mental energy lately, or maybe you've just been killing it in the gym. Practice identifying the causes of both true hunger and emotional eating.

Instead of obsessing over getting all my workouts in, staying in my calorie zones, tracking every step, and feeling defeated when the scale went up instead of down, I learned to be kind to myself, customize the process, and still lose weight. **—KAREN W.**

LEAN GREEN

For two days, each week, you will want to eat meals that are high in protein, low in fat, and low/moderate in carbohydrates along with plenty of vegetables. The macronutrient range I suggest is as follows:

10–15% fat

30–50% protein

20–40% carbohydrate

Here's how:

- Eat lean proteins and lots of plants!
- Avoid excess fats on lean green days. Remember that while many foods are high in protein, such as nuts and nut butters, they are also high in fat.
- Use high-quality ingredients to fuel your tank.
- When in doubt about the fat content of a food, check it on an app like MyFitnessPal.

Meal ideas:

- Sweet Potato and Egg Scramble (page 295)
- Egg Muffins (page 276)
- Smoothie with greens, and berries such as blueberries or blackberries, and quality protein powder (see Berry Green Smoothie, page 276)
- Salad with lots of greens and non-starchy vegetables such as celery, mushrooms, cucumbers, brussels sprouts, broccoli, and more
- Roasted cabbage or sautéed greens with protein of choice (such as baked chicken)
- Low-carb coconut wraps (found in many health food stores as well as on Thrive.com and Amazon.com) or lettuce wraps filled with greens and a protein

CARB CHARGE

For the next two days, you will eat high-carb, low-fat, and moderate-protein foods. The ratio is as follows:

15–20% fat

15–25% protein

55–70% carbohydrate

Here's how:

- Choose the healthy carbs that work for you and do not cause you digestive discomfort, bloating, or an inflammatory response, such as sweet potatoes, quinoa, rice, bananas, grapes, other fruits, legumes, and gluten-free pastas.
- Avoid any foods that you know cause you inflammation.

Meal ideas:

- Oatmeal with berries (see Overnight Protein Oats, page 294)
- Egg Muffins (page 276) with toast or fruit on the side
- Smoothies with banana, berries, and protein powder (see Pineapple–Mint Smoothie, page 301)
- Baked potato or Herbed Potato Wedges (page 311) with vegetables and protein of choice
- Leftover low-carb soup like chili with sweet potato or beans added. (see Red Bean and Quinoa Chili, page 307)
- Roasted vegetables, such as sweet potatoes, beets, carrots, or squash of choice and protein of choice with no extra fat added (see Chicken, Quinoa, and Sweet Potato Bowls page 298)
- Quinoa or rice salad with protein of choice

FAT BURNING

For the next three days, you will eat low-carb, high-fat, and moderate-protein foods. The ratio is as follows:

70–80% fat

15–20% protein

5–10% carbohydrate

Here's how:

- Emphasize foods low in carbohydrates and high in healthy fats, much like what you ate during Ignite.
- Limit carb intake to green and nonstarchy vegetables.
- Choose high-quality protein and pasture-raised meats whenever possible. Opt for higher-fat forms of quality meats and fish (such as grass-finished beef, wild-caught salmon).

Meal Ideas:

- Eggs with avocado (see Eggs and Greens, page 314)
- High-fat smoothie with avocado and macadamia nuts
- Almond- or coconut-flour pancakes
- Salad with olives, olive oil dressing, chicken, and low-carb vegetables such as cucumbers, bell peppers, asparagus, mushrooms, zucchini, radishes, etc.
- Non-GMO Tempeh bowl with salsa, guacamole, and low-carb vegetables or Cauliflower Fried Rice (see page 318)
- Baked chicken with roasted cauliflower cooked in coconut oil, dunked in guacamole or macadamia hummus
- Low-carb soup with avocado added, and a side salad dressed with healthy fats

RENEW MEAL PLAN

Here is a sample daily meal plan for one week of Renew. Please refer to Part III for your recipes!

LEAN GREEN DAY

BREAKFAST

Lean Green Breakfast Chili (page 272)

LUNCH

Turkey, Asparagus, and Broccoli (page 283)

DINNER

Garlic Shrimp with Spinach (page 291)

LEAN GREEN DAY

BREAKFAST

Egg, Turkey, and Arugula Breakfast Wrap (page 275)

LUNCH

Salmon Cakes and Spinach Salad (page 278)

DINNER

Turkey Meatballs with Zoodles (page 287)

CARB CHARGE DAY

BREAKFAST

Overnight Protein Oats (page 294)

LUNCH

Chicken, Quinoa, and Sweet Potato Bowl (page 298)

DINNER

Minestrone with Herbed Potato Wedges (pages 306 and 311)

CARB CHARGE DAY

BREAKFAST

Raspberry–Chocolate Breakfast Bowl (page 297)

LUNCH

Root Vegetable Soup (page 302)

DINNER

Sheet Pan Chicken and Vegetables (page 308)

FAT-BURNING DAY

BREAKFAST

Flaxseed–Cinnamon
Muffins (page 312)

LUNCH

Pizza Muffins (page 315)

DINNER

Sea Bass with Mango Salsa
(page 321)

FAT-BURNING DAY

BREAKFAST

Eggs and Greens
(page 314)

LUNCH

Cauliflower Fried Rice
(page 318)

DINNER

Chicken Tenders with
Broccolini with Lemon
and Garlic (pages 225
and 237)

FAT-BURNING DAY

BREAKFAST

Chocolate Peanut Butter
Pancakes (page 198)

LUNCH

BLT Pinwheels (page 218)

DINNER

Turkey Meatloaf with
Buffalo Sauce with Chili-
Lime Brussels Sprouts
(pages 228 and 236)

RENEW TIPS FOR VEGETARIANS AND VEGANS

Some vegetarians find it a challenge to keep carbohydrates low and protein high during Renew. Remember, this is less about precise macronutrient ratios, and more about significant changes in the ranges. Make this plan work for you with the following helpful tips.

LEAN GREEN PROTEIN SUGGESTIONS:

- Egg whites
- Eggs
- Hemp seeds
- High-quality protein powder
- Lentils
- Tempeh

CARB CHARGE PROTEIN SUGGESTIONS:

- Beans and legumes
- Fruits and vegetables, including starchy vegetables such as sweet potatoes or squash
- Lentils
- Quinoa
- Rice or other grains, as tolerated
- Tempeh

FAT-BURNING PROTEIN AND FAT SUGGESTIONS:

- Avocado
- High-quality plant protein powder
- Non-starchy vegetables such as cucumbers, radishes, spinach, kale, mushrooms, zucchini, celery, brussels sprouts
- Nuts and nut butters
- Oils (coconut, MCT, olive, avocado)
- Olives
- Seeds and seed butters
- Tempeh

WEEK 4: FASTING AND REFUELING

Even if you've had success with a previous fast and refuel week during the Ignite and Nourish phases, take the time now to assess your readiness, schedule, stress, and need before beginning one again. Should you choose not to fast, continue macrophasing for the final week of Renew.

MAKE SURE YOU'RE READY!

PRE-FAST SELF-ASSESSMENT CHECKLIST

☐ I have been macrophasing for at least two weeks.

☐ I have followed fat-burning macronutrient ratios for at least three days.

☐ I have followed a daily eating window of eight hours or less for at least one week.

☐ I feel comfortable and confident with this way of eating.

☐ I am not currently under a high level of stress.

☐ I am not sick, pregnant, or nursing; do not have diabetes; and am not on medications that must be taken with food.

☐ I have reviewed the "Who Should Avoid Fasting" list on page 121 to ensure it's safe for me to fast.

☐ I have on hand some optional items to help support my fast, including tea, coffee, water, coconut oil, MCT oil, bone broth, electrolyte mix, ketone supplements, or anything else I plan to use.

☐ I know that if for any reason I don't feel well during a fast, I should end my fast and consult a physician.

☐ I have selected the appropriate level of fast for me at this time.

If you agree with all the statements in the checklist, then go ahead and select another fasting level from Chapter 5, such as Level 4: Three-Day Mini-Fast, for week 4 of Renew. Be sure to carefully follow the fasting and refueling guidelines!

*****

I spent most of the last two decades living in fear of weight gain. I let false beliefs about my faulty body become my reality. I viewed many foods as the enemy and my metabolism as the consolation prize. I punished myself with brutal workouts. I craved the freedom that others had. I wasn't desperate to lose weight; I was desperate to be healthy, a term I associated with being thin. I wanted freedom from the hours of endless exercise and calorie counting. The ever-looming threat of weight gain was robbing me of my joy.

It took a steadfast commitment, at first not to myself but to my family. (Sometimes our own fear is so real, it helps to use the love we have for others to motivate change.) Once I started on this journey, I became my "why." I began to experience for the first time what it felt like to be healthy. I couldn't believe the foods I was able to enjoy or how much better my body felt. I couldn't believe how much better I felt about my body. My body was working with me. It wasn't my enemy; it was my gift.

In the beginning, I struggled with familiar thoughts. Each time I phased my diet, I did so reluctantly, struggling with the belief that I would screw up the success I had finally found. When I started phasing my diet, including macrophasing in what I now call Renew, I remember slipping into my old way of thinking: "Maybe I can tell people to do this, but there's no way it will work for me." It wasn't just my diet that needed to change; I needed to change my thinking.

I reminded myself that I was too smart not to trust the research and the team of crazy-smart experts I had assembled. I chose to challenge that nagging negative belief and embrace Renew. I didn't need to fear carbs or any food, for that matter. I needed to repair my relationship with these foods and trust that my body would not betray me.

Renew is your opportunity to start fresh, a win earned by the work—not perfection—of your two previous phases. The end of Renew signifies the end of your first cycle.

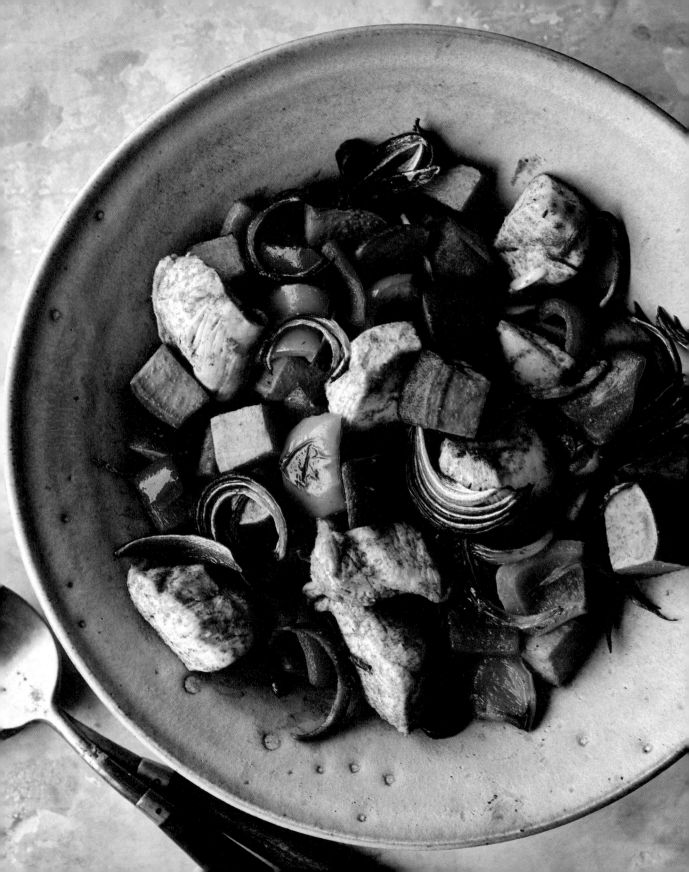

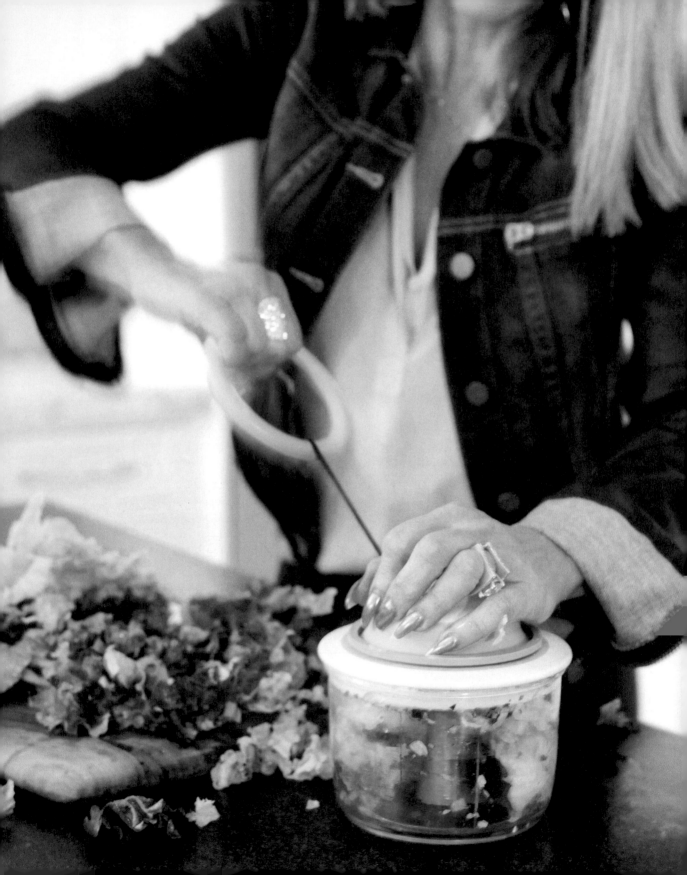

CHAPTER 9

THE LIFESTYLE PHASE

You did it! With the help of the 131 Method, you've ditched the dieter's mentality, mastered the mystery of your metabolism, improved your immune system, and taken ownership of your health. You're well on your way to achieving the healthy, happy life you deserve. I am so freaking proud of you!

Do you remember the initial assessment you completed before you started the program? Grab your measuring tape and smartphone! It's time to take new measurements and progress pics! While you're at it, fill out the following assessment to compare all your results with your initial assessment on page 90:

131 METHOD FINAL ASSESSMENT

Date _____

Weight _____

Optional

Body Fat Percentage _____

Resting Heart Rate _____

Bloating (scale of 1–10) _____

CIRCUMFERENCE MEASUREMENTS:

Waist: _____ Hips: _____ Chest: _____

Biceps: R _____ L _____ Thighs: R _____ L _____ Calves: _____

Rate each area below on a scale of 1 to 10, with 10 being the best:

How do you rate your overall health? _____

Rate the comfort of your clothing fit: _____

Does it change day to day from swelling, bloating, or water retention?

Explain: _____

For women, rate how regular your cycle is: _____

How heavy are your periods? Do you have cyclical cramping, acne, breast tenderness, or headaches?

Explain: _____

How regular is your digestion? _____

If necessary, be more specific about bowel frequency/quality, belching, gas, bloating, pain, etc.

Explain: _____

How well are you able to focus or maintain mental clarity? _____

TO DOWNLOAD AND MAKE COPIES OF THIS FORM, GO TO 131METHOD.COM/FORMS

Do you forget things easily, have brain fog or trouble concentrating, or generally feel anxious and restless?

Explain: _____

Rate your overall energy level: _____

How consistent and sound is your sleep? _____

Include here how many hours of sleep you get each night: _____

Do you wake up several times or sleep straight throughout the night? _____

How is the quality of your skin? _____

Do you have rashes, acne, bumps, reactions, dry or scaly skin?

Explain: _____

Rate any pain: _____

Headaches, joint pain, muscle aches? _____

Explain: _____

Rate the frequency of any food cravings (for example, I crave sweets after dinner every single night, 10): _____

Indicate the type, frequency, and when they most often occur: _____

Explain: _____

Rate the intensity of your cravings (example, I cannot go without having chocolate every night, 10): _____

How easy is it for you to identify true hunger versus cravings? _____

Explain (throughout the day, between meals, etc.):
_____

Rate the depth of your relationship with food: _____

Do you view food as a friend, a crutch, or fuel?

Explain: _____

AN ALL NEW YOU

Anyone can go on a diet and lose weight temporarily, but what you've accomplished is a lasting transformation. You've taken control of your body from the inside out. You put faith in your smarts, prioritized your health, gave yourself permission to be imperfect, and personalized the process. You decided enough was enough and seized the opportunity to demystify the mystery of metabolism. Today you're a different person in more ways than just the physical. You have changed the way you eat, the way you define health, and most importantly the way you think. You no longer think like a dieter. You are no longer focused on perfection, and can enjoy making regular progress.

The maintenance or lifestyle chapter in most diet books is devoted to your nutrition. *The 131 Method* has been different from the start and so too will be this chapter. To help ensure your long-term success, we will address the most important area at this time: your newly improved mind-set.

One of the best ways to identify where you want or need to make progress is through self-awareness and taking pen to paper. Let's do a quick assessment to help you identify any area where you have room for improvement related to healthy mind-set.

Place an X next to any of the following statements that on some level you might still believe or relate to.

- ☐ "I've blown it this week. I'm off my diet."
- ☐ "I can't have carbs."
- ☐ "I bet I'll go back to my old ways."
- ☐ "I'll just do one quick dieting trick, and then I'll go back to doing what I know is best for me."
- ☐ "There must be something wrong with me! I should have lost more weight."
- ☐ "I need to lose five pounds by Saturday, so I'd better start fasting today."

- ☐ "I just don't have what it takes to be a healthy person."
- ☐ "I am destined to struggle with my weight for the rest of my life."
- ☐ "I don't have the discipline that other people have."
- ☐ "I won't remember anything I learned."
- ☐ "I hope I can maintain this when my family comes to visit."

If random thoughts like these still resonate with you, you're still struggling with the residual effects of what I call the "diet mentality." It's okay! Like everything else, you'll do this in stages, and the first step is self-awareness. We've endured a lifetime of this sticky stuff. It's going to take time to reverse those long-held false beliefs. When a magazine cover, social media site, or your well-meaning mom triggers thoughts that don't serve you, ask yourself if the negative thought you're having is the truth or a belief.

You now know too much ever to go back. You've kicked those one-size-fits-all dumb diets, quick fixes, and all-or-nothing mind-set to the curb. Now more than ever it's important you fortify your new way of thinking and that happens when you permanently change beliefs. You must believe you deserve the best.

If you've ever dated someone you knew wasn't good for you, yet you struggled to let go, struggled to believe you deserved better, you understand how this happens. We like familiarity, even when it isn't good for us. And that's where your support system makes the difference. Together, as a community of 131-ers, we stand shoulder to shoulder and redefine what it means to be healthy.

You, my friend, have come to your senses and let go of these once firmly held false beliefs! Never again will you waste time chasing down the latest celebrity meal plan or wondering if that cleanse everyone is talking about really works. You see right through those peddling weight loss pills and magical health shakes.

There is no one-size-fits-all diet that works for everyone.

COMMIT TO BE JUST A LITTLE BETTER TOMORROW

There is no superfood cure-all. Health is not something you do for 21 days or 12 weeks. Health, a strong immune system, balanced hormones, and maintaining a healthy weight, is a journey. It's only when we stop searching for the finish line that we can sit back and enjoy the ride.

WHAT IS THE 131 METHOD LIFESTYLE?

All life revolves around seasons, cycles, and phasing. There are phases of the moon, phases to a woman's hormonal cycle, phases of cell development, and seasonal changes. Nearly all living organisms revolve around phases. Nature works in cycles, seasons, and phases.

Following the 131 Method lifestyle means adopting a framework, a mind-set, a way of life, that you can realistically and effortlessly maintain and improve for the *rest of your life*. You are committed to steady progress. And because you understand there is always room for growth, you're motivated to repeat the process. If you're excited about the prospect of continued improvements to your health and metabolism, I strongly encourage you to repeat another cycle of the 131 Method following the guidelines of Ignite, Nourish, and Renew (in that order).

Myself and thousands of others have adopted the 131 Method as a way of life, phasing our diet every four to six weeks or so, just as you've learned to do in this book.

As our circumstances change, often so too will our diet need to be adjusted. Factors such as our age, environment, stress, illness, infections, childbirth, and menopause (just to name a few) impact our hormones. But these hormonal changes don't have to result in unexplained weight gain and other unpleasant side effects. Your very personal solution lies in your nutrition.

Each time you enter the Ignite phase, continue to refine your macronutrient ratios and revisit why tracking them is so important. Refining and tracking your macronutrients will help keep your hormones in check and recalibrate your engine to work smoothly and efficiently. Each time you follow Ignite you'll be amazed at how much more natural it is to flip the switch and run your body on stored fat. Revisiting Ignite will further refine the work you've done to correct your appetite and keep you on the path to improved gut health.

After Ignite, you'll transition into the Nourish phase and rediscover the power of plant-based foods and macronutrient-dense protein. Each time you revisit Nourish you'll have a better understanding of your realistic protein needs and feel better equipped to identify foods that improve your gut health.

Once you finish Nourish, you'll move on to the Renew phase. Each time you do Renew, you'll experience what it means to be able to eat foods that your body once converted to fat. You'll discover new ways to fine-tune the flexibility of your metabolism and how to use macrophasing to obtain your ideal body composition while enjoying foods that were once off-limits for you. Free! Free! Free at last from fear of food.

I saw results so quickly on Ignite that I was really motivated. I wanted to start the Ignite phase over a few times, but I decided to trust the process by doing the other phases. And I am so glad that I did! **—CINDY H.**

The 131 Method has been an absolute blessing. I can't thank everyone enough for taking the time and dedication to produce the program for us. It is incredible and life changing. **—JESSICA S.**

Diets are unrealistic, unforgiving, and completely unreliable. The 131 Method is not a diet. It's a lifestyle based on a few health-promoting principles.

PULL OUT YOUR
PHONE AND SNAP A
PIC OF THIS PAGE

In summary:

- Focus first on gut health
- Phase your diet every four to six weeks
- Eat less meat
- Eat quality pasture-raised, grass-finished quality animal protein whenever possible
- Eat more plants
- Remember that calories don't matter as much as quality ingredients
- Avoid artificial ingredients
- Eat real food
- Avoid foods that have been processed to remove fat
- Avoid foods that cause inflammation
- Minimize sugar and carbohydrate intake
- Limit alcohol
- Limit emotional stress
- Limit physical stress
- Exercise a minimum of 30 minutes every day
- Get more sleep
- Limit exposure to known toxins
- Drink 75 ounces of water or more per day
- Practice intermittent fasting in phases
- Phase in and out of mild ketosis
- Fast for health several times per year (as appropriate)
- Eat healthy fats
- Track macros each time you repeat Ignite (at least once a quarter)
- Choose high-quality supplements when needed
- Pay attention to how you feel
- Become an expert on your own digestion
- Be a role model for others, not a know-it-all

Allow the principles of the 131 Method to guide, rather than rule, your life. Following these principles will improve your health on a cellular level, correct insulin sensitivity, enhance metabolic flexibility, reduce inflammation, and increase your energy level while helping you to maintain your ideal weight effortlessly.

1 PERCENT BETTER EACH WEEK

It's impossible to hit your mark if you don't have a target. Even the most disciplined of us needs a well-defined goal. Pro athletes, CEOs, and all-around go-getters use clearly defined goals to realize their visions and keep motivation high. A clearly defined goal has a deadline and specific measure. They should be realistic but at the same time challenging.

Maybe you've already established such a specific goal with measure and a deadline. If not, may I suggest you make a goal to improve your efforts by just 1 percent each week— not perfect, just 1 percent better. Embracing the 1 percent better mentality will free you from the pressure we place on ourselves to be perfect and the shame and guilt we feel when we're not. If something doesn't work for you, modify it! Set realistic, achievable daily objectives that move you in the direction of being just a little better every week!

WHAT 1 PERCENT BETTER IS FOR ME

As I sit writing this book in my baby-pink home office, pecking away at my keyboard, I can't help but feel overwhelmed with a sense of relief. I can smell Bret cooking something amazing in the kitchen. All I can think about is taking a break from writing to go enjoy dinner at our dining room table with him and the kids. Just a few years ago the very same scenario would have given me low-grade anxiety. I would have struggled with the shame of allowing myself to eat whatever the rest of the family was eating, or I would have been preoccupied with calculations of how many minutes of exercise I would need to cancel out the calories I had just consumed. It's pretty tough to be present and enjoy life when food feels like the enemy. What a waste of time and energy.

Today I am a different person from the girl who once felt uncomfortable in her own skin, the girl who felt like a fraud talking to people about weight loss or health. To be honest, that girl had some things to learn. We all have things to learn! I'm not looking for a finish line; I'm in this for the long haul, the highs, the lows, the setbacks, and the steps forward. I am here to make the most of this beautiful journey and to change the legacy of health in this world. I am proud to have come so far in my own health and proud of the profound ways I am able to help others find freedom. I am stand-on-a-rooftop-with-a-bullhorn certain this is possible for you, too!

Not every success story includes dramatic weight loss. Your health is the ultimate triumph. Profound transformation doesn't always show up in a smaller pair of jeans. The 131 Method is how you make the very most of the gift of health. With each new cycle you will gain a more profound understanding of and appreciation for your body. You will see food as your healer. You will look forward to every bite and feel a sense of pride with each healthy decision you make. As your gut heals, and your immune system is strengthened, you'll have a hard time remembering the last time you got sick. Your body will grow stronger, pain and swelling will become a thing of the past, and your metabolism will work with you, not against you. Your mind-set will shift. As you apply the 131 principles to your life, your insecurities and self-doubt around nutrition and health will begin to lift, replaced with a bold determination that you will never go back.

THIS DOESN'T HAVE TO BE GOOD-BYE

The tools you've acquired from this book provide you with the foundation you need to phase your diet for the rest of your life. Yet there's no denying the power and accountability that comes from a little structure and the support of a community. If you haven't already spent some time on Google and figured it out yourself, there's a pretty cool 131 Method online community. In fact, it goes beyond community. The 131 Method started out as an online coaching experience: me, online, sharing a virtual coaching experience with thousands of people just like you.

Consider this your formal invitation to kick-start your next cycle of the 131 Method as part of a group that will go through the three phases together in my online 131 Method coaching program. I want 131Method.com to be your reliable, go-to source for all things health and nutrition. It's also where you can sign up to go through your next cycle of the 131 Method with me as your guide. By investing in my online coaching program, you'll experience a deeper level of accountability and community.

The principals of the 131 Method book and online program are consistent. The online program is for those looking for a more interactive experience, an in-depth understanding of the science, and a deep dive into the 131 mind-set. I walk you through every week of the 12-week program through a series of audio and video lessons you can access from your phone (or any device, for that matter). You'll have access to hundreds of helpful handouts, 12 weeks of meal plans, shopping guides, cooking tutorials, motivational and mind-set coaching, interviews with the experts, plus 200 new recipes. I'm not even kidding when I say the variety and simplicity of the recipes will blow you away. We have the ability to offer you far more variety online, from meal plans for breastfeeding new moms to recipes that work for everyone from vegetarians to families of 10. The online recipes have been categorized so that you can quickly click on your current diet phase and create delicious meals to fit your personalized plan.

BUT WAIT, THERE'S MORE!

Going through the 131 Method as part of an online program is ideal for those who need the support of a community. In addition to the support of your fellow participants in the program, you will have access to my team of experts, including registered dietitians, through our "Ask the Dietitian" forum, live tutorials, and hundreds of educational resources. You'll hear from leading experts and scientists and always be up to date on the latest healthy weight-related findings.

A new group starts every Monday. To learn more, visit www.131Method.com/book. BTW, if you do decide to join me, be sure to swing by my Instagram (www.instagram .com/chalenejohnson) and use the hashtag #131Movement in your comment to let me know!

YOU HAVE EVERYTHING YOU NEED

"It's hard to beat a person who never gives up."

—Babe Ruth

Believe in yourself and you can move mountains. You can do anything. Don't forget how much you've already done. Take pride in yourself and your accomplishments. You've accomplished amazing things and you'll continue to do awesome things! Never forget that. Oh and don't tell anyone but I have a special place in my heart for people who read. Do you realize how few people pick up a book and read it? I mean really read it like cover to cover. Readers, like letter writers and landlines, are a dying breed of special peeps. Gosh I hope this doesn't hurt the feeling of audiobook listeners but I'm pretty sure book readers have superior IQs. I don't like to play favorites, but I can't help myself. I want to celebrate and support you! I've prepared an audio recording to help strengthen your new mind-set. It's my gift to you. To download and listen go to www.131method.com/audiogift.

And in case I haven't told you, I'm proud of you. I believe in you. I love you!

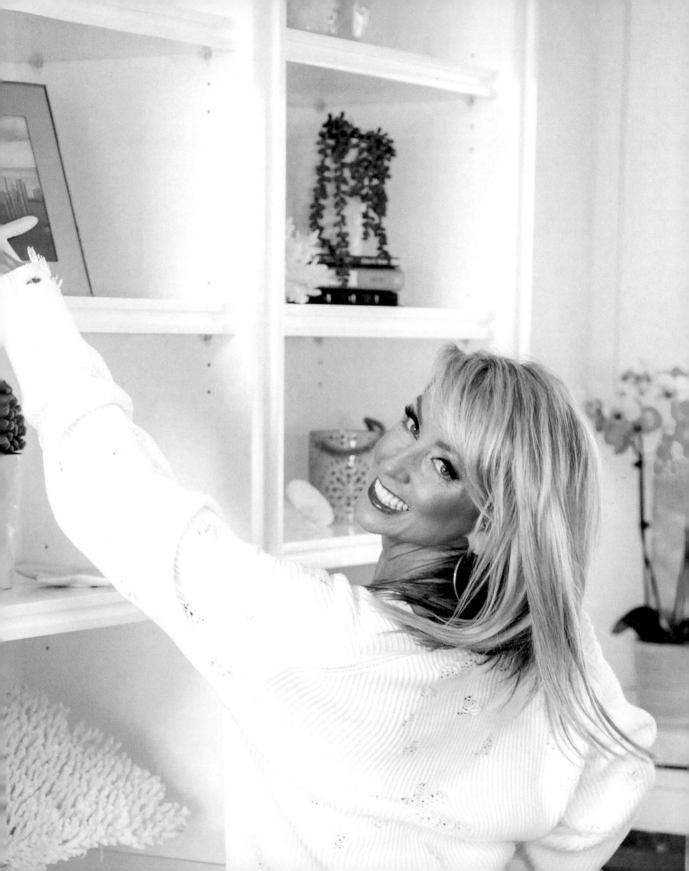

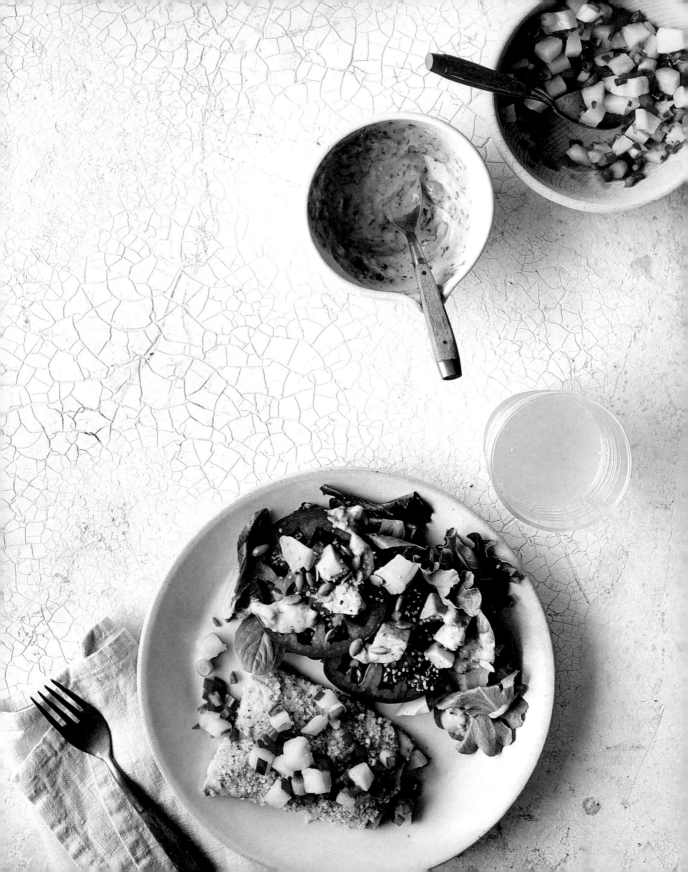

PART III

THE 131 RECIPES

Note to Reader: Some of our recipes contain a sweetener by the brand name Swerve, which is a natural sweetener made from non-GMO ingredients. It's composed of oligosaccharides and erythritol (a sugar alcohol or polyol) found naturally in some fruits, vegetables and fermented foods. Neither affect blood sugar or insulin levels. Swerve is a zero-calorie sweetener; however, its label lists 4g carbohydrates per serving. Since these are not absorbed, they're not included in the nutrition information. Other similar brands include: Pyure, Lakanto, Norbu, and ZSweet. All can be used cup for cup like sugar. If you prefer to sweeten with stevia, adjust the quantity since stevia is concentrated and much sweeter.

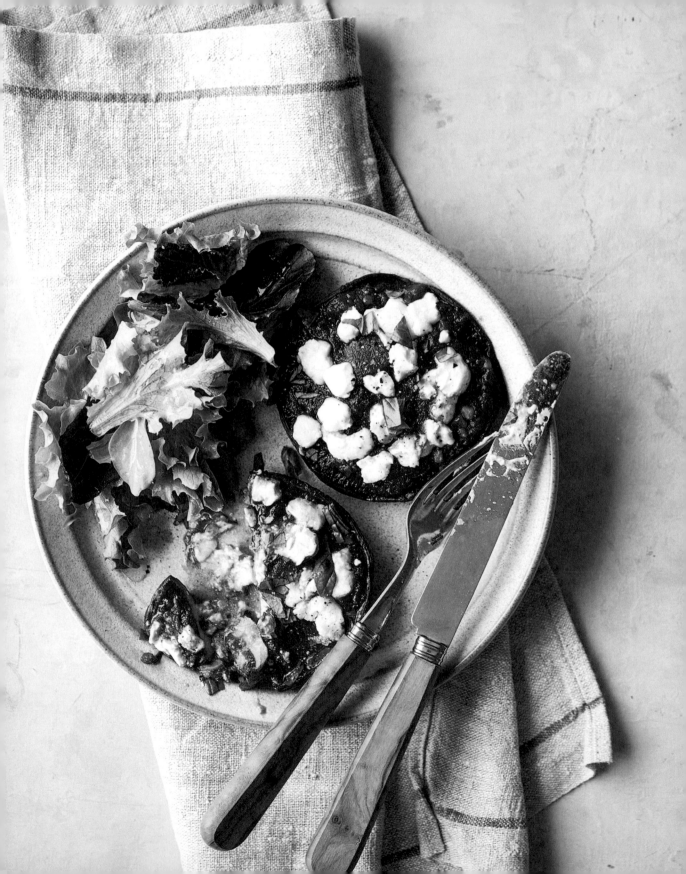

IGNITE RECIPES

CHOCOLATE–PEANUT BUTTER PANCAKES

How good do these chocolaty, peanutty pancakes sound? Here's a morning recipe that you can share with the rest of your family. If you want to. MAKES 4 SERVINGS (12 PANCAKES)

PANCAKES:

2 large organic eggs, lightly beaten

⅔ cup almond meal

2 tablespoons Swerve Sweetener Confectioners

2 tablespoons nondairy milk

1 tablespoon coconut flour

1 tablespoon cacao powder

1 tablespoon salted natural peanut butter

1 teaspoon pure vanilla extract

1 teaspoon aluminum-free baking powder

Coconut oil cooking spray

TOPPING:

2 tablespoons salted peanut butter

2 tablespoons coconut oil

1 tablespoon nondairy milk

2 tablespoons Swerve Sweetener Confectioners

1 tablespoon cacao powder

Pinch fine sea salt

To make the pancakes: Whisk together the eggs, almond meal, Swerve, milk, coconut flour, cacao powder, peanut butter, vanilla extract, and baking powder in a bowl until smooth. Let the batter sit for 3 minutes.

Coat a skillet or griddle with cooking spray and heat over medium-low heat. Using a tablespoon measure, add the batter to the skillet to form pancakes. This may have to be done in batches. Cook until the edges become firm and golden (about 3 minutes), then flip and cook until the undersides are lightly browned and the pancakes are cooked through, 1 to 2 minutes.

To make the topping: Put the peanut butter, coconut oil, and milk in a small bowl and microwave for 20 seconds. Stir in the Swerve, cacao powder, and salt until smooth. Divide the 12 pancakes among 4 plates and drizzle with the warm topping.

CALORIES: 304 | PROTEIN: 11.5G | FAT: 26G | CARBS: 8.5G | FIBER: 4G | NET CARBS: 4.5G

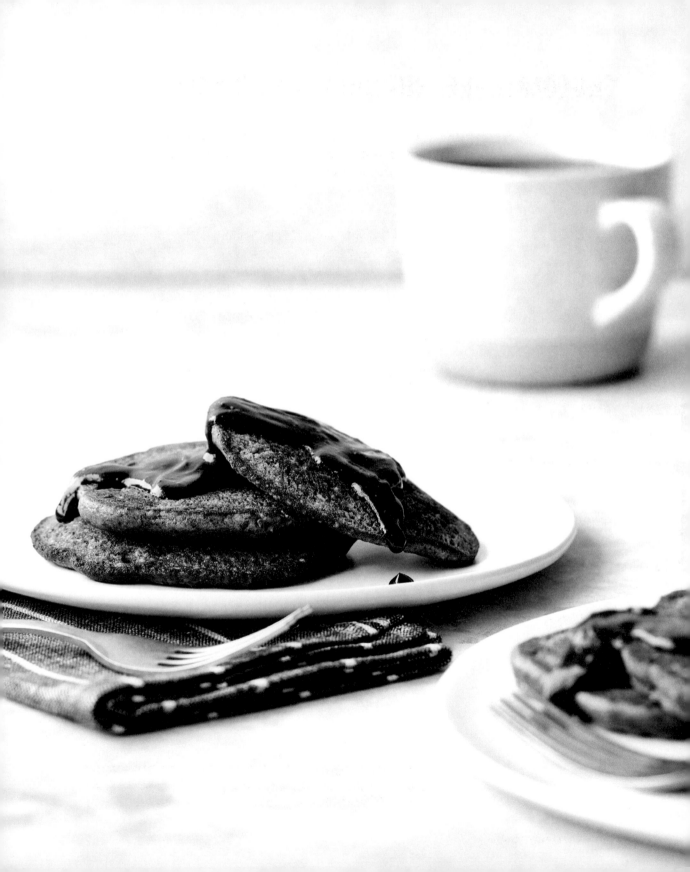

SOUTHWESTERN PANCAKES

These savory pancakes pair well with eggs or can be served as a side to a burger. They're also great on their own, drizzled with butter or salsa.

MAKES 2 SERVINGS (8 PANCAKES)

4 large organic eggs

¼ cup coconut flour

2 tablespoons nondairy milk

1 tablespoon avocado oil

1 teaspoon aluminum-free baking powder

1 teaspoon ground cumin

1 teaspoon chili powder

¼ teaspoon sea salt

Pinch cayenne pepper, optional

¼ cup chopped cilantro

2 tablespoons ghee

Whisk the eggs in a bowl. Whisk in the coconut flour, milk, oil, baking powder, cumin, chili powder, salt, and cayenne, if using, until combined. Let the batter stand for 5 minutes. Once the batter has thickened slightly, use a spatula to fold in the cilantro.

Working in batches, melt 2 to 3 teaspoons of the ghee in a large nonstick skillet over medium-low heat. Using a tablespoon measure, add the batter to the pan to form pancakes (you should be able to make 2 to 4 at a time) and cook for 3 minutes, flipping when the edges appear firm. Cook for 1 to 2 minutes longer, until golden brown. Repeat with the remaining ghee and batter. Divide the pancakes between 2 plates.

CALORIES: 410 | PROTEIN: 15G | FAT: 34.5G | CARBS: 9G | FIBER: 5.5G | NET CARBS: 3.5G

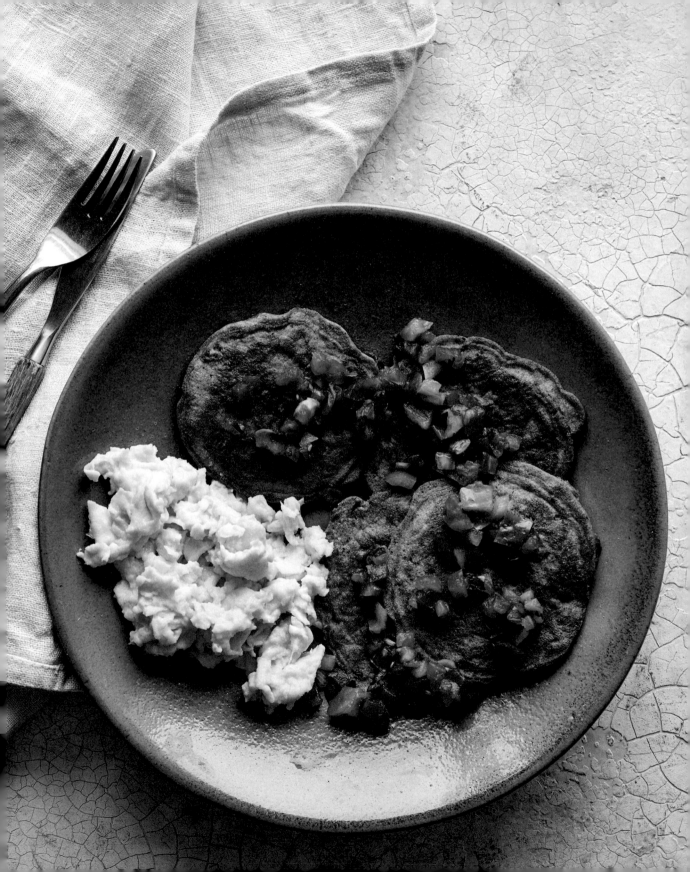

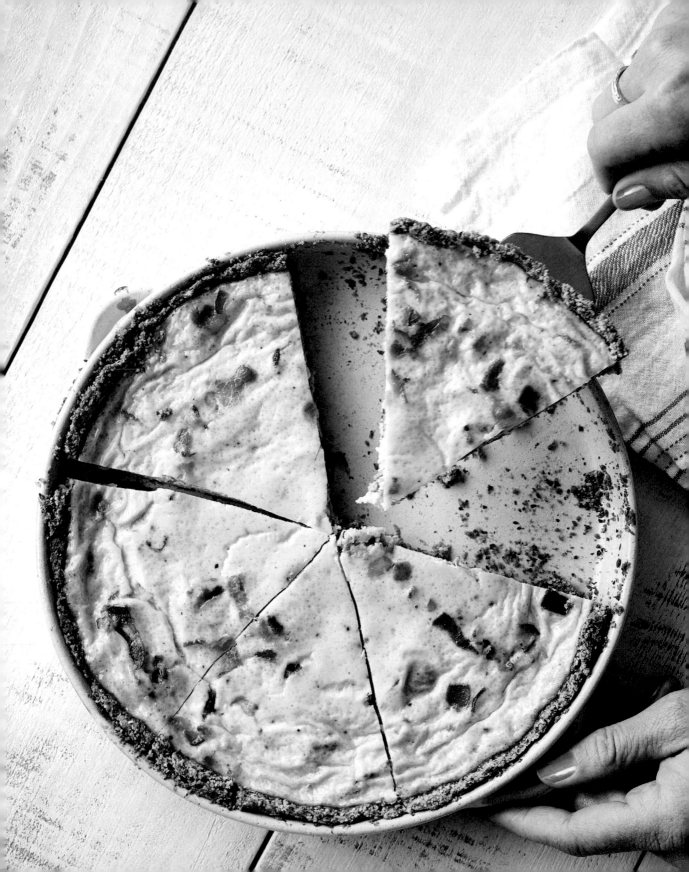

BACON QUICHE

If you prefer, use heavy cream instead of coconut milk for a more neutral flavor.

MAKES 6 SERVINGS

CRUST:

Coconut oil cooking spray

2 cups almond flour

1 large egg

2 tablespoons coconut oil, melted

1 teaspoon fine sea salt

FILLING:

6 strips 100% grass-fed, pastured, and nitrate-free bacon

1½ cups (12 ounces) canned full-fat coconut milk or heavy cream

4 large organic eggs

¼ teaspoon fine sea salt

¼ teaspoon freshly ground black pepper

Heat the oven to 350°F. Coat a 9-inch round pie plate with cooking spray.

To make the crust: Whisk together the almond flour, egg, coconut oil, and sea salt in a bowl until fully combined. Press the dough into the pie plate, pushing it evenly up the sides. Bake for 13 to 15 minutes, until the crust is lightly golden.

To make the filling: Fry the bacon strips in a large skillet over medium heat until crisp on both sides. Put the bacon on paper towels and, when cool enough to handle, blot well, then crumble.

Whisk together the coconut milk, eggs, salt, and pepper in a bowl. Stir in ¾ of the crumbled bacon. Pour the egg mixture into the baked crust and top with the remaining bacon.

Bake for 35 to 38 minutes, until the top is lightly golden, and the eggs are set. Cover with aluminum foil if the crust begins to brown too much. Cool for 15 minutes before slicing.

CALORIES: 460 | PROTEIN: 16G | FAT: 40G | CARBS: 9G | FIBER: 4G | NET CARBS: 5G

SAUSAGE AND GOAT CHEESE FRITTATA

A frittata, an Italian open-faced omelet, is deliciously satisfying. For variety, substitute any ingredients from the list on page 176 for the pork and goat cheese. MAKES 6 SERVINGS

1 tablespoon avocado oil

1 pound 100% organic ground pork

1 small red onion, thinly sliced

4 cups fresh spinach

8 large organic eggs

½ cup canned full-fat coconut milk

½ teaspoon garlic powder

¼ teaspoon ground nutmeg

½ teaspoon sea salt

¼ teaspoon freshly ground black pepper

3 tablespoons chopped chives

4 ounces soft goat cheese, crumbled

Heat the oven to broil. Heat a cast-iron or other ovenproof skillet over medium heat. Add the avocado oil and pork and cook the pork until browned, about 5 minutes. Use a slotted spoon to remove the pork from the pan, leaving the drippings.

Add the onion to the same pan and sauté until translucent, about 5 minutes. Add the spinach and stir until wilted.

Whisk together the eggs, milk, garlic powder, nutmeg, salt, and pepper in a medium bowl.

Return the sausage to the skillet and spread evenly on the bottom. Pour the eggs on top and cook without stirring until nearly set, about 5 minutes. Sprinkle with chives and goat cheese.

Put the skillet in the oven and cook just until the top is set and the cheese is melted, 3 to 4 minutes. Slice into 6 portions. Leftovers can be refrigerated for up to 4 days.

CALORIES: 424 | PROTEIN: 26G | FAT: 33G | CARBS: 5G | FIBER: 0.5G | NET CARBS: 4.5G

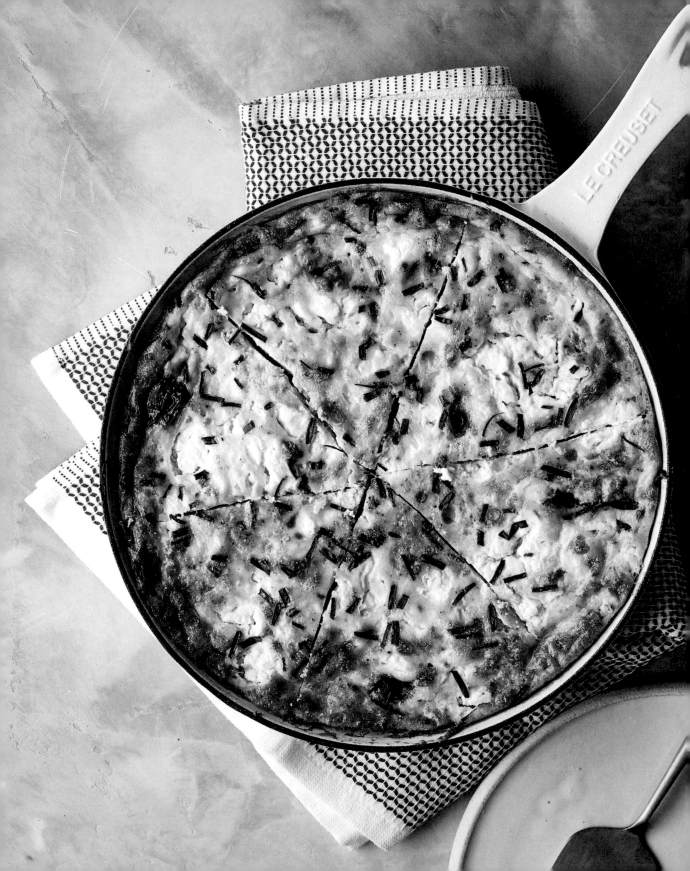

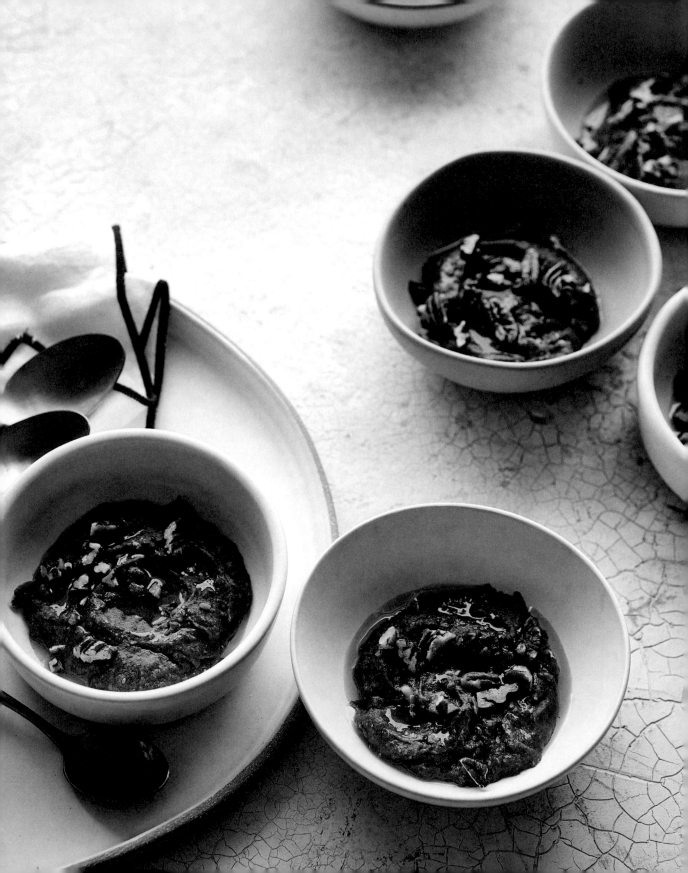

SLOW COOKER PUMPKIN BREAKFAST PUDDING

Since this takes 4 hours to prepare, I suggest making it ahead. Be sure to buy 100% pure canned pumpkin, not canned pumpkin pie filling, which contains sugar.

Refrigerate any leftover pudding in a covered container for up to 5 days. Reheat, stirring in a few tablespoons of nondairy milk, if desired, then top with the ghee and nuts. The pudding is also delicious cold. Another option is to omit the ghee and stir in some almond butter instead. MAKES 6 SERVINGS

Coconut oil cooking spray

1 15-ounce can pure pumpkin

1 13.5-ounce can full-fat coconut milk

½ cup Swerve Sweetener Confectioners

3 tablespoons coconut flour

3 tablespoons ground flaxseed

2 tablespoons chia seeds

1½ tablespoons pumpkin pie spice

1 teaspoon maple extract

½ cup chopped walnuts or pecans

¼ cup ghee or coconut butter

Lightly coat the inside of a slow cooker with the cooking spray.

Put the pumpkin, coconut milk, Swerve, coconut flour, flaxseed, chia seeds, pumpkin pie spice, and maple extract in the slow cooker and stir to combine. Cover and cook on low for 4 hours.

When done, stir well. Divide into portions and serve hot, topping each serving with approximately 1 tablespoon chopped walnuts and ½ tablespoon ghee.

CALORIES: 357 | PROTEIN: 6G | FAT: 31G | CARBS: 14G | FIBER: 7G | NET CARBS: 7G

GRANOLA BITES

These delicious breakfast treats are packed with collagen, nuts, seeds, and other nutritious ingredients. (If you're allergic to nuts, omit them and use hulled pumpkin and sesame seeds instead.) Collagen, the body's most abundant protein, is essential for supporting skin, hair, and nail growth and maintaining bone and joint health. Most of us don't get enough collagen from our food sources, so it's important to supplement our diets with some. When purchasing collagen peptides at a health food store or from an online source, choose those made from 100% grass-fed cows. MAKES 8 SERVINGS (4 CUPS)

Coconut oil cooking spray

½ cup coconut oil, melted

½ cup unflavored collagen peptides

½ cup Swerve Sweetener Confectioners

1 large organic egg, at room temperature

2 tablespoons ground cinnamon

2 teaspoons pure vanilla extract

¼ teaspoon fine sea salt

¾ cup unsweetened coconut flakes

½ cup hemp seeds

½ cup chopped walnuts

½ cup chopped almonds or pecans

2 tablespoons chia seeds

Heat the oven to 300°F. Coat a 9x13-inch pan with the cooking spray.

Whisk together the coconut oil, collagen peptides, Swerve, egg, cinnamon, vanilla, and salt in a bowl.

Combine the coconut flakes, hemp seeds, walnuts, almonds, and chia seeds in another bowl. Pour the nut mixture into the collagen mixture and use a spatula to stir until well combined. (The mixture will be thick and sticky.) Pour the batter into the prepared pan and use a spatula to spread thinly and evenly. Bake for 22 to 24 minutes, until lightly golden.

Remove the pan from the oven and lower the oven temperature to 200°F. Using a metal spatula, turn 2-inch pieces of the granola, trying to maintain small clusters. (The mixture will be soft at this point.) Return the pan to the oven and bake for 18 to 20 minutes more, until browned. Watch carefully so the granola doesn't burn.

Turn the oven off, but leave the granola inside for 1 hour. Remove from the oven. Cool in pan for another hour. The granola will become crisp as it sits. Store in an airtight container for up to 5 days, or in the freezer.

CALORIES: 340 | PROTEIN: 11.5G | FAT: 30.5G | CARBS: 7G | FIBER: 3.5G | NET CARBS: 3.5G

IGNITE HOT CACAO

Untreated, unheated, unprocessed, and unsweetened cacao beans are pure chocolate, right from the seeds of the cacao tree. Cacao nibs, the broken bits of cacao tree seeds, are loaded with antioxidants, essential fatty acids, and other nutrients, especially magnesium. Cacao is also available as a powder. In contrast, cocoa powder undergoes chemical processing to make it less acidic. During processing, nutrients are lost, which is why cacao powder is preferred.

MAKES 1 SERVING

1¼ cups nondairy milk

¼ cup canned full-fat coconut milk

1 tablespoon cacao powder

2 tablespoons Swerve Sweetener Confectioners

1 teaspoon pure vanilla extract

¼ teaspoon ground cinnamon, optional

Pinch fine sea salt

Whisk together the nondairy and coconut milks, cacao powder, Swerve, vanilla extract, cinnamon, if using, and sea salt in a saucepan over medium heat. When the beverage is hot, 2 to 3 minutes, pour into a mug. Drink while hot.

CALORIES: 168 | PROTEIN: 3G | FAT: 15G | CARBS: 6G | FIBER: 2G | NET CARBS: 4G

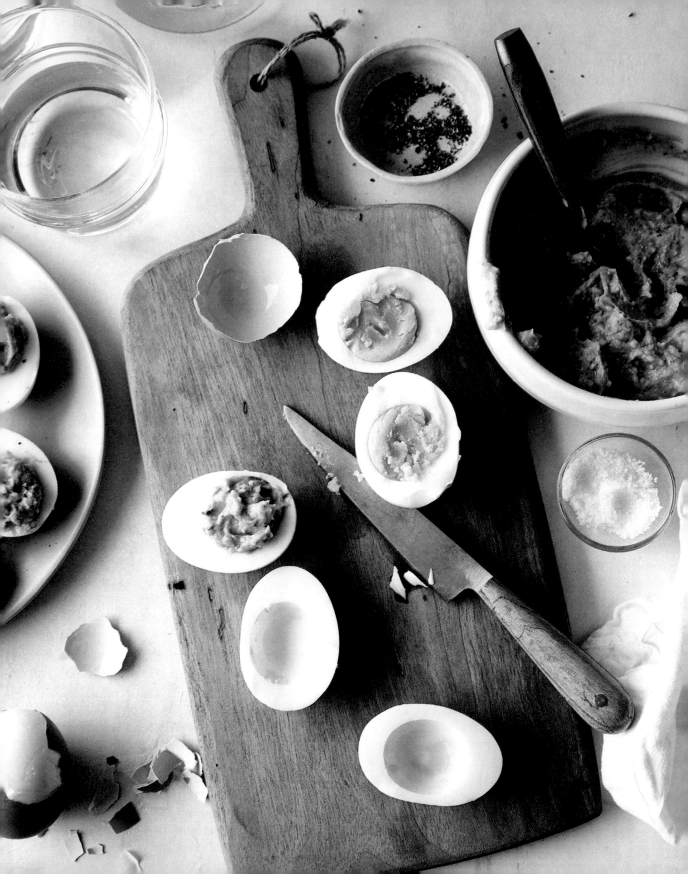

AVOCADO–BASIL DEVILED EGGS

In this recipe, egg yolks are mixed with avocado and basil rather than with mayonnaise. Avocado contains a healthy fat that you can enjoy. Spoon the egg yolk filling into the whites or use a pastry bag for a fancier presentation.

MAKES 2 SERVINGS (8 HALVES)

4 large organic eggs, hard-boiled

6 tablespoons Avocado–Basil Spread (page 334)

½ teaspoon fine sea salt

Freshly cracked black pepper, to taste

Slice each egg in half. Put the yolks, Avocado–Basil Spread, and salt in a bowl, and mash until combined. Fill each egg white with the mixture, and sprinkle with pepper.

CALORIES: 350 | PROTEIN: 16G | FAT: 28.5G | CARBS: 7G | FIBER: 2G | NET CARBS: 5G

MINI BELL PEPPERS WITH GOAT CHEESE AND OLIVES

Bags of mini sweet peppers can be found in supermarkets everywhere. Here, they are sliced lengthwise; filled with creamy goat cheese, olives, and flavorings; and then baked just until the peppers soften. Enjoy for a light lunch with a green salad or serve as an appetizer. MAKES 4 SERVINGS

4 ounces organic soft goat cheese

24 pitted kalamata olives, chopped

2 tablespoons chopped basil

1 teaspoon extra-virgin olive oil

1 green onion, chopped

Zest of 1 medium lemon, optional

2 teaspoons fresh lemon juice

1 teaspoon garlic powder

½ teaspoon sea salt

12 mini bell peppers, halved lengthwise and seeded

Heat the oven to 350°F. Put the goat cheese, olives, basil, olive oil, green onion, lemon zest (if using), lemon juice, garlic powder, and sea salt in a bowl. Use a fork to mash the mixture until well combined.

Arrange the mini pepper halves in a single layer, cut sides up, in a baking dish. Fill each half with the goat cheese mixture.

Bake for 15 to 17 minutes, until bell peppers are soft when pierced with a knife. Serve warm.

CALORIES: 178 | PROTEIN: 7G | FAT: 14.5G | CARBS: 7G | FIBER: 1.5G | NET CARBS: 5.5G

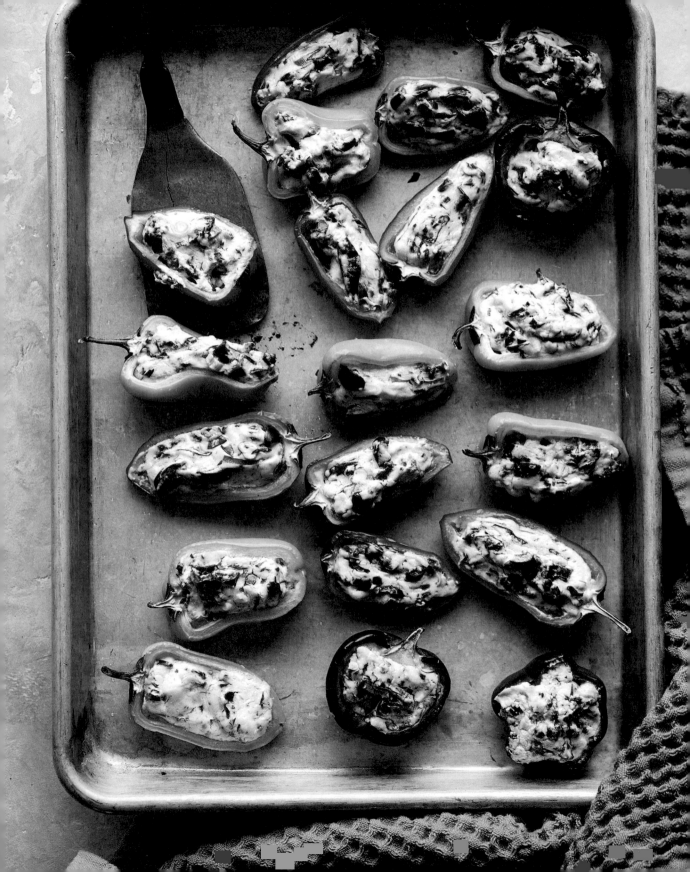

STUFFED PORTOBELLO MUSHROOMS WITH GOAT CHEESE

Large portobello mushrooms make great "bowls" for all kinds of fillings and sauces. This mix of goat cheese and marinara sauce is one of my faves. A green salad makes this a satisfying lunch. MAKES 2 SERVINGS

4 medium portobello mushroom caps

4 teaspoons extra-virgin olive oil

¼ cup low-carb marinara sauce

2 ounces organic soft goat cheese

4 tablespoons chopped basil leaves

Pinch sea salt

Pinch freshly ground black pepper

Heat the oven to 375°F. Place a wire rack on a sheet pan to prevent the mushrooms from becoming soggy.

Set the mushroom caps on the wire rack and brush each one with 1 teaspoon of the olive oil. Spoon 1 tablespoon of marinara in the center of each mushroom, then crumble the goat cheese on top.

Bake for 15 to 18 minutes, until the mushrooms are tender when pierced with a fork. Remove from the oven and sprinkle on the basil, salt, and pepper.

CALORIES: 252 | PROTEIN: 11G | FAT: 19G | CARBS: 7.5G | FIBER: 1G | NET CARBS: 6.5G

CAULIFLOWER–BROCCOLI SOUP

When made in a pressure cooker, this hearty vegetable soup is ready in just 30 minutes. You can also make it in a slow cooker. MAKES 4 1¾-CUP SERVINGS

2 cups broccoli florets

2 cups cauliflower florets

2 shallots, chopped

1 large carrot, sliced

3 cups Vegetable Broth (page 346) or bone broth

1 cup canned full-fat coconut milk

⅓ cup raw cashew pieces

1 teaspoon sea salt

1 teaspoon garlic powder

¼ teaspoon freshly ground black pepper

¼ cup nutritional yeast

1½ tablespoons MCT oil

Put the broccoli, cauliflower, shallots, carrot, broth, coconut milk, cashews, salt, garlic powder, and pepper in a pressure cooker or slow cooker. If using a pressure cooker, set on "soup" setting (30 minutes). If using a slow cooker, set on high for 3 hours. Cook until the vegetables are tender.

Let cool for 5 minutes; then place in a blender and process on high until smooth. You may have to puree the soup in batches. Add the nutritional yeast and MCT oil and blend again. Reheat in a saucepan, if necessary. Season to taste and serve.

CALORIES: 274 | PROTEIN: 8G | FAT: 21G | CARBS: 16G | FIBER: 4G | NET CARBS: 12G

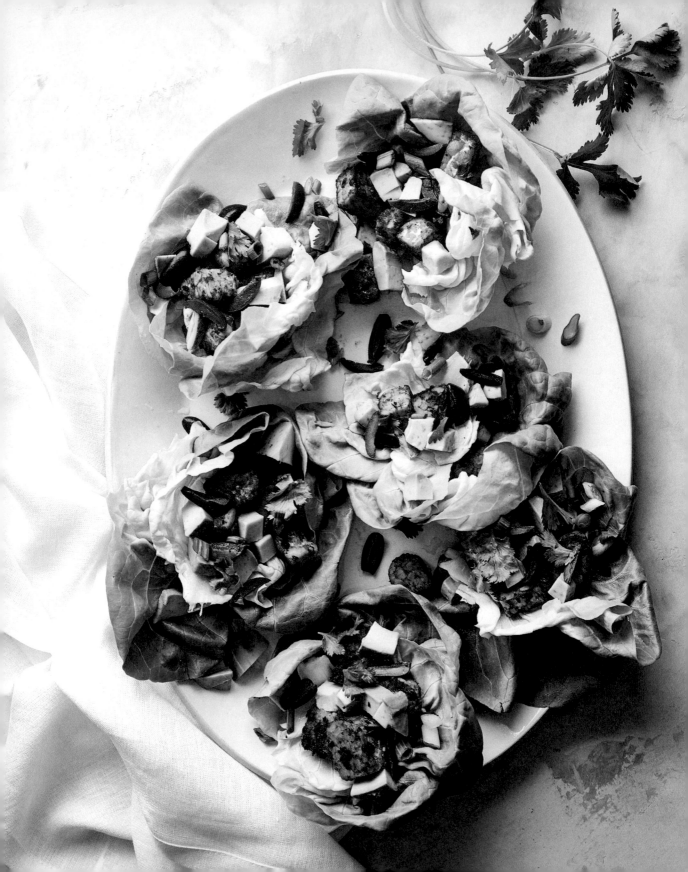

TEMPEH–SALSA LETTUCE WRAPS

Tempeh is made from fermented soybeans. Did you know that more than 90% of soybeans are genetically modified? Purchase tempeh made from 100% organic soybeans. Enjoy this fat-burning vegan meal when you want something light. MAKES 4 SERVINGS (8 WRAPS)

1 8-ounce package tempeh, diced

1 cup Salsa (page 325)

1 tablespoon Taco Seasoning (page 333)

3 tablespoons avocado oil

16 butter lettuce leaves, for serving

1 avocado, peeled, pitted, and chopped

½ cup pitted and sliced black olives

Hot sauce, optional

Put the tempeh in a shallow bowl. Add the salsa and taco seasoning and toss gently. Marinate for 6 hours.

Heat the avocado oil over medium heat. Add the tempeh and sauté until crisp on all sides.

Put 2 lettuce leaves together to form a cup; repeat with remaining lettuce. Spoon the tempeh into the 8 lettuce cups.

Top with avocado, olives, and hot sauce, if using.

Garnish with any low-calorie vegetables you desire, such as sliced bell peppers or green onions, or herbs, such as cilantro or parsley.

CALORIES: 305 | PROTEIN: 12G | FAT: 21G | CARBS: 15.5G | FIBER: 8G | NET CARBS: 7.5G

BLT PINWHEELS

The 131 Method's satisfying version of a turkey club triple decker. Gluten-free almond tortillas replace the usual three slices of bread and guacamole, instead of mayonnaise, provides creaminess. MAKES 4 SERVINGS

4 Almond Flour Tortillas (page 340)

¼ cup Guacamole (page 326)

4 ounces sliced organic turkey breast

4 heritage breed, nitrate-free, uncured bacon strips, cooked

4 lettuce leaves, chopped

1 small tomato, thinly sliced

Spread each tortilla with 1 tablespoon of guacamole. Layer each with 2 ounces of turkey, 1 slice of bacon, lettuce, and tomato slices, along one side of each tortilla. Begin rolling the tortilla from the filled side until it looks like a small burrito. Slice each one into pinwheels and use toothpicks to secure, if necessary.

CALORIES: 267 | PROTEIN: 15.4G | FAT: 19G | CARBS: 9G | FIBER: 3G | NET CARBS: 6G

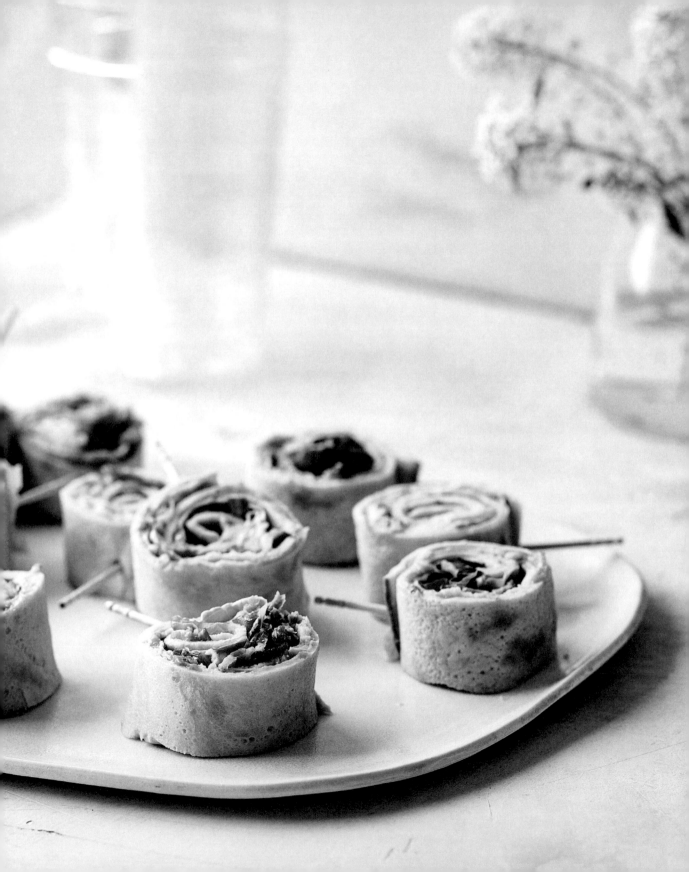

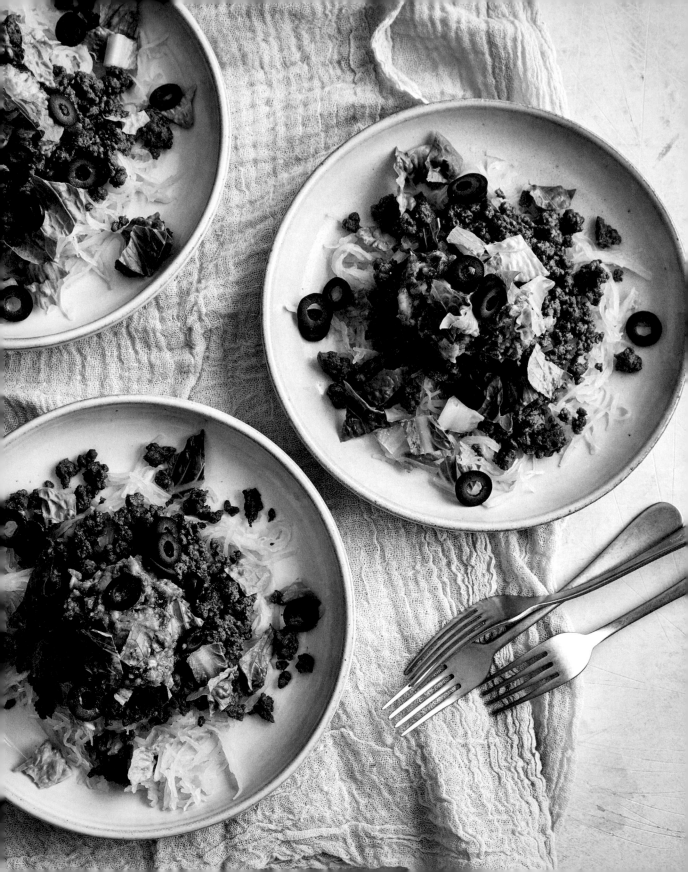

SPAGHETTI SQUASH BOWLS

Oval spaghetti squash looks like other winter squashes when it's raw. Once you bake it and pull the interior away from the sides with a fork, it looks like strands of spaghetti! Here, the squash shells serve as bowls for the beef and other ingredients. MAKES 2 SERVINGS

1 small spaghetti squash, halved and seeds removed

Coconut oil cooking spray

¼ teaspoon plus ½ teaspoon sea salt

1 tablespoon Garlic-Infused Olive Oil (page 324)

8 ounces 100% grass-fed ground beef

½ teaspoon smoked paprika

½ teaspoon ground cumin

¼ cup Guacamole (page 326)

¼ cup pitted and sliced black olives

1 cup chopped lettuce

Heat the oven to 450°F.

Place the squash halves cut side up in a large baking dish. Coat the cut sides with the coconut oil spray and sprinkle with ¼ teaspoon sea salt. Roast for 30 to 35 minutes, until the strands are tender and can be pulled apart like spaghetti. (Overcooked squash will become mushy.) Remove 2 cups of the strands to 2 bowls and refrigerate the remaining squash for another use.

Heat the garlic oil in a skillet. Add the beef, paprika, cumin, and remaining ½ teaspoon salt. Cook for 5 to 6 minutes, until meat is well browned and cooked through. Spoon the meat mixture over each serving of spaghetti squash. Garnish with guacamole, olives, and lettuce.

CALORIES: 455 | PROTEIN: 22.5G | FAT: 30.5G | CARBS: 11.5G | FIBER: 3.5G | NET CARBS: 8G

LOW-CARB BARBECUED CHICKEN PIZZA

If cheese doesn't cause you any inflammatory symptoms, then sprinkle about ¾ cup mozzarella on top of the chicken before adding the onions. MAKES 8 SERVINGS

½ cup Low-Carb Barbecue Sauce (page 331), divided

1 recipe Low-Carb Pizza Crust (page 337)

12 ounces cooked chicken breast

½ small red onion, thinly sliced

½ teaspoon crushed red pepper, optional

2 tablespoons fresh cilantro, optional

Heat the oven to 400°F.

Spread 2 to 3 tablespoons barbecue sauce on the pizza crust. Combine the remaining sauce and chicken in a bowl and toss well. Arrange the chicken, onion, and red pepper, if using, on the pizza.

Bake for 10 to 12 minutes, or until the chicken is warm and the onions have softened. Sprinkle with cilantro, if desired, before serving.

CALORIES: 322 | PROTEIN: 22.5G | FAT: 23G | CARBS: 10G | FIBER: 4G | NET CARBS: 6G

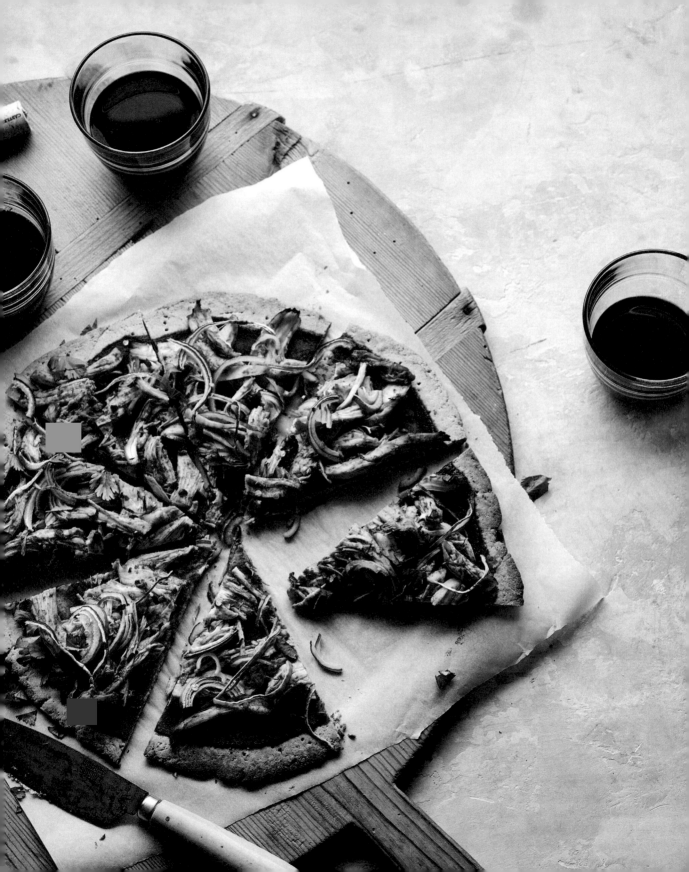

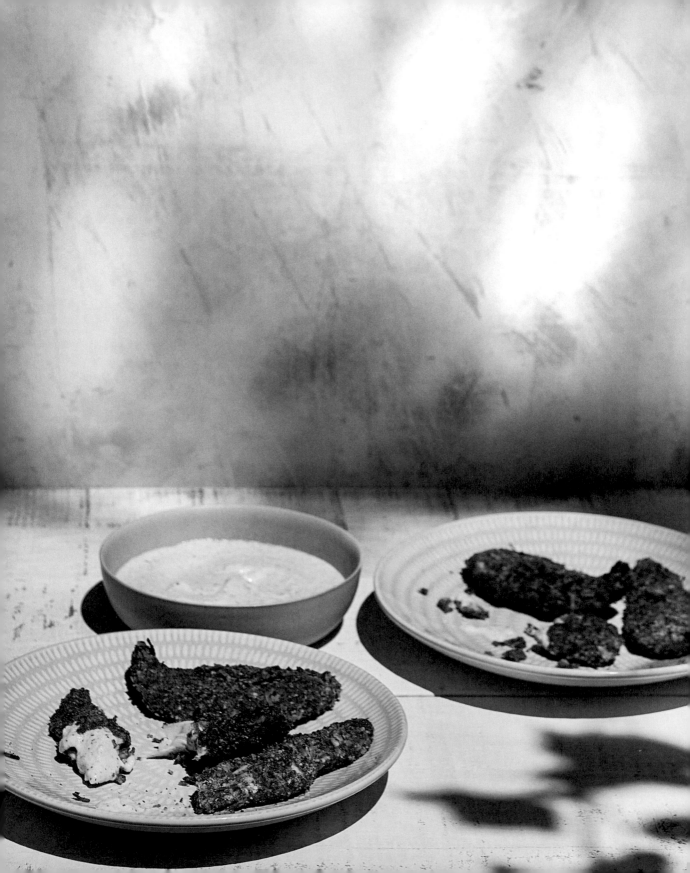

CHICKEN TENDERS

Kids of all ages love these chicken tenders, especially when accompanied by a side of Macadamia Ranch Dressing (page 329) for dipping. The dressing adds healthy fats to keep your fat-burning ratio on track. MAKES 4 SERVINGS

2 teaspoons extra-virgin olive oil

1 pound boneless, skinless organic chicken tenders

½ teaspoon sea salt

¼ teaspoon freshly ground black pepper

1 large organic egg

1 large organic egg yolk

¾ cup almond meal

¼ cup unsweetened shredded coconut

2 tablespoons Taco Seasoning (page 333)

Heat the oven to 350°F. Drizzle a baking dish with the olive oil and set aside.

Season the chicken strips with the salt and pepper.

Whisk together the eggs and egg yolk. Place the almond flour, coconut, and taco seasoning in another shallow bowl. Mix gently.

Dip each chicken strip into the egg and then into the almond flour mixture, coating on all sides. Place the strips in the prepared baking dish and bake for 10 minutes. Turn the chicken and bake for an additional 10 minutes, until lightly golden on the outside and cooked through.

Set the oven to broil, and broil the chicken for 1 to 2 minutes, until browned. Serve immediately.

CALORIES: 309 | PROTEIN: 32G | FAT: 17.5G | CARBS: 7G | FIBER: 2G | NET CARBS: 5G

CHICKEN WITH BACON, MUSHROOMS, AND MACADAMIA RANCH DRESSING

The chicken strips are coated in dressing, topped with bacon, and served with a pile of mushrooms. This recipe serves a family, but you can also divide it into portions, refrigerate, and reheat as necessary. MAKES 6 SERVINGS

CHICKEN:

2 boneless, skinless chicken organic breasts (about 18 ounces), each cut into 4 to 5 long strips

½ teaspoon salt

½ teaspoon freshly ground black pepper

1 cup Macadamia Ranch Dressing (page 329)

5 slices 100% organic bacon, chopped

MUSHROOMS:

2 tablespoons ghee

1 pound cremini mushrooms, sliced

1 green onion, sliced

Pinch of fine sea salt

Pinch of freshly ground black pepper

To make the chicken: Heat the oven to 375°F. Cut the chicken breasts into 4 to 5 long strips; then slice those in half and season with the salt and pepper.

Place the chicken in a bowl and toss with ¾ cup of the Macadamia Ranch Dressing. Refrigerate for 20 minutes.

Arrange the chicken pieces in a 9x9-inch baking pan. Cover with the chopped bacon. Bake for 20 to 25 minutes; then set the oven to broil and broil for 3 minutes, or until the bacon is crisp.

To make the mushrooms: Melt the ghee in a large skillet over medium heat. Add the mushrooms and sauté for 4 minutes, or until tender. Add the green onion, salt, and pepper and cook for 2 minutes longer. Divide the mushrooms among 6 plates and lay chicken pieces on top. Drizzle each serving with about 2 teaspoons of remaining Macadamia Ranch Dressing.

CALORIES: 313 | PROTEIN: 24G | FAT: 22G | CARBS: 5.5G | FIBER: 1.5G | NET CARBS: 4G

SLOW COOKER THAI CHICKEN

If your slow cooker is large enough, you can double this recipe. Serve the chicken over cauliflower rice or shirataki noodles, if desired. You can thin out the sauce by stirring in some additional coconut milk and chicken broth.
MAKES 4 SERVINGS

1 pound boneless, skinless organic chicken thighs

1 cup canned full-fat coconut milk

3 tablespoons natural peanut butter

3 garlic cloves, minced

3 tablespoons Swerve Sweetener Confectioners

2 tablespoons coconut aminos

1 tablespoon fresh lime juice

1 tablespoon curry powder

1 teaspoon ground turmeric

1 teaspoon ground ginger

1 teaspoon sea salt

Pinch cayenne pepper, optional

¼ cup coarsely chopped cilantro leaves

Place the chicken in the slow cooker and set on low. Whisk together the coconut milk, peanut butter, garlic, Swerve, coconut aminos, lime juice, curry, turmeric, ginger, salt, and cayenne pepper, if using, in a medium bowl. Pour over the chicken in the slow cooker. Cover and cook on low for 6 to 8 hours, until the chicken is cooked through. Using 2 forks, shred the chicken in the slow cooker, and serve in bowls with the sauce, sprinkled with chopped cilantro.

CALORIES: 366 | PROTEIN: 24G | FAT: 27.5G | CARBS: 8.5G | FIBER: 2G | NET CARBS: 6.5G

TURKEY MEATLOAF WITH BUFFALO WING SAUCE

Serve with a side of steamed vegetables and some Macadamia Ranch Dressing (page 329). Portion out the meatloaf to enjoy later in the week.

MAKES 5 SERVINGS

Coconut oil cooking spray

1 pound 93% lean ground turkey

½ cup Buffalo Wing Sauce (page 326)

½ cup almond meal

⅓ cup finely chopped onion

¼ cup chopped green bell pepper

1 green onion, sliced

2 ounces fresh organic goat cheese, crumbled

2 tablespoons Taco Seasoning (page 333)

½ teaspoon fine sea salt

Heat the oven to 375°F. Coat an 8x4-inch loaf pan with coconut oil cooking spray.

Combine the ground turkey, wing sauce, almond meal, onion, bell pepper, green onion, goat cheese, seasoning, and sea salt in a large bowl. Using clean hands, mix well and put the mixture into the prepared pan.

Bake for 35 to 40 minutes, until meatloaf is no longer pink in the center.

Slice into 5 pieces, spoon the pan juices on top, and serve.

CALORIES: 328 | PROTEIN: 21G | FAT: 34G | CARBS: 5G | FIBER: 1G | NET CARBS: 4G

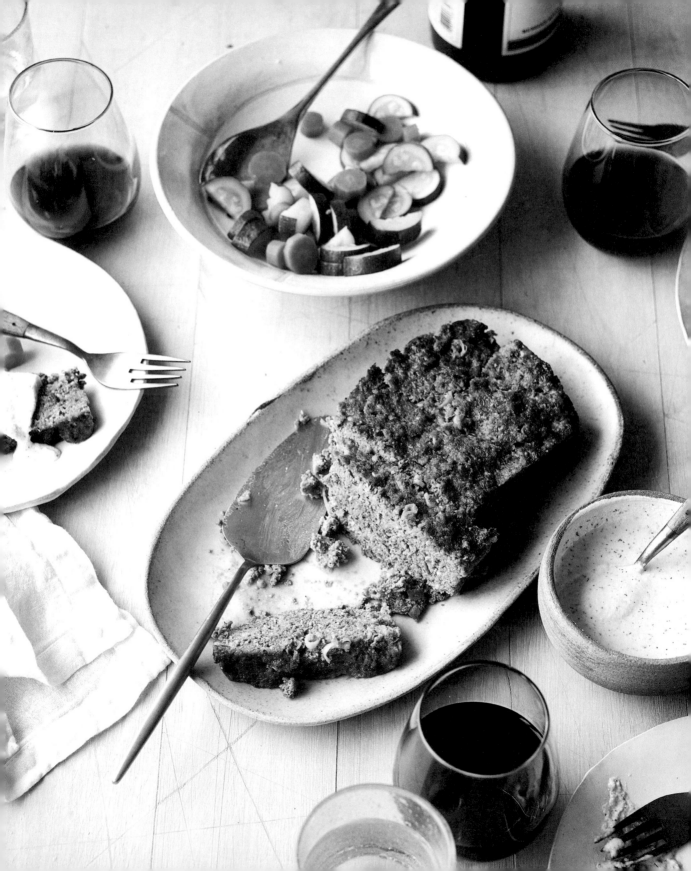

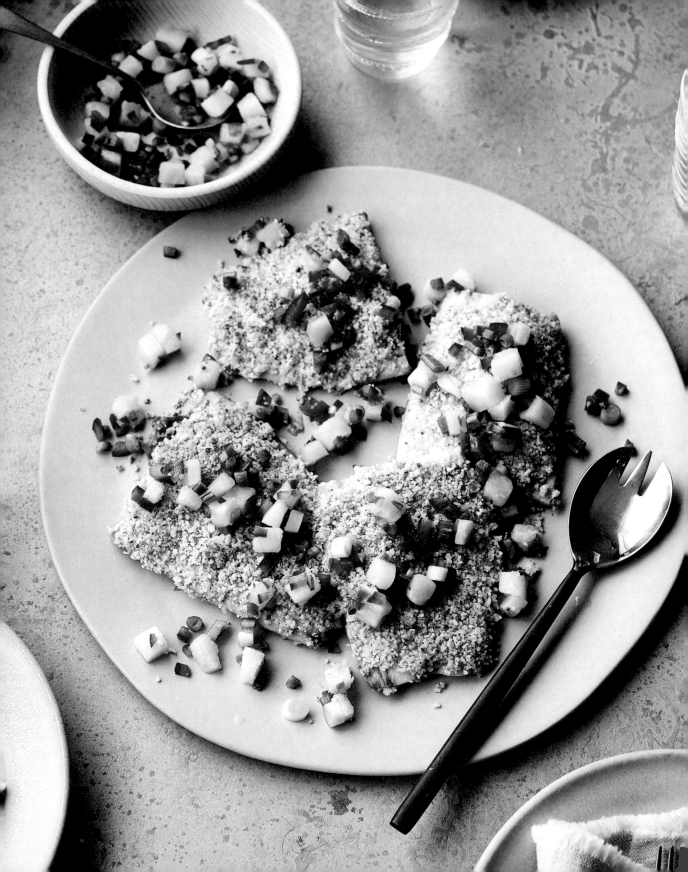

TROPICAL MAHI-MAHI WITH PINEAPPLE SALSA

Macadamia nuts, coconut, cilantro, and seasonings are chopped to make a breadcrumb-like coating for the fish. You can use any kind of white fish for this dish. The salsa mixture used here can also be paired with grilled chicken or steak. MAKES 4 SERVINGS

Four 4-ounce sustainably sourced mahi-mahi or cod fillets

½ teaspoon plus ½ teaspoon fine sea salt

¼ teaspoon freshly ground black pepper

1 cup unsalted macadamia nuts

¼ cup unsweetened shredded coconut

¼ cup chopped cilantro

¼ teaspoon garlic powder

2 teaspoons melted coconut oil

½ cup pineapple tidbits, diced

¼ cup minced red bell pepper

1 green onion, diced

½ medium jalapeño, seeded and minced

Heat the oven to 400°F. Season the fish with ½ teaspoon salt and the pepper. Arrange the fish in a single layer in a baking dish.

Put the macadamia nuts, coconut, cilantro, remaining ½ teaspoon of salt, and garlic powder in a food processor and pulse until the mixture is the consistency of bread crumbs.

Drizzle each fillet with ½ teaspoon melted coconut oil and press the macadamia mixture on top. Bake until the top is crisp and slightly golden, 8 to 10 minutes.

Combine the pineapple, bell pepper, green onion, and jalapeño in a small bowl. Spoon on top of fish and serve.

CALORIES: 399 | PROTEIN: 24G | FAT: 30.5G | CARBS: 11G | FIBER: 4G | NET CARBS: 7G

VEGETARIAN COCONUT CURRY

Loaded with vegetables, this satisfying meal will help you transition away from animal proteins. During a fat-burning phase, eat lower-carb foods like lettuce wraps and brain bombs for the rest of the day. Garnish with chopped cilantro, basil, or green onions or 2 tablespoons of chopped salted peanuts or cashews. You can also spoon each serving of the curry over 1 cup of cooked cauliflower rice. MAKES 4 SERVINGS

2 tablespoons coconut oil

2 garlic cloves, chopped

1 pound mixed mushrooms, sliced

1 cup chopped broccoli,

½ pound green beans, trimmed and chopped into 2-inch pieces

One 13.5-ounce can full-fat coconut milk

1 cup canned diced tomatoes

1½ tablespoons curry powder

2 teaspoons Swerve Sweetener Confectioners

1 teaspoon sea salt

1 teaspoon ground ginger

½ teaspoon ground turmeric

½ teaspoon allspice

Pinch cayenne pepper

Put 1 tablespoon of the coconut oil and the garlic in a large skillet over medium heat. Sauté for 1 minute. Add the remaining 1 tablespoon of oil and the mushrooms and cook for 5 minutes. Stir in the remaining ingredients and simmer, stirring occasionally, for 15 minutes. Divide among 4 bowls and serve.

CALORIES: 332 | PROTEIN: 7G | FAT: 24G | CARBS: 15G | FIBER: 4G | NET CARBS: 11G

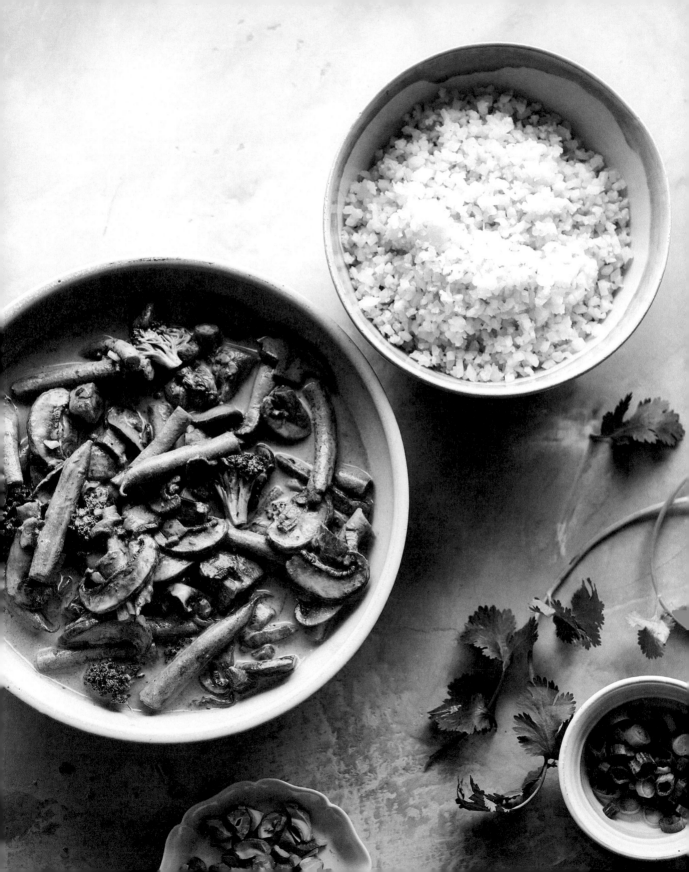

GINGER-VEGETABLE STIR-FRY

Coconut aminos are a great substitute for soy sauce, which contains gluten. To make this condiment, organic coconut sap is aged and blended with sun-dried, mineral-rich sea salt. Don't confuse coconut aminos with liquid aminos, which are made from soybeans. Use it as a substitute for soy in other dishes as well.

MAKES 4 SERVINGS

SAUCE:

⅓ cup canned lite coconut milk

2 avocados, peeled and pitted

2-inch piece ginger, peeled

2 tablespoons fresh lime juice

2 tablespoons coconut aminos

1 tablespoon rice vinegar

5 drops liquid stevia

¼ teaspoon fine sea salt

¼ teaspoon freshly ground pepper

VEGETABLES:

2 tablespoons coconut oil

2 garlic cloves, minced

½ cup diced red onion

2 cups shredded purple or green cabbage

1 cup sliced mushrooms

1 large bunch broccolini, chopped

6 cups arugula or spinach

½ teaspoon fine sea salt

½ teaspoon freshly ground black pepper

To make the sauce: Combine all of the sauce ingredients in a blender and process until thick and creamy.

To make the vegetables: Heat coconut oil in a large skillet over medium heat. Add the garlic and stir for 1 minute. Add the onion and cook for 3 minutes. Add the cabbage, mushrooms, and broccolini and sauté until vegetables are tender, about 5 minutes.

Stir in the sauce and cook for another 2 to 3 minutes to warm the sauce and coat the vegetables. Serve the vegetables over the arugula. Season with salt and pepper.

CALORIES: 209 | PROTEIN: 4G | FAT: 16G | CARBS: 14G | FIBER: 2G | NET CARBS: 12G

LEMON AND HERB CAULIFLOWER RICE

We eat a lot of low-calorie, low-carb cauliflower rice on the 131 Method. Packages of riced cauliflower are now available in many markets, and you can flavor it any way you like with different seasonings, just as you would jazz up rice. Add some sautéed onion and bell pepper for a Spanish touch or some Mexican flavor like lime juice and cilantro. MAKES 4 SERVINGS

1 medium head cauliflower

2 tablespoons avocado oil

1 tablespoon Italian seasoning

1 teaspoon lemon–garlic seasoning powder

Zest of 1 lemon

1 tablespoon fresh lemon juice

½ teaspoon sea salt

Pull the cauliflower apart into 1-to-2-inch florets. Rinse in a colander and shake off any excess water. Put the cauliflower in a food processor. (You can also rice the cauliflower on a box grater, but avoid using a blender, which will result in uneven pieces.) Pulse the cauliflower 3 or 4 times, until it looks like rice.

Heat the avocado oil in a large skillet over medium heat. Add the cauliflower, Italian seasoning, lemon–garlic seasoning, lemon zest, lemon juice, and salt. Cook for 7 to 8 minutes, stirring occasionally, until tender but not soft.

CALORIES: 102 | PROTEIN: 3G | FAT: 8G | CARBS: 8G | FIBER: 3G | NET CARBS: 5G

CHILI-LIME BRUSSELS SPROUTS

The leaves of the sprouts are separated, coated with a bit of oil and seasoning, and then roasted until the edges are crisp. Low-carb, high-fiber, and packed with nutrients, they make a yummy snack. (Note: the actual carb figure will be lower than indicated, depending on how much of each brussels sprout is discarded.) MAKES 2 SERVINGS

1 pound brussels sprouts

2½ tablespoons avocado oil

1 tablespoon fresh lime juice

1 teaspoon fine sea salt

1 teaspoon chili powder

Heat oven to 400°F. Line a sheet pan with parchment paper.

Slice the stems off the brussels sprouts and separate the sprouts into individual leaves. There should be about 2 cups of leaves. Discard inner portions and any limp or damaged outer leaves.

Place the leaves in a large bowl and add the avocado oil, lime juice, salt, and chili powder.

Toss well until the leaves are evenly coated.

Arrange the leaves in a single layer on the sheet pan and roast for 8 to 10 minutes, until the edges are crisp and lightly browned.

CALORIES: 241 | PROTEIN: 5G | FAT: 17.5G | CARBS: 16G | FIBER: 5G | NET CARBS: 11G

BROCCOLINI WITH LEMON AND GARLIC

Broccolini has smaller florets and longer stems than broccoli, so there's no need to cut it up. This method also works well with broccoli, cauliflower, asparagus, and brussels sprouts. Red pepper flakes add some heat; omit them if you prefer. MAKES 4 SERVINGS

2 bunches (about 18 ounces) broccolini

⅓ cup extra-virgin olive oil

2 to 3 garlic cloves, slivered

1 teaspoon red pepper flakes

½ teaspoon fine sea salt

1 tablespoon fresh lemon juice

Heat the oven to 400°F.

Toss the broccolini with the olive oil, garlic, and red pepper flakes in a baking dish large enough to hold the broccolini in a single layer. Bake for 13 to 14 minutes, until the broccolini is soft when pierced with a knife. Sprinkle with salt and squeeze the lemon juice over the broccolini before serving.

CALORIES: 205 | PROTEIN: 4G | FAT: 18G | CARBS: 10G | FIBER: 3G | NET CARBS: 7G

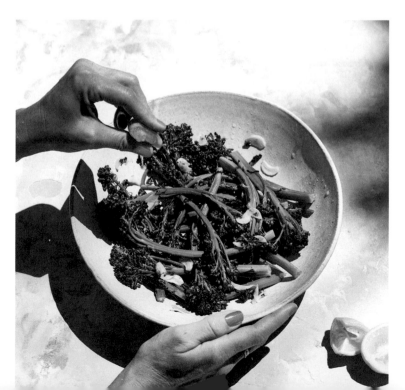

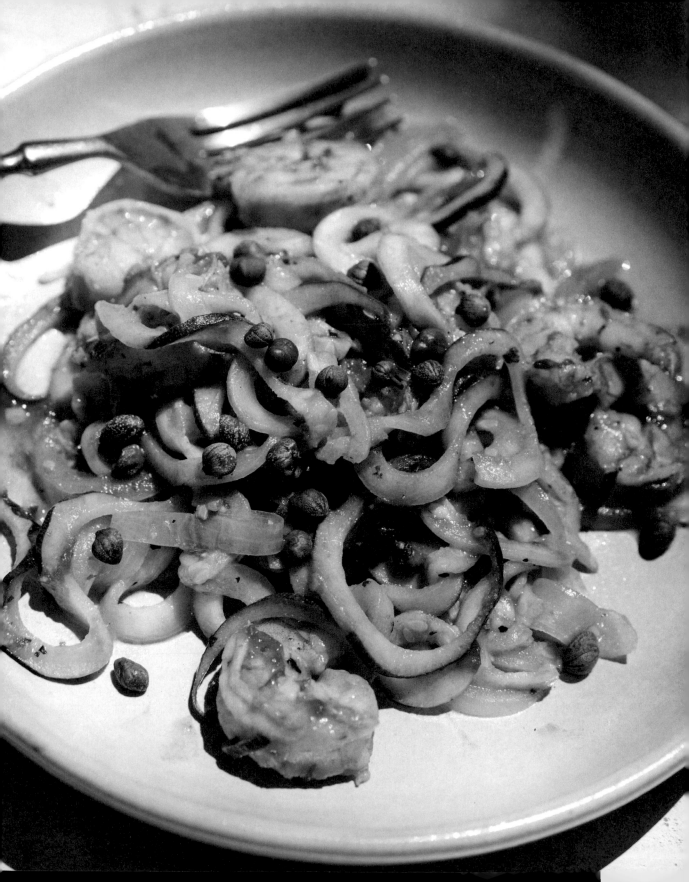

CHAPTER 11

NOURISH RECIPES

BREAKFAST

LUNCH

DINNER

EMERGENCY JUICE "COCKTAIL"

The fiber of fruits and vegetables is significantly reduced when juiced, but you will still receive some of their micronutrients. Make this juice when you're feeling a little under the weather, when you feel a cold coming on, or when you're missing your expensive green juice from the health food store. This process is a lot faster and less messy than juicing at home, too. Feel free to add parsley, kale, or a small apple to change up the flavors. MAKES 1 SERVING

2 cups spinach

2 clementines or
1 large orange, peeled

1 Persian cucumber,
sliced

2 tablespoons fresh
lemon juice

1 teaspoon avocado oil

1-inch piece ginger,
peeled

1-inch piece turmeric,
peeled

Pinch cayenne pepper

5 drops liquid stevia,
optional

Place the spinach, 1 cup water, clementines, cucumber, lemon juice, avocado oil, ginger, turmeric, cayenne pepper, and stevia, if using, into a blender and process for 30 seconds on high. Strain into a glass over ice.

CALORIES: 173 | PROTEIN: 4G | FAT: 6G | CARBS: 29G | FIBER: 1G | NET CARBS: 28G

FROZEN HAZELNUT CACAO COFFEE

For additional protein, add ½ scoop vegan chocolate protein powder or collagen peptides to the blender. MAKES 1 SERVING

1 cup ice

1 cup nondairy milk

1 cup brewed coffee, chilled

¼ cup chopped hazelnuts

10 drops vanilla liquid stevia, or to taste

1 tablespoon cacao nibs

1 tablespoon cacao powder

Put the ice, milk, coffee, hazelnuts, stevia, cacao nibs, and cacao powder in a blender. Process until thick and creamy, adding additional ice if you wish.

CALORIES: 314 | PROTEIN: 8G | FAT: 26G | CARBS: 12G | FIBER: 8G | NET CARBS: 4G

FROZEN SMOOTHIE BOWL

To make this, you'll need to plan ahead and freeze canned coconut milk in ice cube trays, which is a great way to avoid waste when you don't use a full can in recipes. Then you can just pop out the cubes as needed. Most smoothie bowls sold in juice and smoothie bars are over the top when it comes to carbs, sugar, and calorie counts. Make your own at home and customize your flavors depending on which phase of the 131 Method you're in. MAKES 2 SERVINGS

1 cup canned full-fat coconut milk

1 cup spinach

½ cup frozen blueberries

½ cup frozen raspberries

⅓ cup nondairy milk

8 drops liquid stevia, or to taste

¼ cup unsweetened coconut flakes

¼ cup chopped pecans

2 tablespoons ground flaxseed

2 tablespoons hemp seeds

Freeze the coconut milk in an ice cube tray in advance of preparing this recipe for at least 2 hours. Once frozen, add the cubes to a large, high-powered blender with the spinach, blueberries, raspberries, milk, and stevia. Process on low, then high, scraping sides as needed or using a pusher mechanism. Mixture should be quite thick, like soft-serve ice cream, and not a drinkable smoothie.

Spoon into 2 chilled bowls. Divide the coconut, pecans, and flaxseed between the bowls and stir. Sprinkle with hemp seeds and serve immediately.

CALORIES: 495 | PROTEIN: 9G | FAT: 42.5G | CARBS: 19G | FIBER: 8.5G | NET CARBS: 10.5G

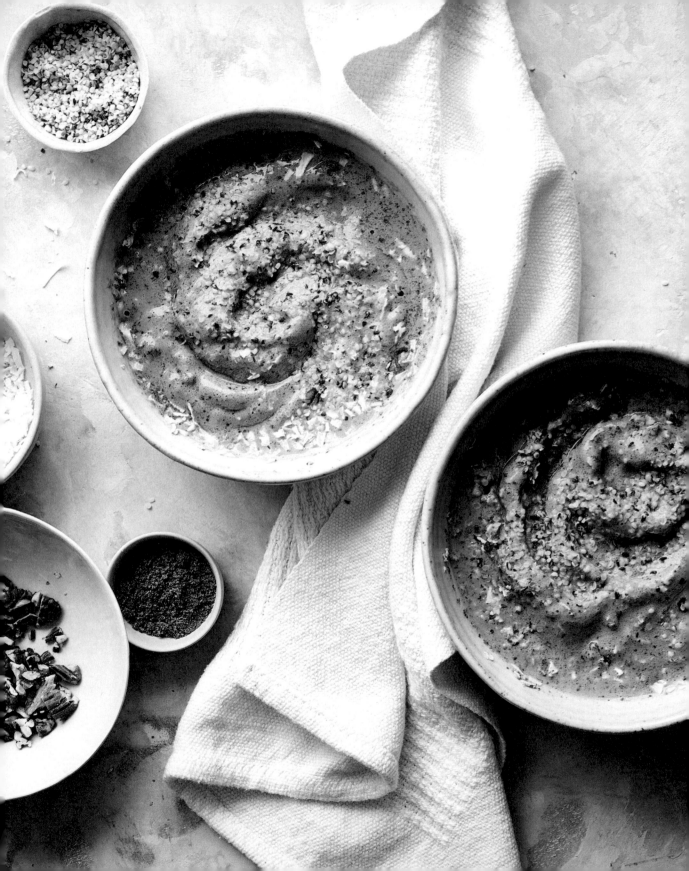

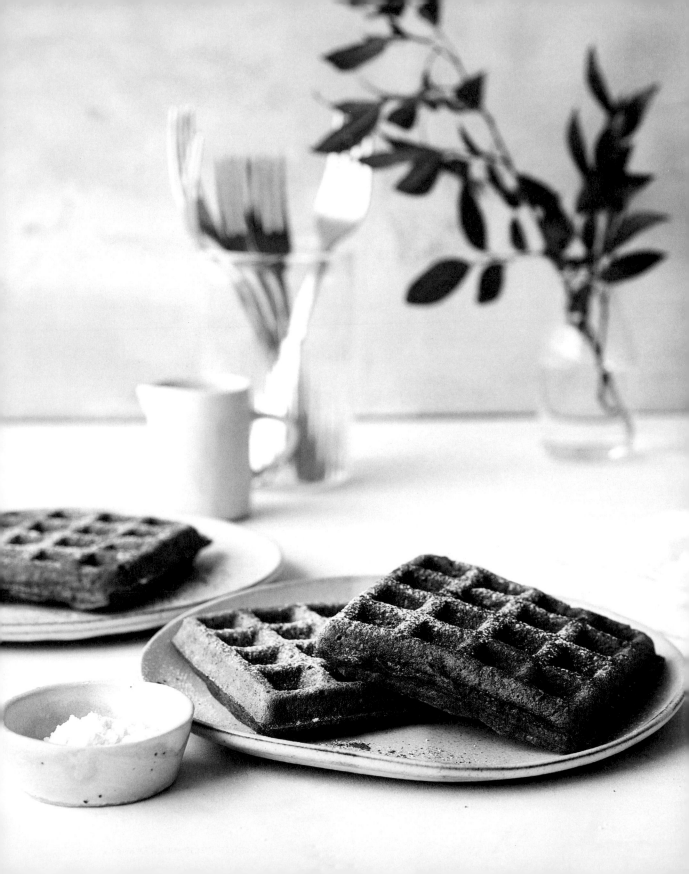

HAZELNUT WAFFLES

While the textures of hazelnut flour and almond flour are the same, hazelnut flour has a richer, nuttier flavor. You can certainly use almond flour if you prefer. If you like super-crisp waffles, heat the oven to 350°F and set a wire rack on top of a baking sheet. Once the waffles are done, put them on the wire rack and bake for 5 minutes. To serve, drizzle with ghee or coconut butter and a sprinkle of ground cinnamon.

With so many different waffle irons on the market, know that some will make 4 waffles, while others may yield 6. MAKES 4 SERVINGS

4 large organic eggs

1½ cups hazelnut flour

¾ cup Swerve Sweetener Confectioners

⅓ cup nondairy milk

3 tablespoons melted coconut oil

3 tablespoons tapioca flour

2 tablespoons cacao powder

1 teaspoon pure vanilla extract

½ teaspoon aluminum-free baking soda

Pinch fine sea salt

Coconut oil cooking spray

Heat an electric waffle iron to medium-high.

Put the eggs, hazelnut flour, ½ cup of the Swerve, milk, coconut oil, tapioca flour, cacao powder, vanilla extract, baking soda, and salt to a blender and process for 20 seconds.

Coat the waffle iron with coconut oil cooking spray. Pour ⅔ to ¾ cup batter into the waffle iron and cook for 3 to 4 minutes, until brown. Repeat with the remaining batter. If the batter thickens while sitting, add 1 tablespoon milk to thin it out. Sift 1 tablespoon of Swerve on top of each hot waffle before serving.

CALORIES: 465 | PROTEIN: 9G | FAT: 41G | CARBS: 15G | FIBER: 5G | NET CARBS: 10G

TACO SALAD

If you like, double the amount of ground beef and seasonings. Freeze in handy 1- or 2-portion containers so you can put a salad together in minutes. If you have the carbs to spare, feel free to add vegetables like sliced cucumbers and red bell pepper. MAKES 4 SERVINGS

1 tablespoon extra-virgin olive oil

½ small white onion, diced

1 garlic clove, minced

1 pound grass-fed, grass-finished ground beef

2 tablespoons Taco Seasoning (page 333)

1 teaspoon fine sea salt

½ teaspoon freshly ground black pepper

1 large head romaine lettuce, coarsely chopped

¼ cup Salsa (page 325)

Juice of 1 lime

1 avocado, peeled, pitted, and chopped

Put the oil in a saucepan over medium heat. Add the onion and garlic and sauté for 4 to 5 minutes, until the onion is softened and translucent.

Add the ground beef and cook, stirring frequently, until browned, about 7 to 10 minutes. Stir in the taco seasoning, salt, and pepper.

Arrange the lettuce, beef, salsa, and lime juice in a bowl and toss to combine. Divide among 4 bowls; top each with some avocado.

CALORIES: 370 | PROTEIN: 22.5G | FAT: 26.5G | CARBS: 10G | FIBER: 4G | NET CARBS: 6G

CANNELLINI, AVOCADO, AND CUCUMBER SALAD

Because this salad is fiber-rich but also heavy in carbs, I suggest you enjoy this during your prep week rather than in the days leading up to your fast, when your carb intake should be lower. MAKES 2 SERVINGS

One 15-ounce can white cannellini beans, rinsed and drained

1 ripe avocado, peeled and pitted

1 large cucumber, diced

3 pickle spears, diced

1½ tablespoons fresh lemon juice

1 teaspoon garlic powder

½ teaspoon onion powder

½ teaspoon fine sea salt

½ teaspoon freshly ground black pepper

8 celery stalks

Mash the white beans with the avocado. Fold in cucumber, pickles, lemon juice, garlic powder, onion powder, salt, and pepper. Divide between 2 plates and serve with celery.

CALORIES: 376 | PROTEIN: 14.5G | FAT: 14G | CARBS: 48G | FIBER: 16.5G | NET CARBS: 31.5G

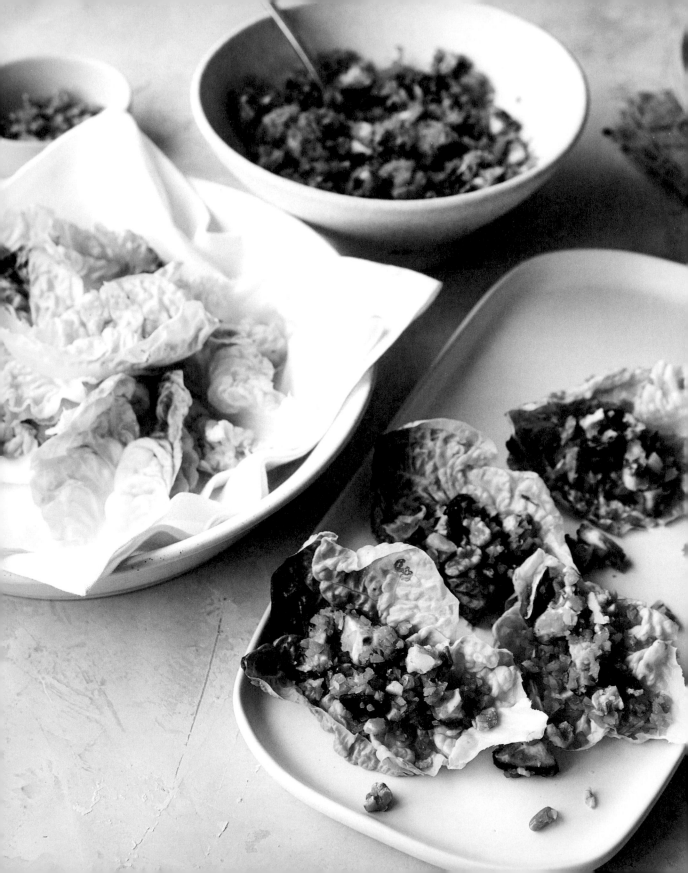

VEGETABLE LETTUCE WRAPS

To add more healthy fat, top each wrap with some chopped avocado. To add a little more protein (and cheesy flavor), sprinkle on 1 tablespoon nutritional yeast per serving. MAKES 4 SERVINGS

2½ cups cubed butternut squash

2 tablespoons extra-virgin olive oil, divided

8 ounces mushrooms, stemmed and chopped

2 garlic cloves, chopped

2 green onions, chopped

2 tablespoons coconut aminos

1 teaspoon sea salt

½ teaspoon garlic powder

Pinch cayenne pepper

¼ cup chopped walnuts

8 to 12 large lettuce leaves

Put the squash in the food processor and pulse until the pieces look like rice.

Heat 1 tablespoon of the oil in a skillet over medium heat. Add the riced squash and sauté for 3 minutes. Push the squash to side of the pan and add the remaining oil, mushrooms, and garlic. Cook and stir for 2 minutes, then mix the squash back in and sauté for an additional minute. Stir in the green onions, coconut aminos, salt, garlic powder, cayenne, and walnuts and sauté for an additional minute or so. Divide the vegetables among the lettuce cups and serve.

CALORIES: 160 | PROTEIN: 5G | FAT: 12G | CARBS: 19G | FIBER: 3G | NET CARBS: 16G

LENTIL-FALAFEL SALAD

Unlike dried beans, lentils don't require soaking, and they cook in just 20 minutes. To cook, put 1 cup brown lentils in a strainer, pick over them to remove any stones, and rinse them well under cool water. Put the lentils in a saucepan with 3 cups water. Bring to a boil, lower the heat to a simmer, and cover and cook for 15 to 20 minutes. Taste a few to see if they're done. The lentils should be cooked through but not mushy. (1 cup dried lentils will yield 2 to 2½ cups cooked.) For this recipe, cook, drain, and chill the lentils ahead of time; the falafels will hold together better.

You can also purchase already steamed and vacuum-packed lentils. Look for them in the produce section of your market. MAKES 4 SERVINGS (ABOUT 20 MINI FALAFELS)

Coconut oil cooking spray

2 cups cooked, cold lentils

1 small red onion, diced

½ cup parsley

2 garlic cloves, minced

½ cup almond meal

¼ cup ground flaxseed

2 teaspoons curry powder

1 teaspoon ground turmeric

1 teaspoon ground cumin

1 teaspoon fine sea salt

¼ teaspoon freshly ground black pepper

4 cups arugula

1 cup Salsa (page 325)

1 medium avocado, peeled, pitted, and diced

Heat oven to 400°F. Line a sheet pan with parchment paper and spray with coconut oil cooking spray.

Put the lentils, onion, parsley, and garlic in a food processor. Pulse until the mixture is light in color and sticky. Transfer the mixture to a bowl and stir in the almond meal, flaxseed, curry powder, turmeric, cumin, sea salt, and pepper. Mix well until the mixture is fully combined and begins to stick and hold shape when pieces are pinched together.

Shape the mixture into 20 balls; then flatten each one to ½-inch thickness. Place on the prepared pan and bake for 12 minutes. Using a spatula, turn the falafels and lightly spray them with cooking spray. Bake an additional 10 to 12 minutes, until the outsides are slightly crisp and the centers are tender when pierced with a knife.

Assemble the arugula on 4 plates and top each with 5 falafels. Top with the salsa and avocado.

CALORIES: 360 | PROTEIN: 16G | FAT: 16G | CARBS: 41.5G | FIBER: 17G | NET CARBS: 24.5G

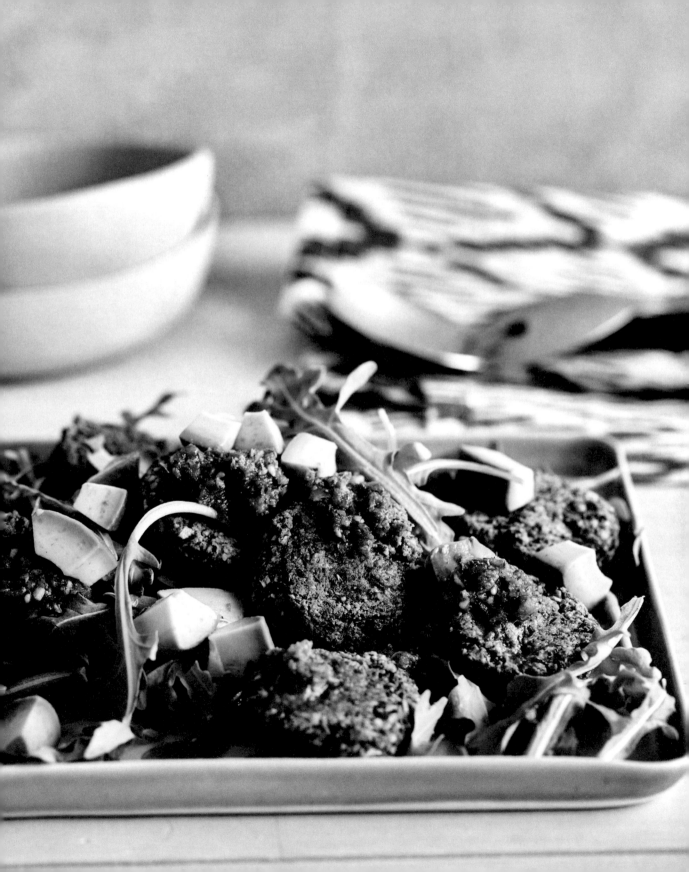

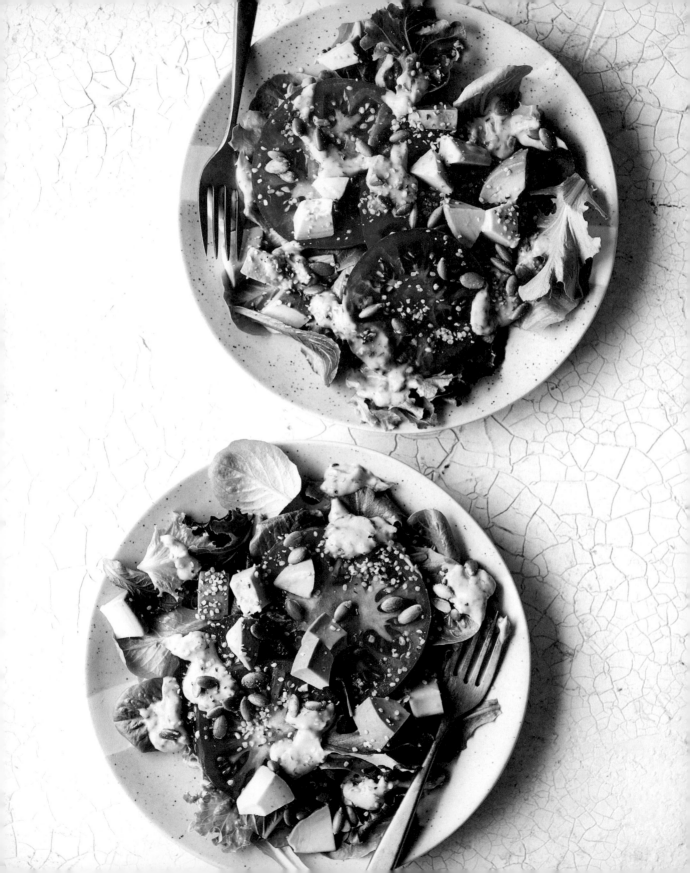

SPICY AVOCADO SALAD WITH PUMPKIN AND HEMP SEEDS

DRESSING:

1 medium avocado, peeled and pitted

½ cup cilantro leaves

⅓ cup full-fat coconut milk

2 tablespoons avocado oil

1 garlic clove

Juice of 1 lime

1 tablespoon apple cider vinegar

1 teaspoon fine sea salt

½ teaspoon ground cumin

½ teaspoon freshly ground black pepper

½ medium jalapeño, seeded and diced

SALAD:

¼ cup hemp seeds

8 cups (12 ounces) spring mix salad greens

2 medium heirloom tomatoes, sliced

1 medium avocado, peeled, pitted, and diced

¼ cup shelled, salted pumpkin seeds

Pumpkin seeds and hemp seeds are nutritional powerhouses wrapped up in tiny packages. They contain a wide array of beneficial plant compounds known as phytosterols and free radical-scavenging antioxidants, which can give your health an added boost. They're great for people with nut allergies. Be sure to use shelled green pumpkin seeds in this and all other salads. You can buy them raw or roasted and salted; I use the latter for salad toppers because they add more crunch and flavor. MAKES 4 SERVINGS

To make the dressing: Put the avocado, cilantro, coconut milk, avocado oil, garlic clove, lime juice, apple cider vinegar, salt, cumin, pepper, and jalapeño in a blender. Process until thick and creamy, about 20 seconds. Pour into a jar.

To make the salad: Put the hemp seeds in a small skillet over medium heat. Toast them, shaking the pan continuously, until they become fragrant and light golden, about 2 minutes. Watch carefully, as they can burn in seconds.

Assemble the salad by dividing the greens, tomato, and diced avocado among 4 plates. Drizzle with the dressing and sprinkle with the toasted hemp seeds and the pumpkin seeds.

CALORIES: 377 | PROTEIN: 9.5G | FAT: 31G | CARBS: 15G | FIBER: 8G | NET CARBS: 7G

CHOCOLATE-MINT PROTEIN SHAKE

Rich and refreshing, this satisfying shake will keep you nourished and well fed for hours. MAKES 2 SERVINGS

1 cup canned full-fat coconut milk

2 cups spinach

1½ cups nondairy milk

2 scoops vegan chocolate protein powder or collagen peptides

2 tablespoons Swerve Sweetener Confectioners

1 tablespoon cacao powder

¾ teaspoon peppermint extract

1 tablespoon cacao nibs

5 to 6 ice cubes

Pour coconut milk into ice cube trays and freeze for 2 hours, or until firm.

Place the coconut milk ice cubes in a high-powered blender and add the spinach, milk, protein powder, Swerve, cacao powder, peppermint extract, cacao nibs, and ice. Process until smooth and creamy.

CALORIES: 346 | PROTEIN: 13.5G | FAT: 27.5G | CARBS: 11G | FIBER: 5G | NET CARBS: 6G

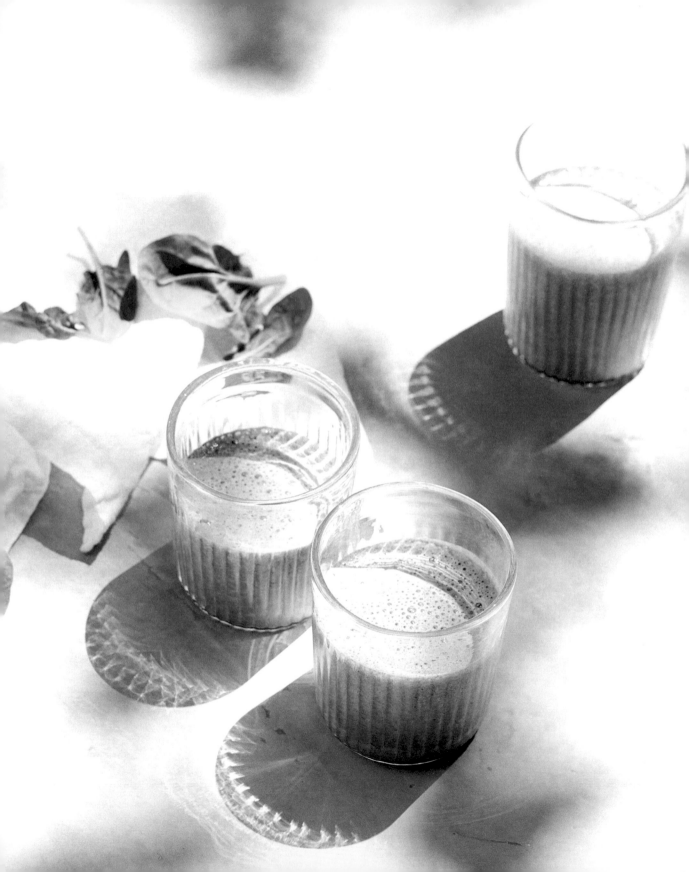

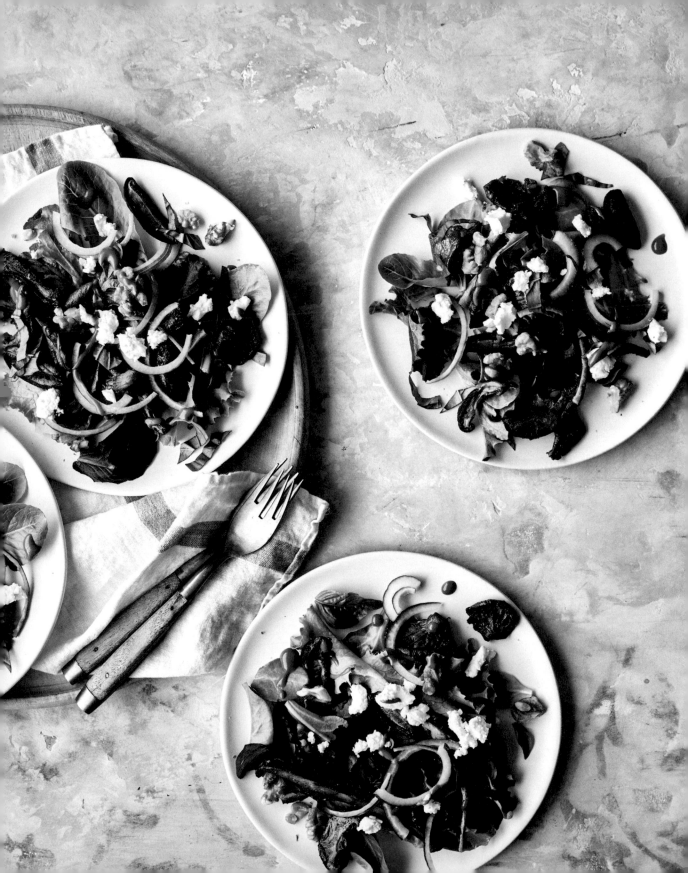

WARM MUSHROOM, GOAT CHEESE, AND WALNUT SALAD

Mushrooms are a meaty, hearty substitute for beef and other proteins. While this salad calls for portobellos, feel free to use a mix of button, cremini, shiitake, and other mushrooms. MAKES 4 SERVINGS

DRESSING:

⅓ cup extra-virgin olive oil

¼ cup balsamic vinegar

2 tablespoons Dijon mustard

1½ teaspoons Swerve Sweetener Confectioners

½ teaspoon garlic powder

¼ teaspoon sea salt

¼ teaspoon freshly ground black pepper

SALAD:

4 large portobello mushrooms

½ cup coarsely walnuts or pecans

8 cups baby spinach or mixed greens

⅓ cup sliced basil leaves

½ small red onion, sliced

2 ounces goat cheese, optional

To make the dressing: Put the oil, balsamic vinegar, mustard, Swerve, garlic powder, salt, and pepper in a mini food processor and process until smooth. Reserve ¼ cup and pour the rest into a shallow dish. Place reserved dressing in a container in the refrigerator.

To make the salad: Remove mushroom stems and discard. Slice into 1-inch strips. Add to the dish with the dressing and marinate for 1 hour to overnight in the refrigerator.

Heat the oven to 375°F. Remove the mushrooms from the marinade and place them on a baking sheet. Bake for 20 minutes, until slightly softened.

Toast the walnuts in a small skillet over medium heat until they become fragrant, about 2 to 3 minutes. Give the skillet a good shake every so often so the walnuts don't burn.

Divide the spinach among 4 plates. Arrange the mushrooms on top. Sprinkle with the basil, onion, walnuts, and goat cheese, if using. Drizzle with the reserved dressing.

CALORIES: 377 | PROTEIN: 10G | FAT: 32.5G | CARBS: 11G | FIBER: 3G | NET CARBS: 8G

MUSHROOM BOLOGNESE

Mushrooms, cauliflower, and other vegetables along with walnuts impart a meaty texture to this sauce. Ladle over the spiral-cut zucchini for a hearty meal. MAKES 4 SERVINGS

4 medium zucchini

2 teaspoons fine sea salt

4 cups Cauliflower Rice (page 344)

1 pound sliced cremini mushrooms

1 large carrot, chopped

½ medium yellow onion, minced

3 garlic cloves, minced

1 cup walnut pieces

⅓ cup nutritional yeast

2 tablespoons avocado oil

2 teaspoons dried oregano

2½ cups tomato sauce

2 teaspoons Swerve Sweetener Confectioners

Pinch cayenne pepper

Spiral cut the zucchini. (If you don't own a spiralizer, simply use a vegetable peeler to create ribbons.) Place in a colander and sprinkle with 1 teaspoon of the salt to help the liquid release. Let it rest for 15 minutes, then blot dry with a clean dish towel or paper towels.

Put the cauliflower rice in a large cast-iron skillet. Put the mushrooms and carrot in a food processor and pulse until the pieces are the size of rice. Add the mushrooms, carrot, onion, and garlic to the skillet. Heat to medium and cook for 6 to 8 minutes until vegetables can be pierced with a fork. The mushrooms will give up and then reabsorb their liquid.

Add the walnuts to the food processor and pulse a few times until they resemble coarse meal. Add the ground walnuts, ¼ cup of the nutritional yeast, avocado oil, and oregano to the skillet and stir well. Stir in the tomato sauce, Swerve, remaining salt, and cayenne pepper and sauté for 8 to 10 minutes, until all of the liquid has evaporated.

Heat the zucchini noodles in a skillet over medium heat for 2 to 3 minutes, until just warmed. Divide the noodles among 4 plates and top with the sauce. Sprinkle each serving with 1 teaspoon of nutritional yeast.

CALORIES: 460 | PROTEIN: 18G | FAT: 28G | CARBS: 34G | FIBER: 10G | NET CARBS: 24G

VEGETABLE FAJITAS

Large portobello mushrooms are seasoned and sautéed with other vegetables, then rolled up in lettuce leaves or tortillas. Again, you can use a blend of any fresh mushrooms. MAKES 4 SERVINGS

4 large portobello mushrooms, stems removed

3 tablespoons avocado oil

⅓ cup fresh lime juice

1 teaspoon dried oregano

1 teaspoon ground cumin

1 teaspoon garlic powder

½ teaspoon chili powder

½ teaspoon sea salt

½ teaspoon ground pepper

1 large red bell pepper, seeded and sliced

1 large orange bell pepper, seeded and sliced

1 small yellow onion, thinly sliced

4 large lettuce leaves or Almond Flour Tortillas (page 340)

2 medium avocados, peeled, pitted, and chopped

¼ cup Salsa (page 325)

Use a spoon to gently scrape out the insides of the mushrooms to remove the gills. Slice the mushrooms into long, ¼ -inch strips.

Put 2 tablespoons of the avocado oil, the lime juice, oregano, cumin, garlic powder, chili powder, salt, and pepper in a large, shallow dish. Add the mushrooms and turn to coat well. Marinate for 30 minutes or overnight in the refrigerator.

Heat the remaining avocado oil in a large skillet over medium heat. Add the bell peppers and onion and sauté for 5 minutes. Add the mushroom slices to the pan and discard the marinade. Cook for about 5 minutes, stirring frequently, until mushrooms are tender.

Serve the mushrooms spooned into the wraps of your choice. Spoon on the avocado and top with the salsa.

CALORIES: 319 | PROTEIN: 6G | FAT: 23G | CARBS: 22G | FIBER: 8G | NET CARBS: 14G

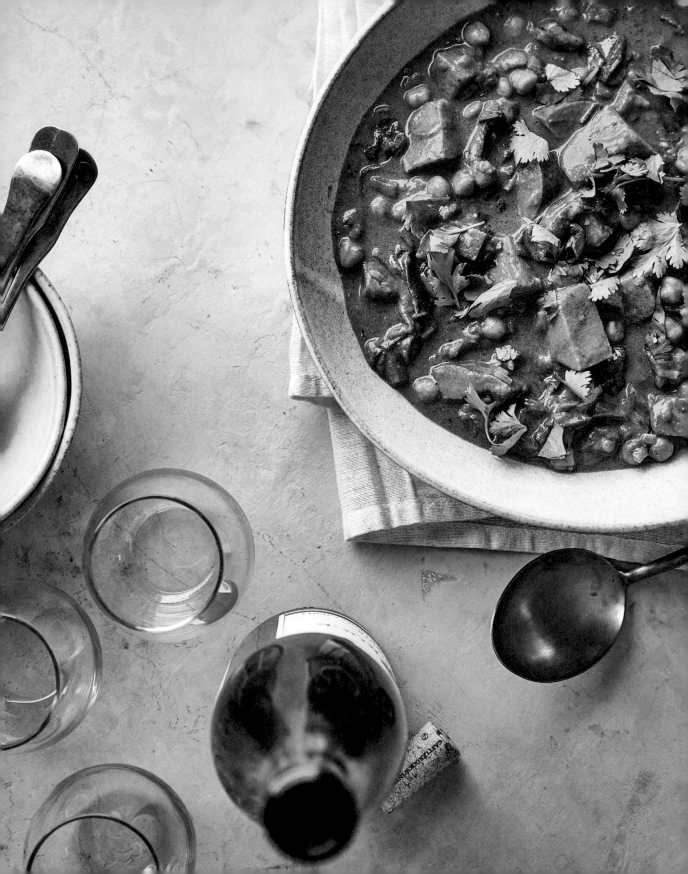

MOROCCAN VEGETABLE STEW

Warming spices and colorful vegetables are combined in this delicious stew, which is just the thing for a chilly evening. If you like, serve over cauliflower rice. If making in a slow cooker, add everything except the spinach and cilantro and cook on low for 6 hours or on high for 4. Then proceed with the last step below. MAKES 4 SERVINGS (4 CUPS)

Coconut oil cooking spray

1 small yellow onion, minced

2 garlic cloves, minced

2 cups Vegetable Broth (page 346)

One 15-ounce can chickpeas, rinsed and drained

One 14.5-ounce can fire-roasted tomatoes, with juices

½ cup natural almond butter

1 medium sweet potato, cut into 2-inch pieces

1 red bell pepper, seeded and diced

1 teaspoon chili powder

1 teaspoon fine sea salt

½ teaspoon ground cinnamon

½ teaspoon ground cumin

½ teaspoon ground cloves

½ teaspoon ground ginger

¼ teaspoon cayenne pepper

2 cups baby spinach

¼ cup chopped cilantro

Coat a Dutch oven with cooking spray. Add the onion and garlic and sauté for 3 minutes, until softened. Add the broth, chickpeas, tomatoes, almond butter, sweet potato, bell pepper, chili powder, salt, cinnamon, cumin, cloves, ginger, and cayenne pepper. Stir to combine.

Bring to a boil over medium-high heat, then reduce heat and simmer, covered, until the vegetables are tender, about 1 hour.

Stir in the spinach until wilts, then divide among 4 bowls. Top with cilantro and serve.

CALORIES: 432 | PROTEIN: 14G | FAT: 21G | CARBS: 48G | FIBER: 11G | NET CARBS: 37G

CHICKEN LO MEIN

MARINADE:

3 tablespoons coconut aminos

2 tablespoons sriracha

1 tablespoon toasted sesame oil

2 green onions, sliced

2 garlic cloves, minced

1-inch piece ginger, minced

1 pound boneless, skinless organic chicken, thinly sliced

STIR-FRY:

2 tablespoons coconut or avocado oil

1 pound cremini mushrooms, sliced

2 large celery stalks, sliced into ⅛-inch pieces

1 medium red bell pepper, seeded and thinly sliced

1 cup fresh bean sprouts, rinsed, drained, and dried

¼ cup Chicken Broth (page 345)

Four 7-ounce bags shirataki noodles, such as Miracle Noodles, drained and rinsed

2 green onions, sliced

½ teaspoon sea salt

½ teaspoon crushed red pepper flakes, optional

¼ cup chopped cilantro

1 tablespoon toasted sesame seeds

1 tablespoon toasted sesame oil

Shirataki noodles, made from the konjac plant, have been part of the Japanese diet for a thousand years. They are vegan, gluten-free, and low-carb and can be found in the produce section of supermarkets and health food stores. My go-to brand is Miracle Noodle. MAKES 4 SERVINGS

To make the marinade: Put the coconut aminos, sriracha, sesame oil, green onions, garlic, and ginger in a shallow dish. Add the sliced chicken and marinate, turning once, for at least 1 hour or overnight in the refrigerator.

To make the stir-fry: Heat 1 tablespoon of the coconut oil in a large skillet over medium heat. Add the chicken and sauté for 5 minutes, until browned. Remove the chicken to a plate.

Add the remaining 1 tablespoon coconut oil to the skillet. Add the mushrooms, celery, bell pepper, and bean sprouts and sauté over medium heat for 5 minutes. Add the broth, and simmer until reduced by half, about 5 minutes. Add the shirataki noodles, green onions, salt, and crushed red pepper, if using, and cook, stirring occasionally, for 3 minutes.

Divide the stir-fry among 4 plates. Sprinkle each serving with the cilantro and sesame seeds and a drizzle of sesame oil.

CALORIES: 370 | PROTEIN: 31G | FAT: 19G | CARBS: 15G | FIBER: 3G | NET CARBS: 12G

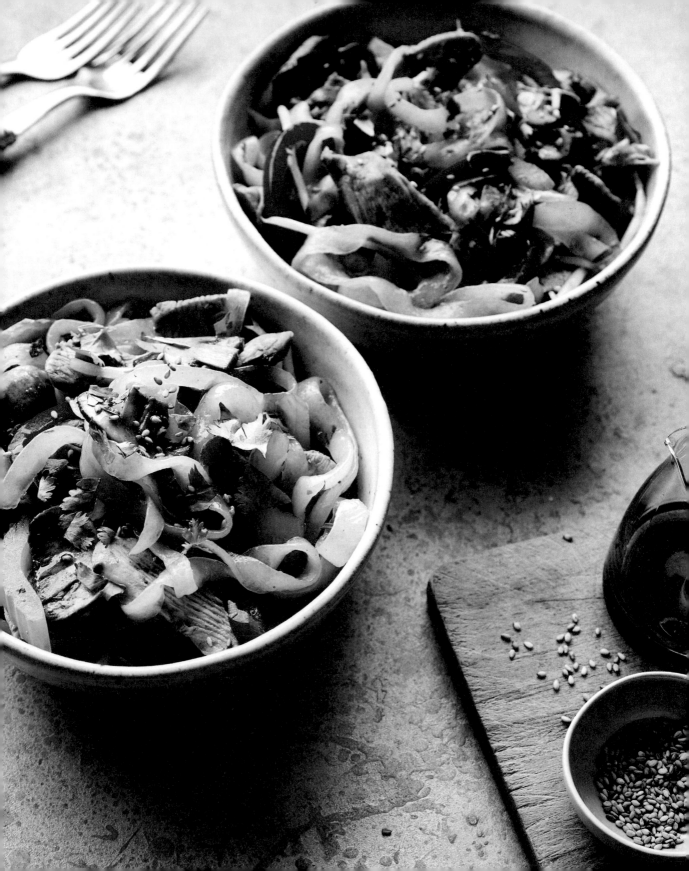

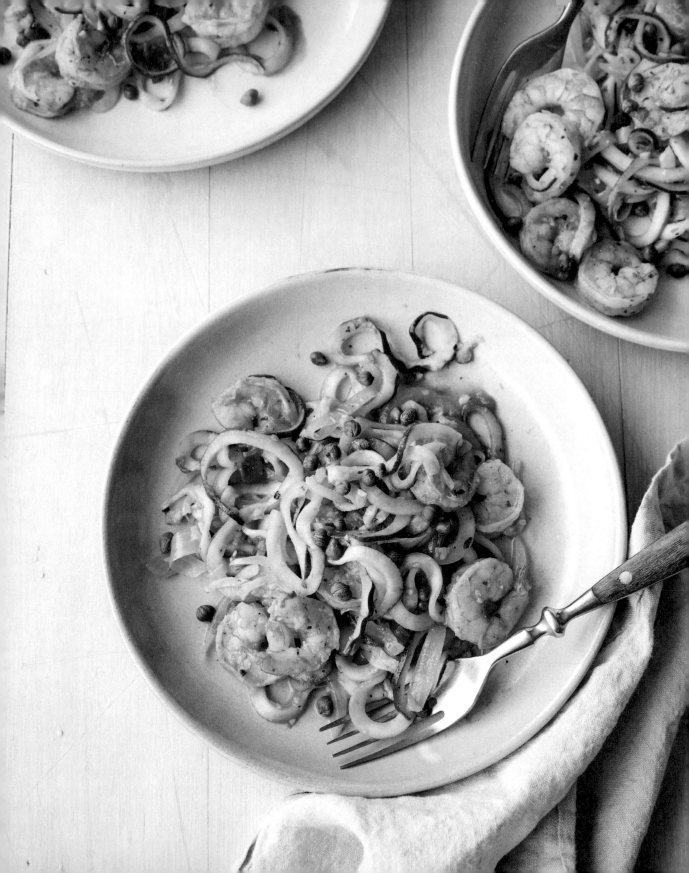

SHRIMP WITH ZUCCHINI NOODLES

Zoodles, or spiral-cut zucchini noodles, can be found in the produce sections of many markets if you don't want to spiral cut the zucchini yourself. If you like, you can stir in some Pesto (page 330) to add another level of flavor to this dish. MAKES 4 SERVINGS

4 medium zucchini

2 teaspoons fine sea salt

¼ cup extra-virgin olive oil

1 pound large shrimp, peeled, deveined, and dried

¼ teaspoon freshly ground black pepper

1 large yellow onion, thinly sliced

1 tablespoon minced garlic

½ cup white wine

1 large tomato, chopped

2 tablespoons unsalted organic butter or ghee

2 teaspoons Italian seasoning

2 tablespoons capers, rinsed and drained, optional

Spiral cut the zucchini. (If you don't own a spiralizer, simply use a vegetable peeler to create ribbons.) Place in a colander and sprinkle with 1 teaspoon of the salt to help the liquid release. Let it rest for 15 minutes, then blot dry with a clean dish towel or paper towels.

Put 2 tablespoons of the olive oil in a large skillet. Heat the oil over medium-high heat until shimmering. Season the shrimp with the remaining salt and the pepper. Add the shrimp in a single layer and let them cook without stirring until pink on one side, about 1 minute. Turn the shrimp and continue to cook until pink, about 1 minute. Shrimp do not have to be fully cooked through at this point. Transfer to a plate.

Add the remaining 2 tablespoons olive oil to the same pan. Add the onion and garlic, stirring occasionally, until the onion begins to soften, about 3 minutes. Deglaze the pan with 2 tablespoons of the wine; then add the tomato and remaining wine. Increase the heat slightly and simmer until the liquid is reduced by half, about 5 to 7 minutes. Add the butter, shrimp, and Italian seasoning and toss to coat the shrimp. Cook for 2 minutes.

Add the zucchini noodles to the skillet and cook for 30 seconds, tossing to combine. Garnish with the capers before serving.

CALORIES: 350 | PROTEIN: 28G | FAT: 21G | CARBS: 12G | FIBER: 3G | NET CARBS: 9G

CAULIFLOWER BITES WITH BUFFALO WING SAUCE

Cauliflower florets are tossed with Buffalo Wing Sauce and are roasted until tender and dripping with flavor. I like to serve mine with a side of our Macadamia Ranch Dressing (page 329). Who needs chicken wings? MAKES 6 SERVINGS

1 large head cauliflower

1 cup Buffalo Wing Sauce (page 326)

1 teaspoon garlic powder

½ teaspoon fine sea salt

Macadamia Ranch Dressing (page 329)

Heat the oven to 450°F. Line a baking sheet with parchment paper.

Separate the cauliflower florets from the stems and place the florets in a bowl. (Discard the stems.) Add the wing sauce, garlic powder, and salt, tossing to coat well. Arrange the cauliflower in a single layer on the prepared pan. Roast for 18 to 20 minutes, until tender when pierced with a knife. Set oven to broil. Broil the cauliflower for 2 minutes. Serve with Macadamia Ranch Dressing, if desired.

CALORIES: 388 | PROTEIN: 3G | FAT: 40G | CARBS: 7G | FIBER: 3G | NET CARBS: 4G

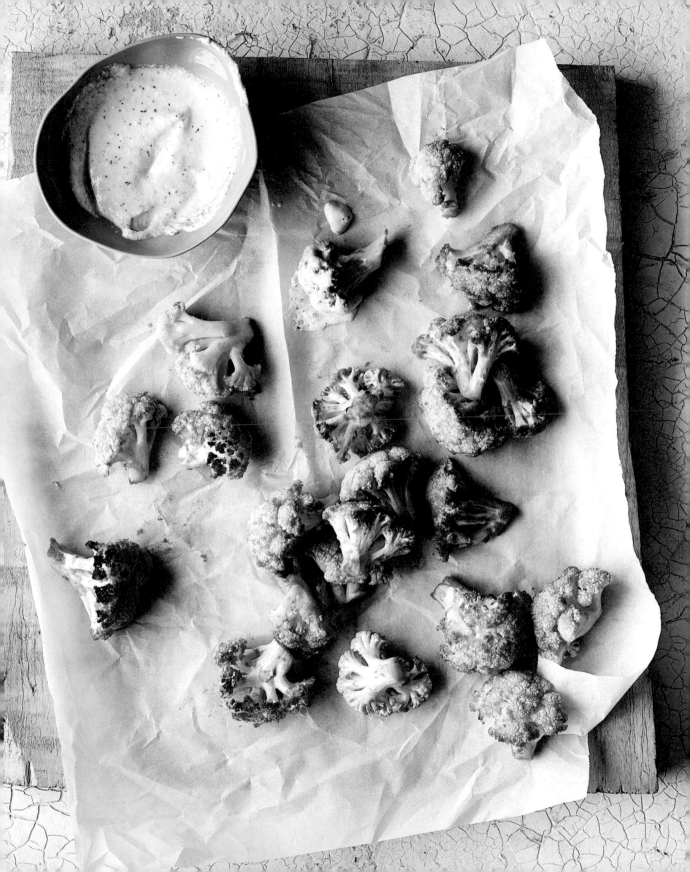

GOLDEN CAULIFLOWER RICE

Organic cauliflower rice can be found in markets everywhere. Serve hot as a side dish or add cooked tempeh or chicken for a hearty meal. MAKES 4 SERVINGS

1 tablespoon ghee

½ medium yellow onion, diced

2 garlic cloves, minced

4 cups Cauliflower Rice (page 344)

½ green bell pepper, seeded and chopped

1 13.5-ounce can full-fat coconut milk

2 tablespoons curry powder

2 teaspoons ground turmeric

2 teaspoons Swerve Sweetener Confectioners

½ teaspoon fine sea salt

¼ teaspoon freshly ground black pepper

Melt the ghee in a large skillet over medium heat. Add the onion and garlic. Sauté for 4 to 5 minutes, until the onion is softened and translucent. Add the cauliflower and bell pepper and sauté for 5 minutes. Stir in the coconut milk, curry powder, turmeric, Swerve, salt, and pepper. Simmer for 5 minutes to allow the flavors to combine.

CALORIES: 280 | PROTEIN: 5G | FAT: 23G | CARBS: 13G | FIBER: 5G | NET CARBS: 8G

NUTTY ROASTED BRUSSELS SPROUTS

Almond meal stands in for bread crumbs or Parmesan cheese and adds a toasty crunch. MAKES 4 SERVINGS

1 pound brussels sprouts, stemmed and halved

3 tablespoons avocado oil

¼ cup almond meal

1 teaspoon garlic powder

½ teaspoon fine sea salt

½ teaspoon freshly ground black pepper

Put the brussels sprouts and 2 tablespoons of the avocado oil in a bowl and toss well. Heat a large skillet over medium heat and add the brussels sprouts, cut side down. Cook for 6 to 8 minutes, without stirring, until golden brown.

Mix the almond meal, garlic powder, salt, and pepper in a bowl.

Add the remaining oil to the skillet and stir in the almond meal mixture, tossing with brussels sprouts to coat. Cook, stirring occasionally, until sprouts are brown on all sides. Serve immediately.

CALORIES: 190 | PROTEIN: 5G | FAT: 14G | CARBS: 11G | FIBER: 4G | NET CARBS: 7G

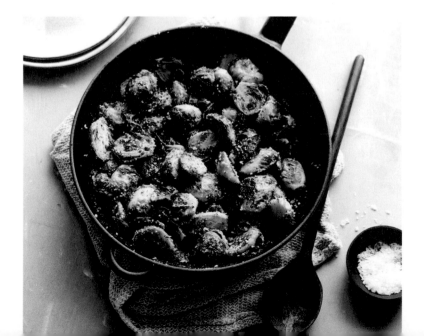

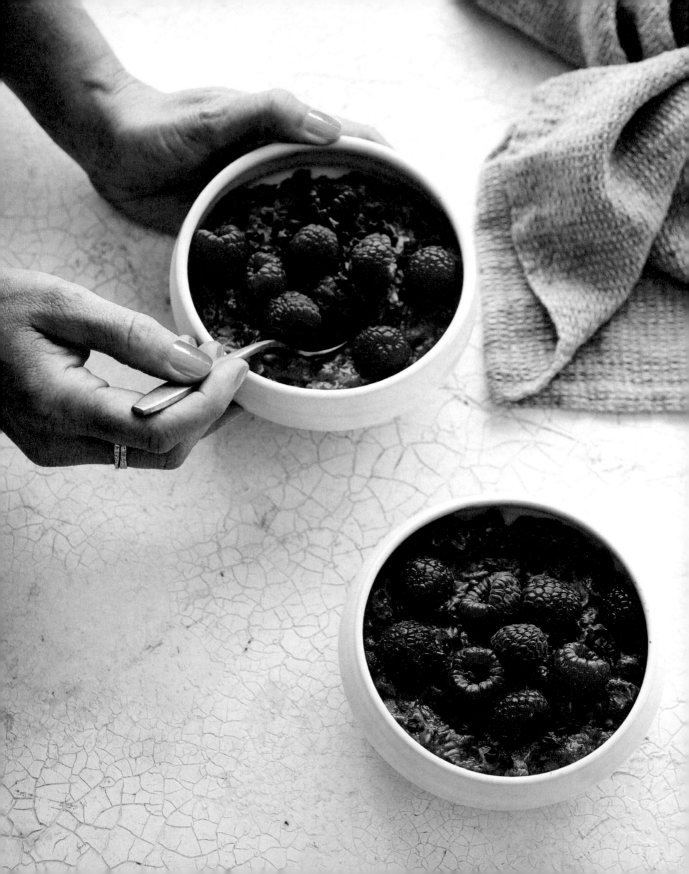

RENEW RECIPES

LEAN GREEN BREAKFAST CHILI

Chili for breakfast? Why not? This 131 Method chili is made with lean protein (turkey) and plenty of vegetables to get your day started. For an even heartier meal, top with an over-easy egg or scrambled egg whites. There's enough here to share with your family or portion out for meals later in the week.

MAKES 4 SERVINGS

1 tablespoon
avocado oil

½ cup diced red onion

1 pound 99% lean
ground turkey

1 cup salsa verde

1 cup shredded
cabbage

½ cup Chicken Broth
(page 345)

½ cup canned black
beans, drained and
rinsed

1 tablespoon Taco
Seasoning (page 333)

1 teaspoon fine
sea salt

Pinch cayenne pepper,
optional

¼ cup chopped
cilantro

Heat the oil in a Dutch oven over medium heat. Add the onion and sauté for 3 minutes. Add the turkey and cook, stirring frequently, about 5 minutes, until brown on all sides.

Add the salsa, cabbage, broth, beans, taco seasoning, salt, and cayenne pepper, if using, and stir well.

Reduce the heat and simmer for 5 minutes. Garnish with the cilantro before serving.

CALORIES: 217 | PROTEIN: 29G | FAT: 5G | CARBS: 10.5G | FIBER: 3G |
NET CARBS: 7.5G

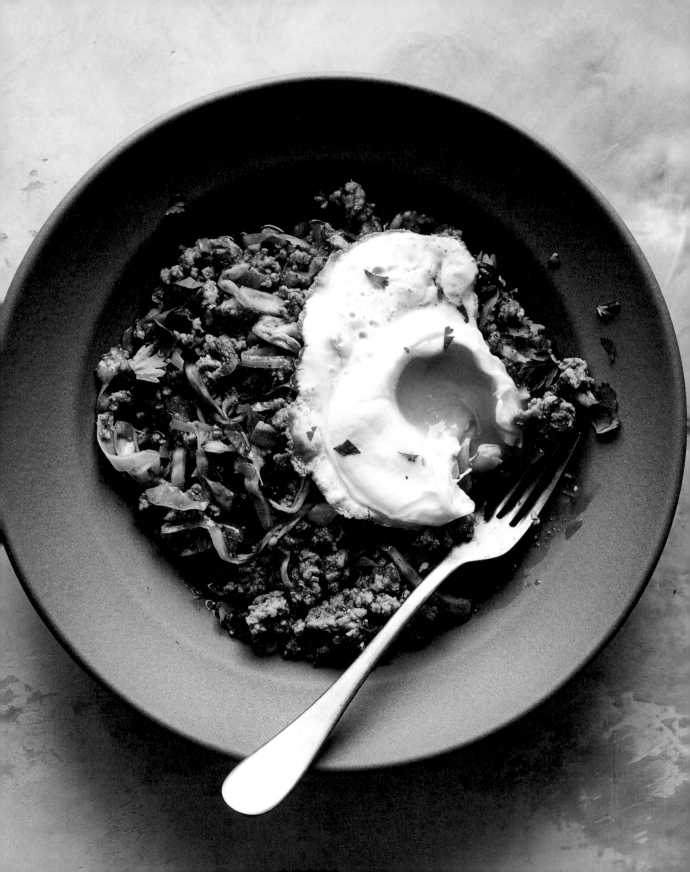

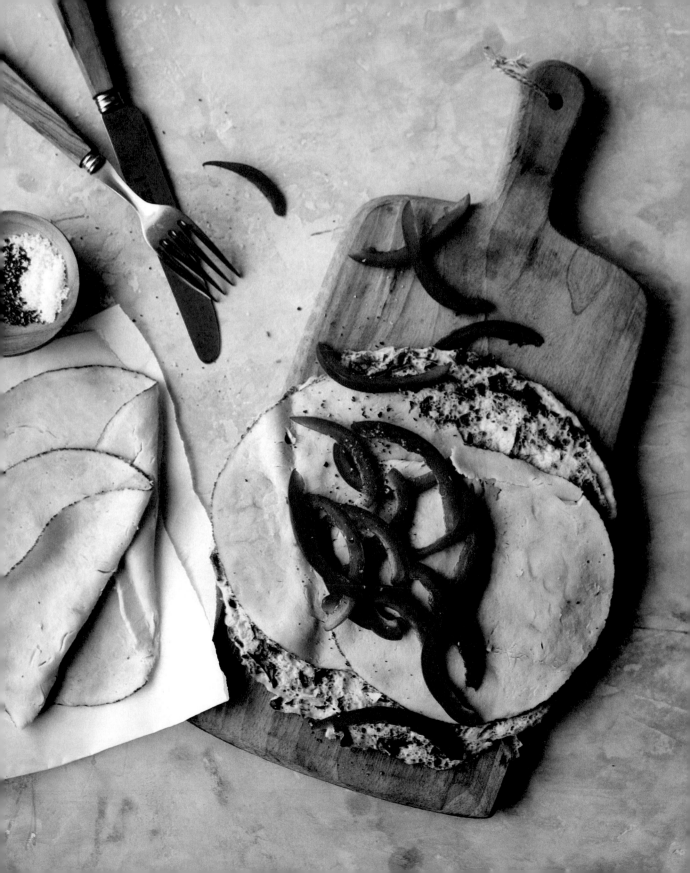

EGG, TURKEY, AND ARUGULA BREAKFAST WRAP

An omelet serves as the wrap for a filling loaded with protein and vegetables.

MAKES 1 SERVING

Coconut oil cooking spray

1 large organic egg

2 large organic egg whites

1 cup chopped arugula

Pinch fine sea salt

Pinch pepper

2 ounces sliced organic turkey

¼ red bell pepper, seeded and thinly sliced

Coat a small skillet with cooking spray. Heat the skillet over medium heat. Whisk together the egg, egg whites, arugula, salt, and pepper in a small bowl. Add to the skillet and swirl so the mixture covers the bottom. Cook until a little liquid remains; then use a spatula to turn and cook for 1 minute more. Remove from the pan and arrange the turkey slices on top. Top with the pepper slices. Sprinkle with additional salt and pepper, if desired. Roll into a long wrap.

CALORIES: 208 | PROTEIN: 31G | FAT: 6G | CARBS: 4G | FIBER: 1G | NET CARBS: 3G

EGG MUFFINS

These can be made ahead, then frozen and reheated for an easy on-the-go breakfast. MAKES 2 SERVINGS

Coconut oil cooking spray

3 large organic eggs

3 large organic egg whites

2 cups chopped spinach

½ cup chopped bell pepper, any color

2 tablespoons nondairy milk

1 green onion, chopped

½ teaspoon garlic powder

¼ teaspoon fine sea salt

Pinch freshly ground black pepper

Heat the oven to 350°F. Coat 6 cups of a muffin tin with cooking spray.

Whisk together the eggs, egg whites, spinach, bell pepper, milk, green onion, garlic powder, salt, and pepper in a medium bowl. Divide the mixture among the prepared muffin cups.

Bake until eggs are cooked through, about 22 to 24 minutes.

CALORIES: 153 | PROTEIN: 16G | FAT: 7.5G | CARBS: 5G | FIBER: 1.5G | NET CARBS: 3.5G

BERRY GREEN SMOOTHIE

Spinach and berries provide a healthy dose of antioxidants, while the collagen peptides offer necessary protein. MAKES 1 SERVING

1½ cups nondairy milk

1 cup spinach

2½ scoops unflavored collagen peptides

½ cup frozen mixed berries

4 to 5 ice cubes

5 drops liquid stevia

Put the milk, spinach, collagen peptides, berries, ice cubes, and stevia in a blender. Process until smooth and creamy, adding more ice, if needed, to reach desired consistency.

CALORIES: 180 | PROTEIN: 25G | FAT: 4G | CARBS: 11G | FIBER: 5G | NET CARBS: 6G

MOCHA SMOOTHIE

Frozen cauliflower rice provides a creamy texture with added fiber and no detectable flavor. Check the frozen food aisle for frozen organic cauliflower rice, or freeze extra cooked cauliflower rice when you make your own.

MAKES 1 SERVING

¾ cup nondairy milk

¾ cup frozen cauliflower rice

½ cup brewed coffee, chilled

1 tablespoon cacao powder

2 teaspoons almond butter

1 scoop chocolate bone broth protein powder or collagen protein powder

10 to 12 ice cubes

2 tablespoons Swerve Sweetener Confectioners

Put the milk, cauliflower, coffee, cacao powder, almond butter, protein powder, ice cubes, and Swerve in a large blender. Process until smooth and creamy.

CALORIES: 239 | PROTEIN: 26G | FAT: 10G | CARBS: 12G | FIBER: 5G | NET CARBS: 7G

SALMON CAKES AND SPINACH SALAD

Moist and flavorful salmon cakes are served on a bed of spinach and other vegetables drizzled with a lemony dressing. MAKES 2 SERVINGS

SALMON CAKES:

One 6-ounce can salmon, well drained

1 large organic egg

1 tablespoon almond meal

½ tablespoon coconut flour

¼ cup diced red onion

2 tablespoons diced red bell pepper

2 tablespoons chopped parsley

1 tablespoon Dijon mustard

2 teaspoons fresh lemon juice

½ teaspoon onion powder

½ teaspoon sea salt

¼ teaspoon freshly ground black pepper

Coconut oil cooking spray

SALAD:

2 cups spinach

½ large cucumber, diced

1 green onion, sliced

2 tablespoons Dijon mustard

1½ tablespoons fresh lemon juice

1½ tablespoons nondairy milk

1 teaspoon avocado oil

Pinch stevia

To make the salmon cakes: Put the salmon, egg, almond meal, coconut flour, onion, bell pepper, parsley, Dijon mustard, lemon juice, onion powder, salt, and pepper in a bowl. Mash with a fork to combine.

Divide the mixture and shape it into 4 patties. Coat a medium skillet with cooking spray. Heat the skillet over medium-low heat. Add the patties and cook for 5 minutes. Turn and cook for an additional 4 to 5 minutes until golden.

To make the salad: Divide the spinach, cucumber, and green onion between 2 plates. Whisk together the mustard, lemon juice, milk, oil, and stevia in a bowl. Drizzle the dressing on the greens and top each serving with 2 salmon cakes.

CALORIES: 231 | PROTEIN: 26G | FAT: 9G | CARBS: 10G | FIBER: 3G | NET CARBS: 7G

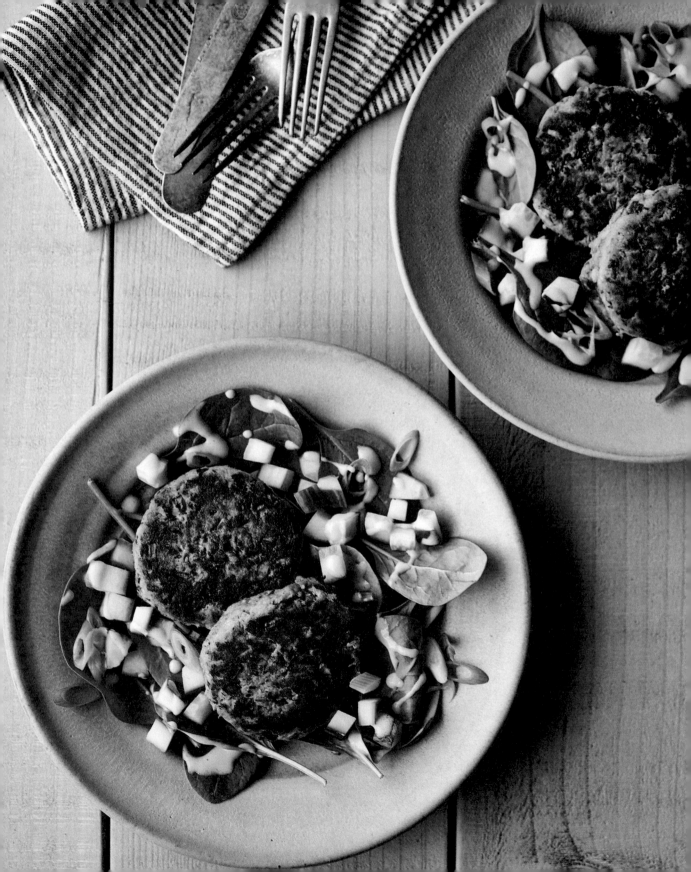

TUNA SALAD WITH DILL

Tuna salad is often the same old blend of fish and celery, but my version includes cucumber, avocado, capers, and more, making it new! MAKES 1 SERVING

One 5-ounce can solid white tuna packed in water, well drained

1 mini Persian cucumber, diced

¼ small avocado, mashed

1 tablespoon lemon juice

1 tablespoon capers

2 sprigs fresh dill, chopped

½ teaspoon garlic powder

Pinch fine sea salt

Pinch black pepper

2 cups fresh spinach

1 roma tomato, chopped

Put the tuna, cucumber, avocado, lemon juice, capers, dill, garlic powder, salt, and pepper in a bowl and mix well. Plate the spinach and tomato and top with the tuna mixture.

CALORIES: 273 | PROTEIN: 37.5G | FAT: 9.5G | CARBS: 13G | FIBER: 7G | NET CARBS: 6G

CREAMY CELERY SOUP

If you want more protein, use bone broth in place of the vegetable broth.

MAKES 4 SERVINGS

1 tablespoon butter-flavored coconut oil or ghee

1 small yellow onion, chopped

¾ cup sliced leeks (white parts only)

3 garlic cloves, minced

2½ cups chopped celery (about 8 stalks)

2 cups Vegetable Broth (page 346)

One 13.5-ounce can lite coconut milk

3 cups spinach

4 scoops collagen peptides

1 teaspoon fine sea salt

½ teaspoon black pepper

Put the oil and onion in a large saucepan over medium heat. Sauté for 4 minutes; then add the leeks and garlic and sauté for 3 minutes. Add the celery and sauté for 2 minutes. Add the broth and simmer for 15 minutes.

Transfer the mixture to a blender. Add the coconut milk, spinach, collagen peptides, salt, and pepper. Blend on low for 30 seconds, then on high for 1 minute, until smooth. Return the soup to the saucepan and reheat before serving.

CALORIES: 175 | PROTEIN: 10G | FAT: 10G | CARBS: 9.5G | FIBER: 1.5G | NET CARBS: 8G

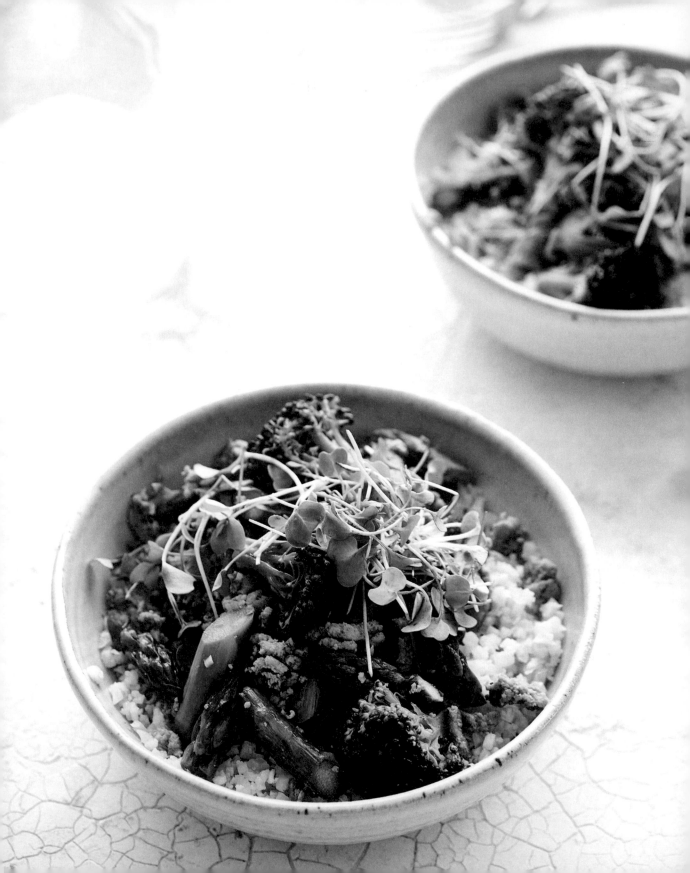

TURKEY, ASPARAGUS, AND BROCCOLI

Serve this over some cauliflower rice for a satisfying meal. MAKES 4 SERVINGS

2 tablespoons
avocado oil

20 asparagus,
trimmed and cut into
1-inch pieces

2 garlic cloves, minced

1 pound 99% lean
ground turkey

1 tablespoon hot sauce

⅓ cup Chicken Broth
(page 345)

2 cups broccoli florets

½ teaspoon fine
sea salt

½ teaspoon freshly
ground black pepper

2 ounces microgreens

Put 1 tablespoon of the avocado oil in a large skillet over medium heat. Add the asparagus and garlic and stir-fry for 3 minutes. Transfer the asparagus to a plate.

Add the remaining oil, turkey, and hot sauce to the skillet. Cook until the turkey is brown on all sides, about 5 to 6 minutes, breaking up the turkey as it cooks.

Stir in the broth and broccoli and cook until the broccoli begins to soften. Return the asparagus to the skillet. Season with salt and pepper. Simmer for 2 to 3 minutes, until all vegetables are tender.

Divide the turkey and vegetables among 4 bowls and top with microgreens.

CALORIES: 229 | PROTEIN: 31G | FAT: 9G | CARBS: 9G | FIBER: 4G |
NET CARBS: 5G

GREEN CHILE CHICKEN CASSEROLE

This easy casserole tastes like it was made with loads of butter and cream, but it's sneaky cauliflower that provides the rich, Alfredo-like taste and texture. You can substitute heavy cream for the coconut cream, if desired.
MAKES 4 SERVINGS

2 cups cauliflower florets

⅓ cup Chicken Broth (page 345)

3 tablespoons canned coconut cream

3 tablespoons nutritional yeast

1½ teaspoons garlic powder

1 teaspoon fine sea salt

½ teaspoon freshly ground black pepper

One 4-ounce can diced fire-roasted green chiles

4 large (about 1½ pounds) boneless, skinless organic chicken breasts

Heat the oven to 375°F. Place cauliflower florets and broth in a small saucepan. Simmer for 6 to 7 minutes, covered, until cauliflower is very soft. Pour into a blender.

Add the coconut cream, nutritional yeast, garlic powder, ½ teaspoon of the sea salt, and ¼ teaspoon of the black pepper to the blender and process until smooth, about 20 seconds. Stir in 2 ounces of the green chiles with the juices.

Put the chicken in an 8x11-inch casserole dish. Season with remaining salt and pepper.

Pour the cauliflower cream sauce on top of the chicken. Arrange the remaining chiles across the top. Bake uncovered for 30 to 35 minutes.

CALORIES: 352 | PROTEIN: 58G | FAT: 10G | CARBS: 5.5G | FIBER: 2G | NET CARBS: 3.5G

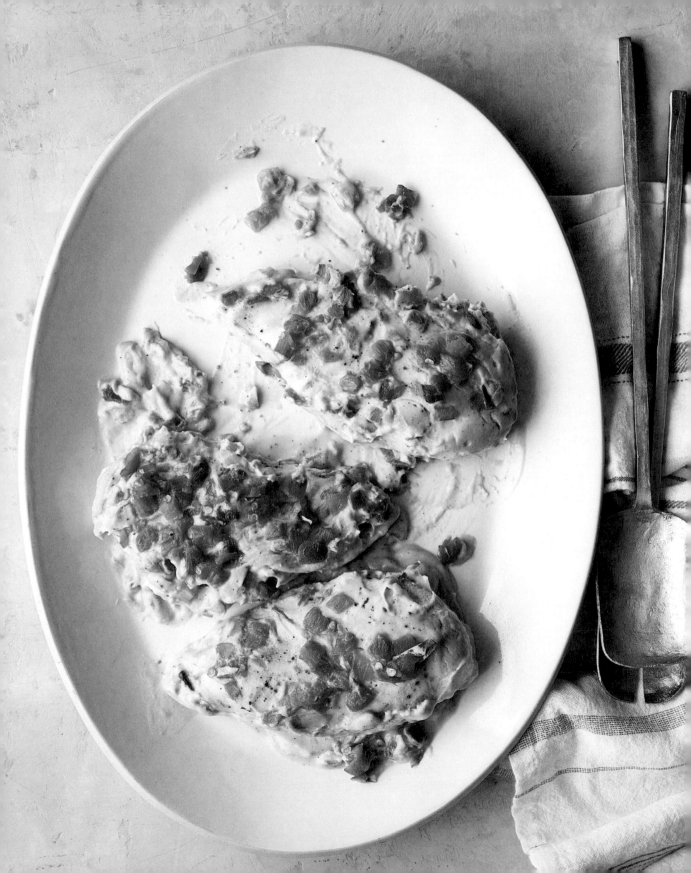

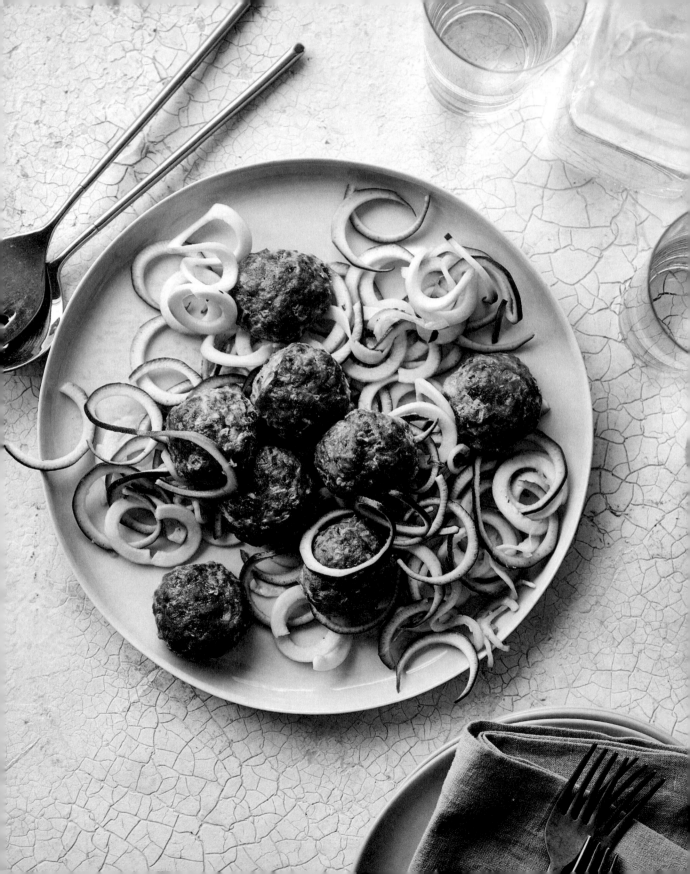

TURKEY MEATBALLS WITH ZOODLES

I suggest doubling and freezing the recipe for the meatballs, so you'll have another meal just minutes away. MAKES 4 SERVINGS

1 pound 93% lean ground turkey

½ small red onion, diced

½ green bell pepper, seeded and finely chopped

¼ cup chopped cilantro

1 jalapeño, seeded and diced

2 tablespoons tomato paste

2 large organic egg whites

1 teaspoon garlic powder

1 teaspoon fine sea salt

4 medium zucchini, spiral cut

Juice of 1 lime

Heat the oven to 350°F. Mix the turkey, onion, bell pepper, cilantro, jalapeño, tomato paste, egg whites, garlic powder, and salt in a medium bowl.

Shape into 16 meatballs. Freeze for at least 60 minutes. Place on a rimmed baking sheet lined with parchment paper. Bake for 30 minutes, until meat is no longer pink inside when you cut into a meatball.

Place the zucchini noodles on a paper towel–lined plate and add the lime juice. Cover the noodles with another paper towel and microwave for 1 minute. Divide the zucchini noodles among 4 plates, top with the meatballs, and serve.

CALORIES: 232 | PROTEIN: 27G | FAT: 9G | CARBS: 11G | FIBER: 3G | NET CARBS: 8G

BEEF AND VEGETABLE STIR-FRY

Ladle this warming stir-fry over some steaming cauliflower rice or shirataki noodles. MAKES 4 SERVINGS

1 tablespoon
avocado oil

1 pound 100% grass-
fed beef sirloin tip
steak, thinly sliced

3 tablespoons coconut
aminos

4 baby bok choy,
trimmed and cut into
bite-size pieces

½ yellow onion,
finely chopped

1 large red bell pepper,
seeded and chopped

2 garlic cloves, minced

1 teaspoon freshly
grated ginger

1 teaspoon fine
sea salt

1 tablespoon toasted
sesame seeds

Heat the sesame oil in a large skillet over medium heat. Add the steak slices and stir-fry until browned, about 3 minutes.

Stir in the coconut aminos, bok choy, onion, bell pepper, garlic, ginger, and salt. Stir fry for about 5 minutes, until vegetables are tender. Sprinkle on the sesame seeds to serve.

CALORIES: 246 | PROTEIN: 29G | FAT: 9G | CARBS: 11G | FIBER: 3G |
NET CARBS: 8G

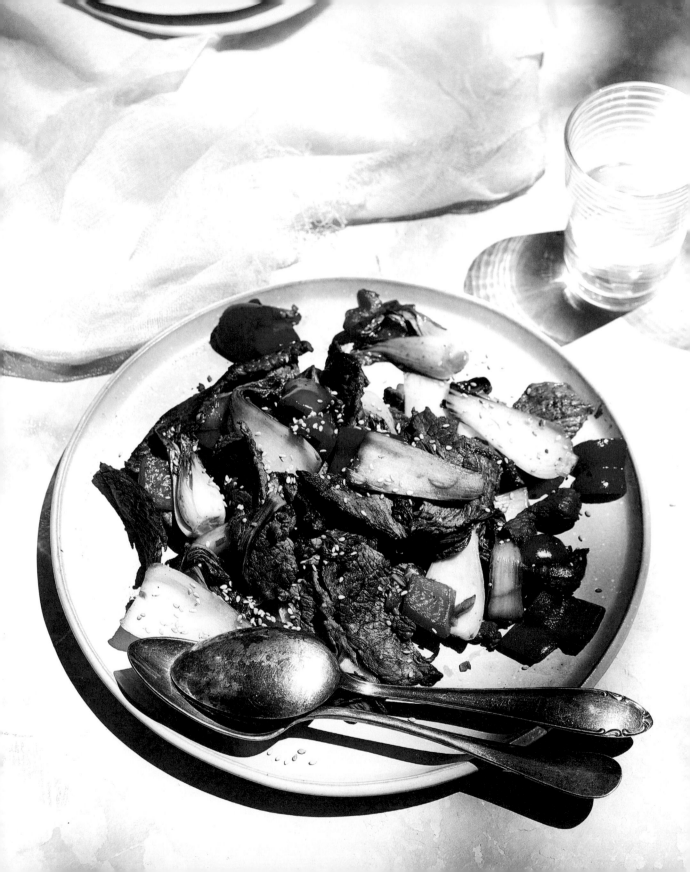

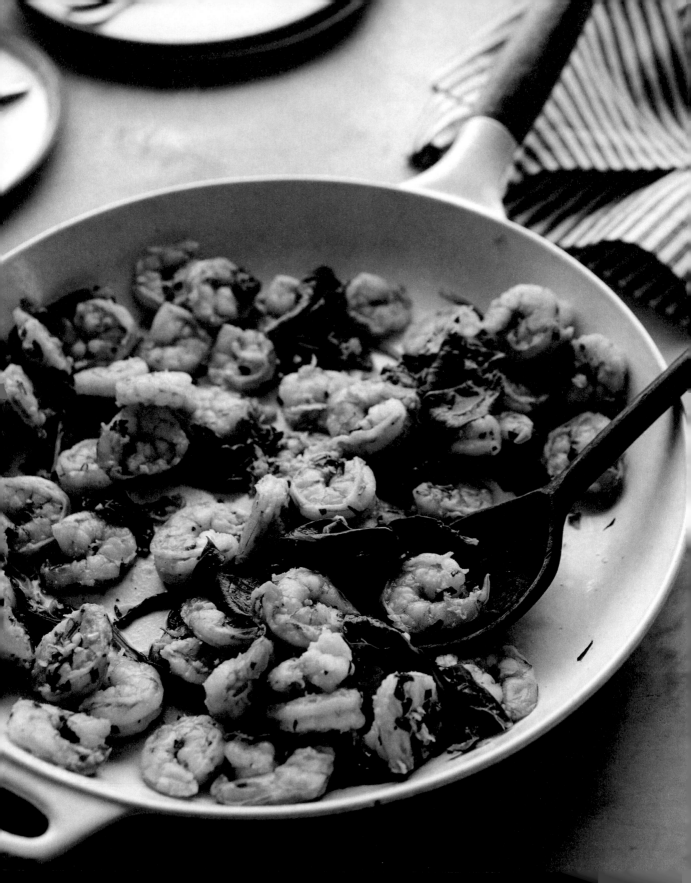

GARLIC SHRIMP WITH SPINACH

If you like, arrange these quickly cooked, garlicky shrimp tossed with spinach and seasonings on a bed of shirataki noodles. MAKES 4 SERVINGS

1 tablespoon ghee

1½ pounds wild-caught shrimp, peeled and deveined

1 teaspoon fine sea salt

½ teaspoon freshly ground black pepper

2 garlic cloves, minced

2 tablespoons fresh lemon juice

¼ cup chopped fresh parsley

¼ teaspoon crushed red pepper

4 cups spinach

Heat the ghee in a large skillet over medium heat. Season shrimp with salt and pepper. Add to the skillet along with the garlic and cook undisturbed for 2 minutes. Turn shrimp and add the lemon juice, parsley, and red pepper. Cook for about 1 minute, until the shrimp turn pink and firm.

Add spinach. Cover and allow greens to wilt, about 1 minute, then stir to combine. Divide among plates and serve.

CALORIES: 209 | PROTEIN: 37.5G | FAT: 6G | CARBS: 3G | FIBER: 0.5G | NET CARBS: 2.5G

FRENCH TOAST WITH BERRY SYRUP

Bread soaked in egg and nondairy milk absorbs the flavors of vanilla and cinnamon. Top with some berries and a drizzle of honey. MAKES 1 SERVING

1 large organic egg

¼ cup nondairy milk

1 teaspoon pure vanilla extract

¼ teaspoon ground cinnamon

2 slices sprouted-grain bread or gluten-free bread

Coconut oil cooking spray

½ cup frozen mixed berries

1 teaspoon organic raw honey

Pinch ground nutmeg

Whisk together the egg, milk, vanilla, and cinnamon in a shallow bowl. Soak the bread in the egg mixture for 30 seconds.

Coat a skillet with cooking spray. Heat over medium heat and put the bread in the skillet. Cook for 2 minutes on each side.

Put the frozen berries and honey in a saucepan. Heat until berries are warmed, then mash to create a compote.

Serve the French toast topped with the berries and a sprinkle of nutmeg.

CALORIES: 316 | PROTEIN: 15G | FAT: 7G | CARBS: 45G | FIBER: 8.5G | NET CARBS: 36.5G

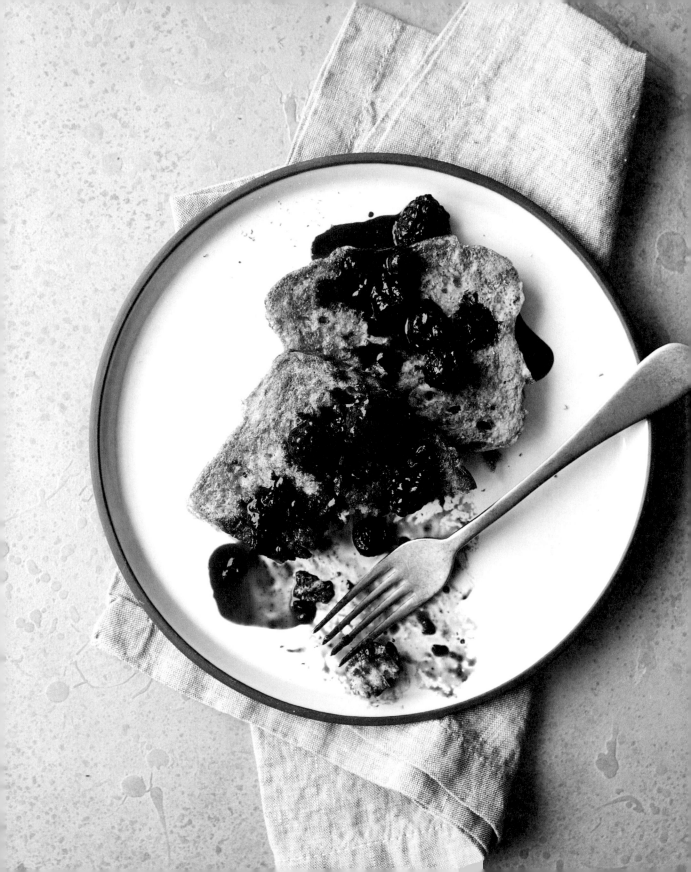

OVERNIGHT PROTEIN OATS

What's great about this power-packed cereal is that you put everything together the night before and then breakfast is ready when you are. You can substitute 2 scoops of collagen peptides for 1 scoop of the bone broth protein powder (or an amount that delivers about 20 grams of protein). Enjoy this right from the glass jar. MAKES 2 SERVINGS

2 cups nondairy milk

1 cup old-fashioned rolled oats

1 scoop vanilla bone broth protein powder

2 tablespoons Swerve Sweetener Confectioners

1½ tablespoons chia seeds

½ teaspoon pure vanilla extract

½ teaspoon cinnamon

1 small banana, sliced

Stir together the milk, oats, protein powder, Swerve, chia seeds, vanilla extract, and cinnamon in a bowl. Divide into 2 glass jars, cover, and refrigerate overnight. Before serving, top each with banana slices.

CALORIES: 334 | PROTEIN: 18G | FAT: 10G | CARBS: 43G | FIBER: 8G | NET CARBS: 35G

SWEET POTATO AND EGG SCRAMBLE

When family members see you eating this egg and vegetable scramble, they'll want some, too. It's easy to double, triple . . . or whatever! MAKES 1 SERVING

1 large organic egg

1 large organic egg white

1 teaspoon ghee

1 small sweet potato, peeled and diced

¼ cup diced yellow onion

¼ cup diced green bell pepper

Pinch fine sea salt

Pinch finely ground black pepper

2 tablespoons Salsa (page 325)

Whisk together the egg and the egg white in a bowl and set aside.

Put the ghee in a skillet over medium-low heat. Add the diced sweet potato and sauté for 6 to 8 minutes, until easily pierced with a fork. Add onion and bell pepper and continue sautéing for about 4 minutes, until all vegetables are tender. Add the eggs and scramble until they are done to your liking. Transfer to a plate, season with salt and pepper, top with salsa, and serve.

CALORIES: 267 | PROTEIN: 13G | FAT: 10G | CARBS: 32G | FIBER: 6G | NET CARBS: 26G

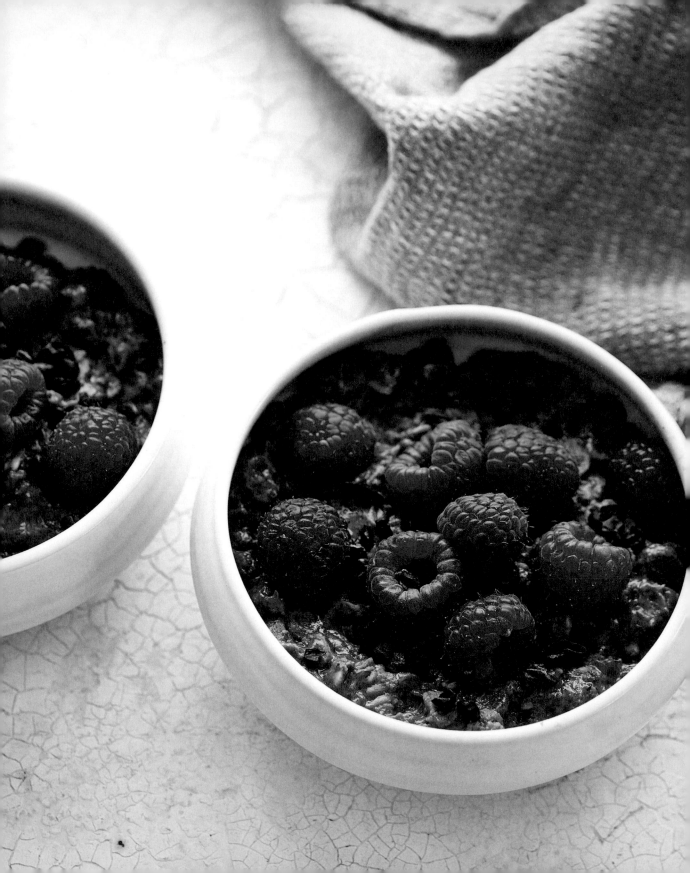

RASPBERRY–CHOCOLATE BREAKFAST BOWL

Chocolate for breakfast? You betcha. This is one of my go-to breakfast bowls.

MAKES 1 SERVING

1 cup nondairy milk

½ cup old-fashioned rolled oats

½ cup raspberries

2 tablespoons Swerve Sweetener Granular

1 tablespoon cacao powder

1 tablespoon ground flaxseed

1 teaspoon pure vanilla extract

1 teaspoon cacao nibs

Heat the milk, oats, ¼ cup of the raspberries, Swerve, cacao powder, flaxseed, and vanilla extract over low heat in a saucepan. Stir until the mixture is fully combined and thickened, about 5 minutes. Top with cacao nibs and the remaining raspberries.

CALORIES: 271 | PROTEIN: 8G | FAT: 9G | CARBS: 39G | FIBER: 10G | NET CARBS: 29G

CHICKEN, QUINOA, AND SWEET POTATO BOWLS

The right kinds of fat, protein, and carbs are balanced in these colorful bowls.

MAKES 4 SERVINGS

2 small sweet potatoes, peeled and cut into 1-inch cubes

Coconut oil cooking spray

Fine sea salt and freshly ground black pepper to taste

2 cups broccoli florets

2 cups cooked quinoa

8 ounces rotisserie chicken breast, chopped

DRESSING:

¼ cup balsamic vinegar

1 tablespoon extra-virgin olive oil

1 tablespoon organic raw honey

1 tablespoon Dijon mustard

½ teaspoon garlic powder

¼ teaspoon sea salt

Heat the oven to 400°F. Arrange the sweet potatoes in a single layer on a sheet pan and coat with coconut oil cooking spray. Sprinkle with salt and pepper. Bake for 10 minutes, then remove from the oven, toss, and add the broccoli to the pan. Coat with coconut oil cooking spray, sprinkle with more salt and pepper, and bake for an additional 10 minutes, until all the vegetables are tender and can be pierced with a knife.

To assemble, divide the quinoa, chicken, and vegetable mixture among 4 bowls.

Put the dressing ingredients in a glass jar, seal, and shake well for 30 seconds. Drizzle some of the dressing over each serving.

CALORIES: 328 | PROTEIN: 22.5G | FAT: 6G | CARBS: 44.5G | FIBER: 6G | NET CARBS: 38.5G

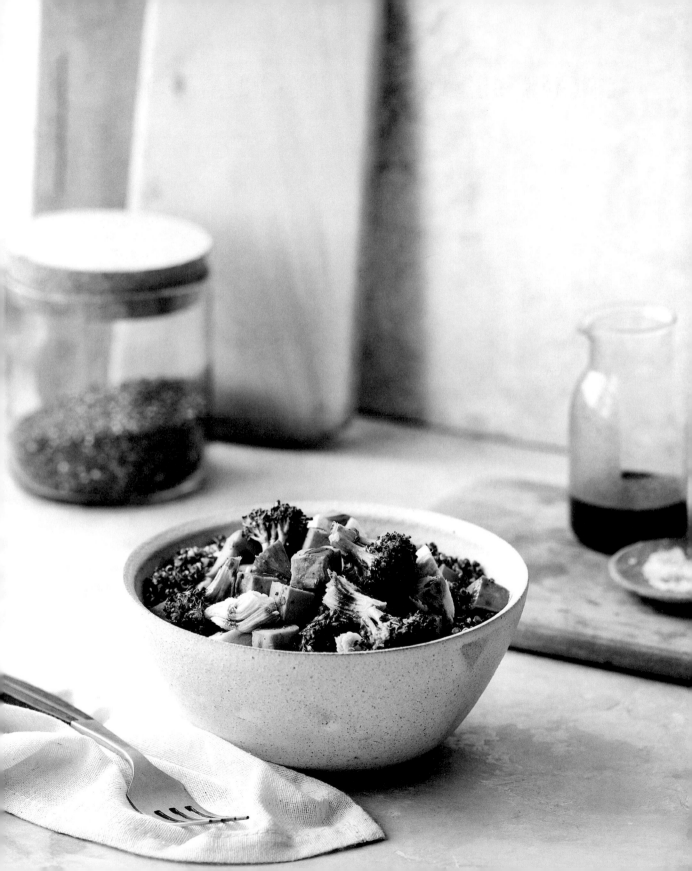

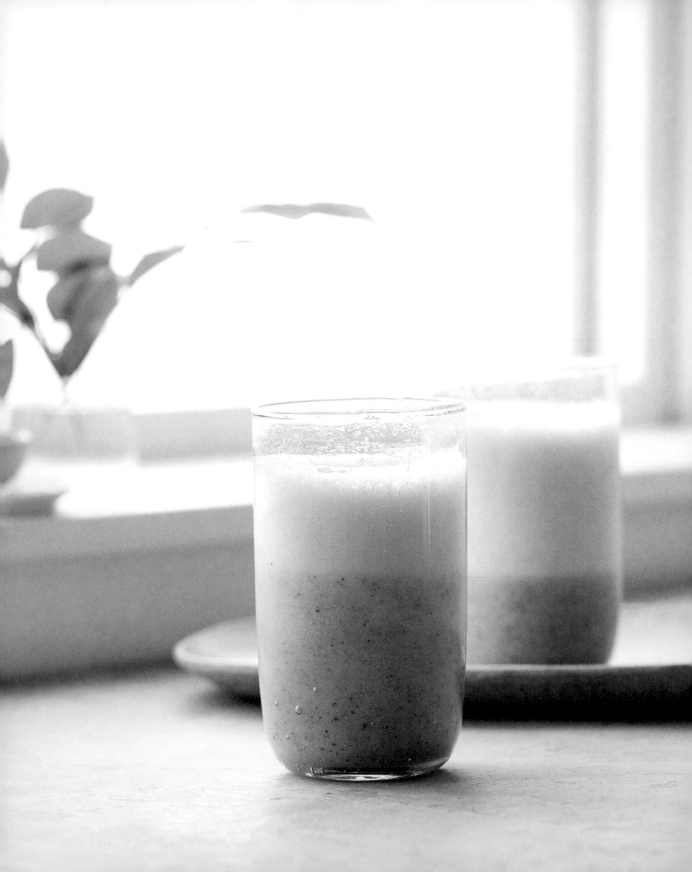

PINEAPPLE-MINT SMOOTHIE

Here's a refreshing smoothie to enjoy for a quick lunch. MAKES 1 SERVING

1½ cups coconut water

1½ cups frozen pineapple tidbits

1 scoop collagen peptides, optional

6 mint leaves

Stevia, to taste

2 to 3 ice cubes, optional

Put the coconut water, pineapple, collagen peptides, if using, mint leaves, and stevia in a blender. Process until thick and smooth (about 30 seconds), adding ice, if desired.

CALORIES: 193 | PROTEIN: 12G | FAT: 1G | CARBS: 36G | FIBER: 5.5G | NET CARBS: 30.5G

ROOT VEGETABLE SOUP

Sweet potato, parsnips, and carrots are combined in this hearty soup. It's just too good not to share with friends and family. How about at Thanksgiving dinner? MAKES 4 SERVINGS

1 tablespoon coconut oil

2 garlic cloves, chopped

1 large onion, quartered

6 cups bone broth or Vegetable Broth (page 346)

1 medium sweet potato, peeled and quartered

2 parsnips, cut into 1-to-2-inch pieces

2 large carrots, cut into 1-to-2-inch pieces

1 teaspoon fine sea salt

½ teaspoon freshly ground black pepper

¼ cup chopped parsley

Put the coconut oil and garlic in a large pot and cook over medium heat for 1 minute. Add the onion and cook, stirring, for 4 minutes. Add the broth, sweet potato, parsnips, carrots, salt, and pepper. Cook on medium heat for 10 minutes, then cover, reduce to medium-low, and simmer for 20 minutes.

Puree in a blender in batches so the soup doesn't overflow or use an immersion blender directly in the pot until the mixture is smooth and creamy. Pour into 4 bowls, garnish with parsley, and serve.

CALORIES: 242 | PROTEIN: 13G | FAT: 3.5G | CARBS: 30.5G | FIBER: 5G | NET CARBS: 25.5G

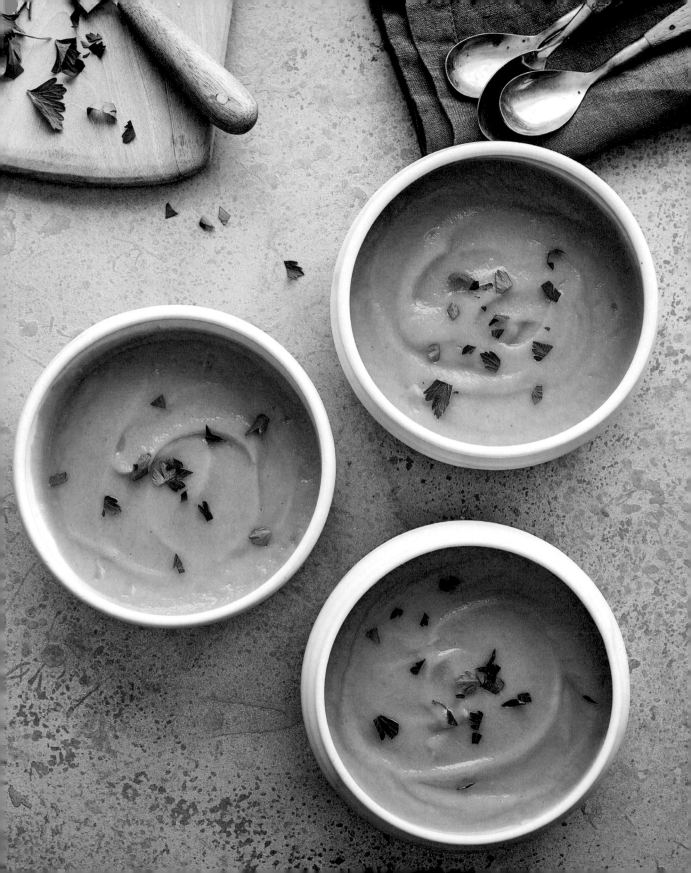

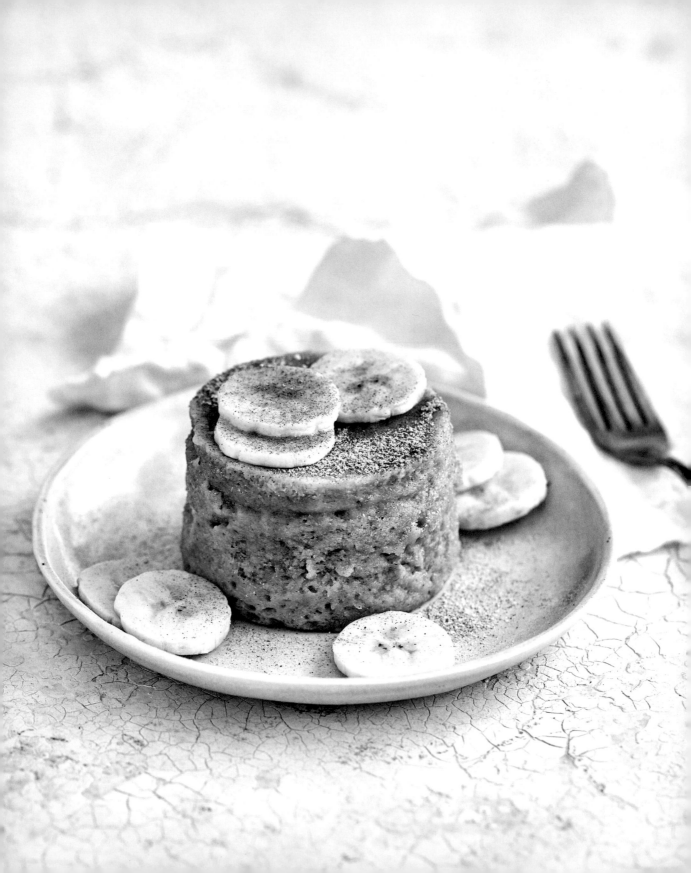

BANANA MUG CAKE

Here's your own individual banana cake microwaved and served in a mug. Kids love these, too. MAKES 1 SERVING

1 large organic egg

1 medium banana

3 tablespoons oat flour

2 tablespoons Swerve Sweetener Granular or coconut sugar

1 tablespoon nondairy milk

½ teaspoon aluminum-free baking powder

½ teaspoon pure vanilla extract

Pinch fine sea salt

Coconut oil cooking spray

1 teaspoon Swerve Sweetener Granular

¼ teaspoon ground cinnamon

Lightly whisk the egg in a small bowl. Slice half of the banana and reserve. Put the remaining half banana in the bowl with the egg and mash together. Add oat flour, Swerve, milk, baking powder, vanilla extract, and salt and stir well.

Coat a large, microwave-safe mug with cooking spray. Pour in the batter and microwave for about 2 minutes, until the cake is set. Invert the cake onto a plate and sprinkle on the Swerve and cinnamon. Top with reserved banana slices.

CALORIES: 256 | PROTEIN: 10G | FAT: 7G | CARBS: 39.5G | FIBER: 5G | NET CARBS: 34.5G

MINESTRONE

Beans and chickpeas are healthy, fiber-rich carbs that will keep you satisfied for hours. This soup is even better the next day when reheated. MAKES 4 SERVINGS, (8 CUPS)

3 tablespoons extra-virgin olive oil

1 small yellow onion, diced

4 large celery stalks, finely diced

2 large carrots, diced

2 garlic cloves, minced

3 cups Vegetable Broth (page 346)

1 28-ounce can fire-roasted tomatoes

1 cup canned white beans, rinsed and drained

1 cup canned chickpeas, rinsed and drained

1 teaspoon dried oregano

1 teaspoon dried thyme

3 cups rainbow chard or spinach leaves, chopped

1 teaspoon fine sea salt

½ teaspoon freshly ground black pepper

Add 1 tablespoon of the olive oil and the onions to a large pot over medium heat. Cook until the onions are soft and translucent, about 5 minutes.

Add the remaining oil, celery, carrots, and garlic and sauté for 5 minutes.

Add the broth, tomatoes, white beans, chickpeas, oregano, and thyme. Simmer uncovered for 5 minutes. Add the chard and cook for about 2 minutes, until wilted. Season with salt and pepper.

CALORIES: 318 | PROTEIN: 7G | FAT: 11G | CARBS: 42G | FIBER: 11G | NET CARBS: 31G

RED BEAN AND QUINOA CHILI

Healthy vegetables, filling beans, quinoa, and warming spices come together in this savory chili. If you don't have kidney beans, substitute black beans or another type. This is another great dish that can be doubled, portioned, and frozen for future meals. MAKES 4 SERVINGS (8 CUPS)

Two 15-ounce cans kidney beans, drained and rinsed

One 15-ounce can tomato sauce

One 14.5-ounce can diced tomatoes with juices

1 cup frozen organic corn

1 medium yellow onion, diced

1 cup Vegetable Broth (page 346) or bone broth

½ cup quinoa, rinsed

1 tablespoon ghee

1 tablespoon chili powder

2 teaspoons ground cumin

1 teaspoon fine sea salt

¼ teaspoon cayenne pepper, optional

Put the beans, tomato sauce, diced tomatoes, corn, onion, broth, quinoa, ghee, chili powder, cumin, salt, and cayenne pepper, if using, in a slow cooker or pressure cooker. Stir to combine.

If using a slow cooker, set to low for 4 hours. If using a pressure cooker, set to the "soup" setting. Stir well before serving.

CALORIES: 416 | PROTEIN: 20.5G | FAT: 6.5G | CARBS: 71.5G | FIBER: 15G | NET CARBS: 56.5G

SHEET PAN CHICKEN AND VEGETABLES

Roasting everything on a sheet pan is the true definition of a one-dish meal. The secret to success is to cut the chicken and vegetables to the same size and arrange them in a single layer on the sheet pans. MAKES 4 SERVINGS

¾ pound boneless, skinless organic chicken breasts, cut into 1-inch pieces

4 medium sweet potatoes, cut into 1-inch pieces

1 red bell pepper, seeded and cut into 1-inch pieces

1 orange bell pepper, seeded and cut into 1-inch pieces

1 small red onion, sliced

6 garlic cloves, sliced

Juice of 1 small lemon

1 teaspoon ground cumin

½ teaspoon fine sea salt

1½ tablespoons extra-virgin olive oil

Heat the oven to 375°F. Line 2 sheet pans with parchment paper.

Arrange the chicken, potatoes, bell peppers, onion, and garlic on the prepared pans. Drizzle the lemon juice over the chicken and vegetables. Season with the cumin and salt. Drizzle with the olive oil and bake for 25 minutes, until the chicken is cooked through and the vegetables are tender when pierced with a knife.

CALORIES: 310 | PROTEIN: 23G | FAT: 6.5G | CARBS: 39G | FIBER: 7G | NET CARBS: 32G

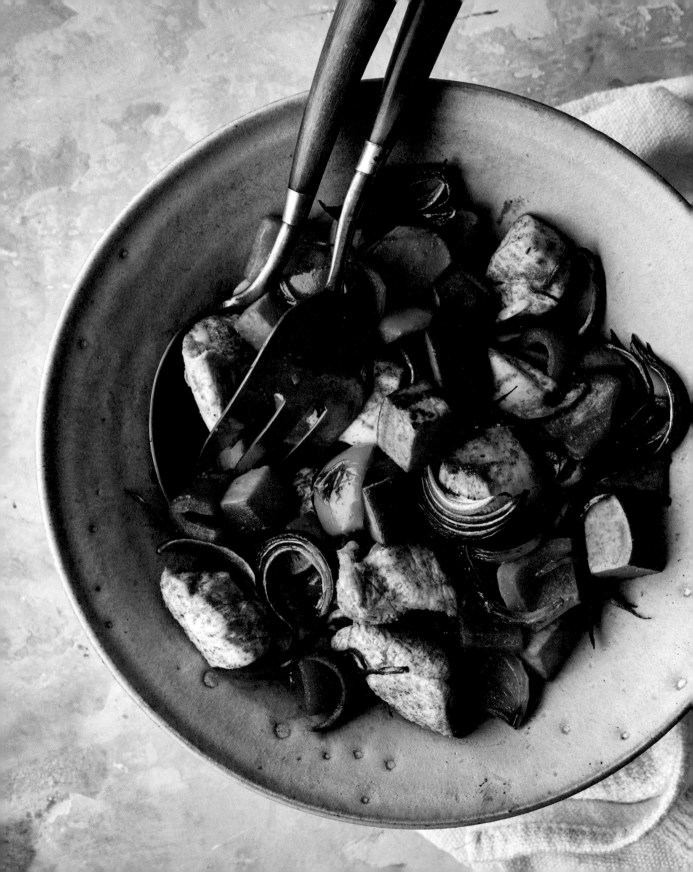

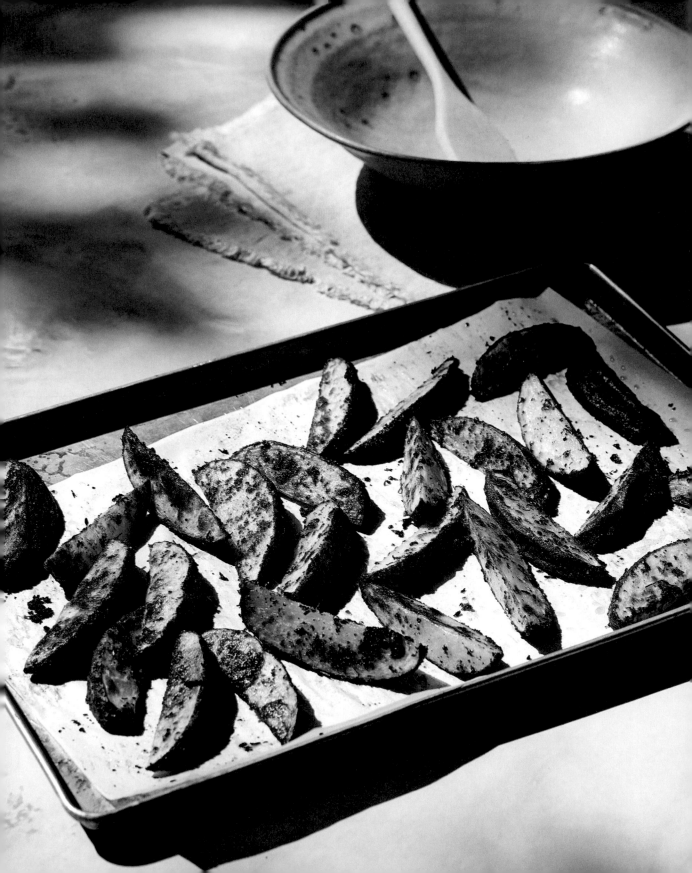

HERBED POTATO WEDGES

Cut-up potatoes are tossed with herbs and spices, then roasted until tender on the inside and crunchy on the outside. Pair them with a lean grilled steak, fish fillet, or chicken breast. MAKES 4 SERVINGS

5 medium russet potatoes

3 tablespoons extra-virgin olive oil

1 tablespoon dried parsley

1 teaspoon garlic powder

1 teaspoon sea salt

½ teaspoon onion powder

½ teaspoon freshly ground black pepper

Heat oven to 425°F. Line a sheet pan with parchment paper.

Cut each potato into 1-inch thick wedges and place in a large bowl. Add olive oil, parsley, garlic powder, salt, onion powder, and pepper and toss well to coat. Arrange the wedges in a single layer on the prepared pan. Bake for about 30 minutes, until wedges are soft on the inside and crisp on the outside.

CALORIES: 229 | PROTEIN: 5G | FAT: 10G | CARBS: 33G | FIBER: 4G | NET CARBS: 29G

FLAXSEED–CINNAMON MUFFINS

Yes, when muffins are made with healthy ingredients, they contribute to your fat-burning goals. You can enjoy these with a cinnamon icing or an almond butter drizzle, or on their own if you prefer. It's your program, so it's all up to you. MAKES 12 SERVINGS

MUFFINS:

2 cups ground flaxseed

½ cup Swerve Sweetener Confectioners

3 tablespoons ground cinnamon

1 tablespoon aluminum-free baking powder

½ teaspoon sea salt

5 large organic eggs

½ cup melted coconut oil or avocado oil

2 teaspoons pure vanilla extract

CINNAMON BUN ICING:

⅓ cup coconut butter

2 teaspoons MCT oil

2 tablespoons Swerve Sweetener Confectioners

1 teaspoon pure vanilla extract

1 teaspoon ground cinnamon

ALMOND BUTTER DRIZZLE:

2 tablespoons natural, salted almond butter

2 tablespoons coconut oil

2 tablespoons Swerve Sweetener Confectioners

Heat oven to 350°F. Line a 12-count muffin pan with paper liners.

To make the muffins: Whisk together the flaxseed, Swerve, cinnamon, baking powder, and salt in a bowl. Place the eggs, coconut oil, and vanilla in a blender with ½ cup room-temperature water and blend on high speed for about 30 seconds, until foamy. Pour the egg mixture over the flaxseed mixture and stir well with a spatula just until incorporated. The batter will be fluffy. Let sit for 3 minutes. Divide the batter among the paper liners. Bake for 17 to 19 minutes, until a toothpick inserted in the middle of a muffin comes out clean. Turn the muffins out on a rack and let cool for at least 20 minutes.

To make the icing: Place the coconut butter and MCT oil in a microwave-safe bowl. Microwave for about 30 seconds, until melted and smooth. Stir in the Swerve, vanilla extract, and cinnamon. Use a knife to spread the icing on each muffin.

To make the drizzle: Place the almond butter, coconut oil, and Swerve in a microwave-safe bowl. Microwave for 20 seconds. Drizzle on top of each muffin.

MUFFIN WITH CINNAMON BUN ICING: CALORIES: 242 | PROTEIN: 7G | FAT: 22G | CARBS: 7G | FIBER: 6.5G | NET CARBS: 0.5G

MUFFIN WITH ALMOND BUTTER DRIZZLE: CALORIES: 226 | PROTEIN: 6.5G | FAT: 21G | CARBS: 6.5G | FIBER: 6G | NET CARBS: 0.5G

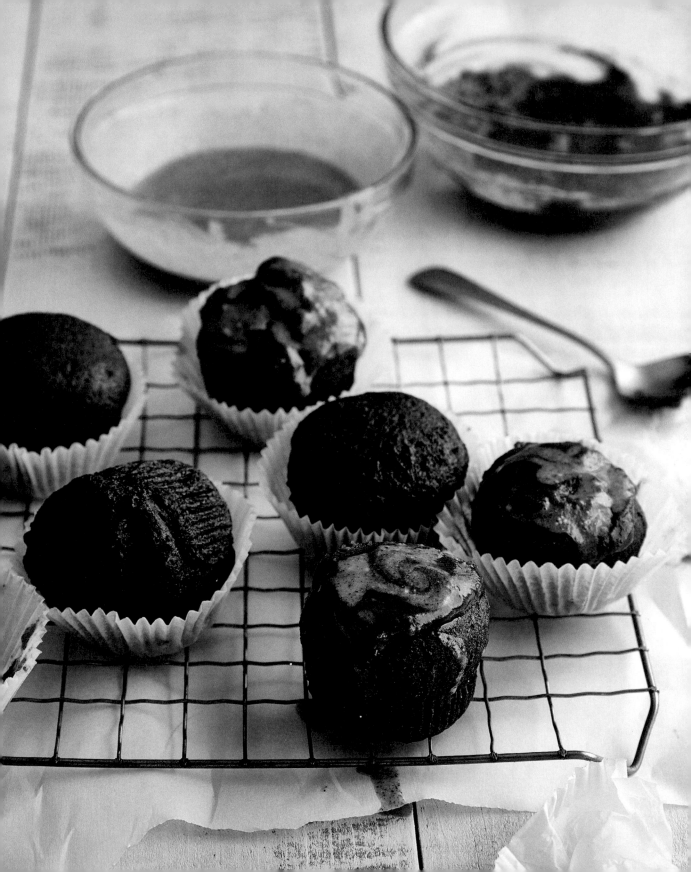

EGGS AND GREENS

Fried eggs and sliced avocado sit on top of cooked broccolini and spinach for a balanced meal rich in protein and healthy carbs. MAKES 2 SERVINGS

2 tablespoons ghee

½ bunch broccolini, chopped

2 garlic cloves, minced

2 cups baby spinach

½ teaspoon sea salt

¼ teaspoon freshly ground black pepper

4 large organic eggs

1 small avocado, peeled, pitted, and sliced

Melt 1 tablespoon of the ghee in a large skillet over medium-high heat. Add broccolini and garlic, stirring occasionally, until softened, about 4 minutes.

Add the spinach, salt, and pepper and stir to combine. Remove from the skillet and cover to keep warm.

Heat remaining ghee in the same skillet. Crack the eggs into the skillet and cook sunny side up or over easy.

Divide the greens between 2 plates. Top each with 2 eggs and some sliced avocado.

CALORIES: 435 | PROTEIN: 18G | FAT: 32.5G | CARBS: 15G | FIBER: 7G | NET CARBS: 8G

PIZZA MUFFINS

Slices of ham or turkey take the place of pizza dough in these little cups. When you line the muffin tins, drape the ham or turkey so there are no gaps or holes, or the egg mixture will slip through. Alternatively, chop the ham, whisk everything together and pour into muffin cups and proceed as directed. MAKES 2 SERVINGS

Coconut oil cooking spray

4 thin slices organic ham or turkey

2 large organic eggs

4 large organic egg yolks

½ cup shredded mozzarella

10 basil leaves, chopped

1 tablespoon tomato paste

1 tablespoon MCT oil

1 teaspoon Italian seasoning

¼ teaspoon fine sea salt

Heat the oven to 350°F. Coat 4 muffin cups with cooking spray or use silicone muffin cups. Press 1 slice of ham into each well.

Whisk together the eggs, yolks, ¼ cup of the mozzarella, basil, tomato paste, MCT oil, Italian seasoning, and salt in a bowl.

Divide the mixture among the four muffin cups and top with the remaining mozzarella. Bake for 22 to 25 minutes, until the filling is set.

CALORIES: 358 | PROTEIN: 24G | FAT: 27.5G | CARBS: 5G | FIBER: 0G | NET CARBS: 5G

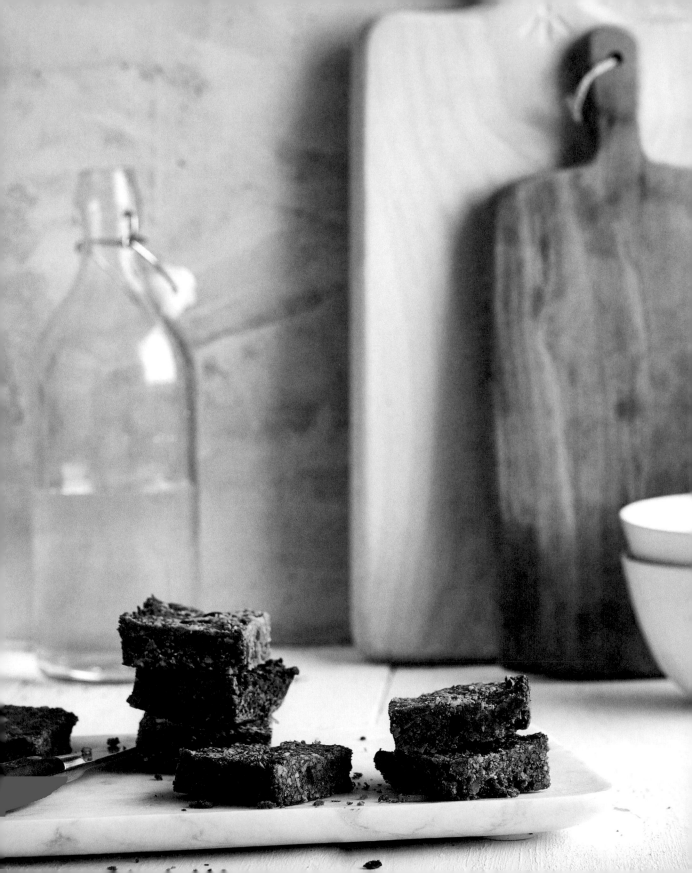

CHOCOLATE CHIP "GRANOLA" SQUARES

You won't believe how good—and good for you—these treats are. Nuts, coconut flakes, chocolate chips, and almond butter make them the perfect snack when you want something sweet.

Lily's is our go-to brand for sugar-free chocolate chips. If you cannot find stevia-sweetened chocolate, use 85% dark chocolate and add extra sweetener.

MAKES 16 SERVINGS

1 cup almonds

1 cup pecans

1 cup unsweetened coconut flakes

5 tablespoons Swerve Sweetener Confectioners

¼ cup melted coconut oil

¼ cup unsweetened almond butter

1 large organic egg, lightly beaten

3 tablespoons sugar-free chocolate chips

2 teaspoons ground cinnamon

1 teaspoon pure vanilla extract

¼ teaspoon fine sea salt

Heat the oven to 350°F.

Put the almonds and pecans in a food processor. Pulse several times to coarsely chop. Transfer to a bowl.

Add the coconut, Swerve, coconut oil, almond butter, and egg to the ground nuts and stir. Add the chocolate chips, cinnamon, vanilla extract, and salt and combine well. Pour the batter into an 8x8-inch square baking dish and gently press into an even layer. Bake for about 18 minutes, until the edges are golden brown. Cool and cut into 16 squares. Refrigerate in an airtight container for up to 2 weeks.

CALORIES: 204 | PROTEIN: 4G | FAT: 19G | CARBS: 6G | FIBER: 3G | NET CARBS: 3

CAULIFLOWER FRIED RICE

Cauliflower rice and other vegetables are stir-fried, then tossed with scrambled eggs. For a final touch, sliced green onions and sesame seeds are sprinkled on top. MAKES 4 SERVINGS

2 tablespoons coconut oil

½ small yellow onion, diced

1 medium green or red bell pepper, seeded and diced

1 cup sliced mushrooms

1 garlic clove, minced

5 cups uncooked cauliflower rice

3 tablespoons coconut aminos

2 tablespoons toasted sesame oil or extra-virgin olive oil

Coconut oil cooking spray

4 large organic eggs, lightly beaten

½ teaspoon fine sea salt

¼ teaspoon black pepper

2 green onions, sliced

1 tablespoon toasted sesame seeds

Heat 1 tablespoon of the coconut oil over medium heat in a large skillet. Add the onion and cook for 3 to 5 minutes.

Add the bell pepper, mushrooms, and garlic. Cook for 5 minutes, stirring frequently.

Add the remaining coconut oil and the cauliflower rice and cook for 5 to 7 minutes, until tender. Stir in the coconut aminos and sesame oil.

While the cauliflower rice cooks, scramble the eggs in a separate skillet coated with cooking spray. Using a spatula, add the eggs to the cauliflower and stir to combine, breaking up the eggs as you stir. Season with salt and pepper. Divide among 4 bowls and garnish with green onions and sesame seeds.

CALORIES: 283 | PROTEIN: 12G | FAT: 20.5G | CARBS: 15G | FIBER: 5G | NET CARBS: 10G

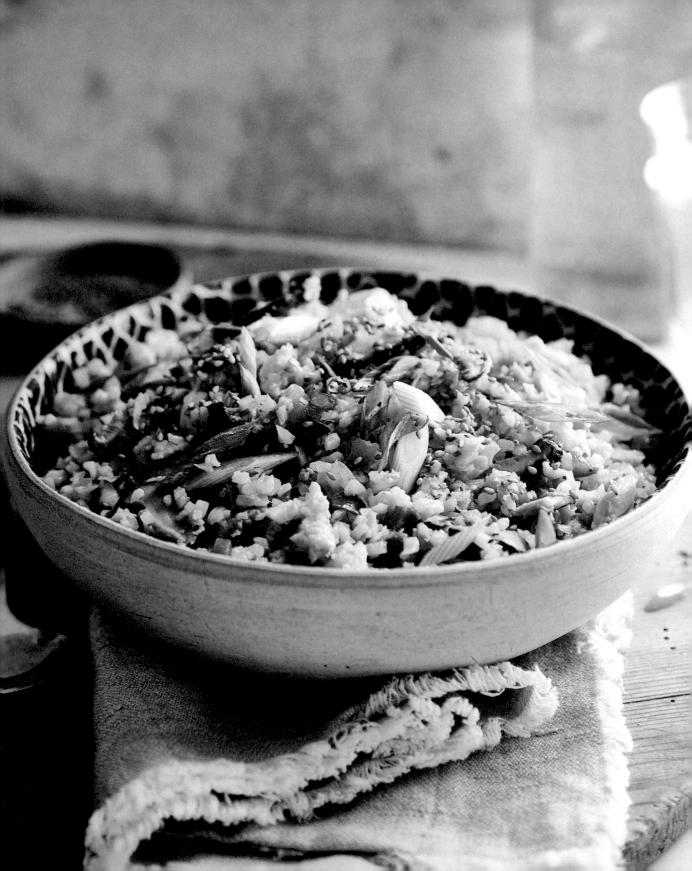

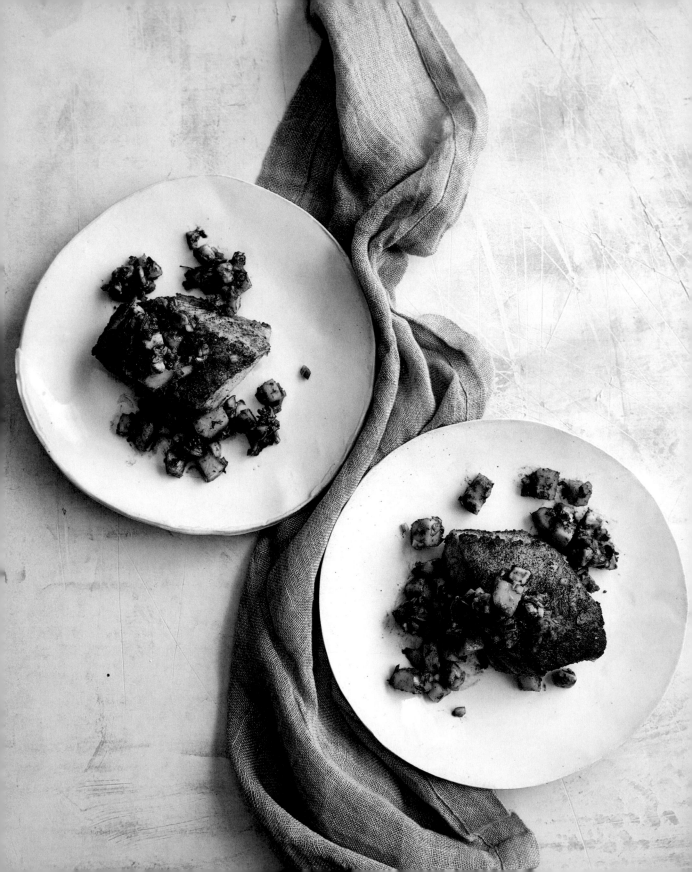

SEA BASS WITH MANGO SALSA

Fish and fruit always make a great pairing, especially when a meaty fish like sea bass or halibut is topped with a colorful mango-avocado salsa. Red onion, lime juice, and a bit of jalapeño add more layers of flavor. MAKES 4 SERVINGS

SALSA:

½ cup coarsely chopped cilantro leaves

½ mango, peeled and diced

1 large avocado, peeled, pitted, and diced

¼ cup diced red onion

2 tablespoons extra-virgin olive oil

1 tablespoon fresh lime juice

½ medium jalapeño, seeded and minced

1 teaspoon chili powder

½ teaspoon fine sea salt

FISH:

Four 3-ounce sea bass or halibut fillets

1 teaspoon sea salt

1 teaspoon paprika

¼ teaspoon freshly ground black pepper

2 tablespoons ghee

To make the salsa: Combine the cilantro, mango, avocado, onion, olive oil, lime juice, jalapeño, chili powder, and salt in a bowl. Mix well and set aside.

To make the fish: Season the sea bass fillets with the salt, paprika, and pepper. Heat the ghee over medium-high heat in a skillet until shimmering. Put the fillets in the skillet in a single layer, skin side up, and cook about 3 minutes. Using a spatula, turn the fillets, turn off the heat, and allow the fish to finish cooking until just flaky, about 2 minutes.

Divide the fish among 4 plates and spoon the salsa on top.

CALORIES: 311 | PROTEIN: 17G | FAT: 23G | CARBS: 9G | FIBER: 3G | NET CARBS: 6G

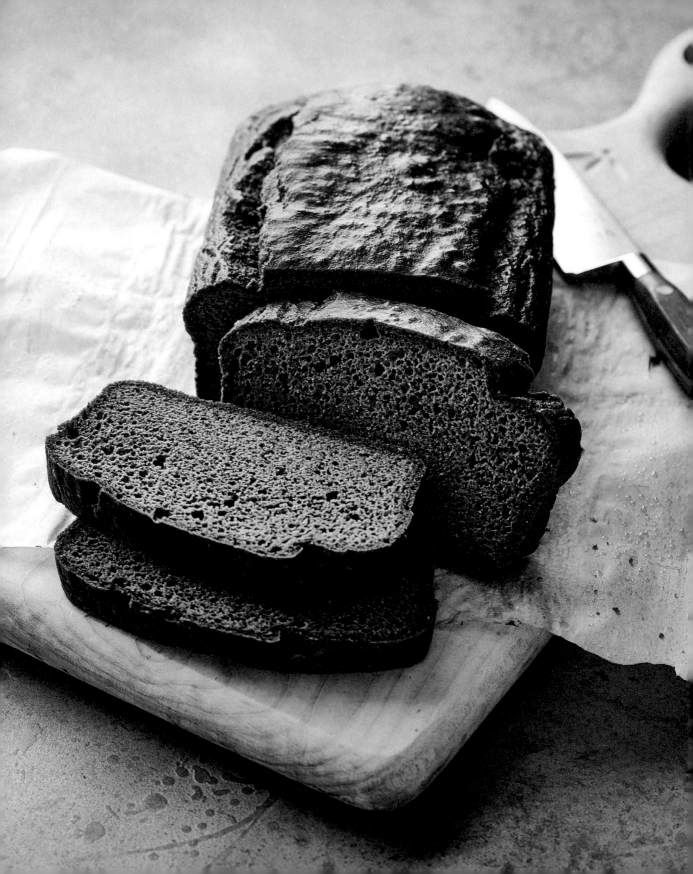

CHAPTER 13

BASIC RECIPES

These are the salsas, dressings, snacks, and other condiments that you will use again and again to add flavor to many of the recipes in this book or to those that you create yourself. Condiments, breads, and tortillas on market shelves are loaded with sugar and gluten, as well as preservatives and other additives to make them shelf stable. Instead of buying those, make these staples and keep them on hand, ready to use.

GARLIC-INFUSED OLIVE OIL

This is perfect on salads or with grilled fish, chicken, and vegetables, and unlike many recipes that contain garlic, infused olive oil is safe for those following a low-FODMAP diet. You can also use this method to infuse olive oil with herbs. Note: This and other infused oils will keep for up to one week in the refrigerator. Bring to room temperature before using. MAKES 16 SERVINGS (1 CUP)

12 garlic cloves, halved lengthwise

1 cup extra-virgin olive oil

Heat the oven to 275°F. Toss the garlic with the olive oil in a small baking dish. Cover and bake for 45 minutes, until garlic is lightly browned.

Remove from oven and, when cool, discard the garlic. Pour the oil into a glass jar and seal. Refrigerate for up to 1 week.

CALORIES: 119 | PROTEIN: 0G | FAT: 13.5G | CARBS: 0G | FIBER: 0G | NET CARBS: 0G

SALSA

Salsa is guacamole's BFF—best friend forever. They are almost inseparable but also shine on their own. Stir a spoonful of salsa into a bowl of soup, or use it as a salad dressing, a sandwich spread, or a dip with some raw vegetables. If you like your guacamole salsa spicier, add more jalapeño.

MAKES 8¼ - CUP SERVINGS

1 cup diced canned tomatoes, drained

1 cup cherry tomatoes, quartered

½ cup minced red onion

¼ cup chopped cilantro leaves

2 tablespoons fresh lime juice

2 garlic cloves, minced

1 tablespoon Taco Seasoning (page 333)

1 medium jalapeño, seeded and minced

½ teaspoon fine sea salt

Put canned tomatoes, cherry tomatoes, onion, cilantro, lime juice, garlic, taco seasoning, jalapeño, and salt into a blender or food processor. Pulse just a few times so the salsa is a little chunky, rather than smooth.

CALORIES: 20 | PROTEIN: 0G | FAT: 0G | CARBS: 4.5G | FIBER: 0.5G | NET CARBS: 4G

GUACAMOLE

There are endless uses for guacamole. Add a spoonful to accompany eggs or grilled fish. Mix a little into salads. Guacamole is the one condiment that is best when freshly made, rather than prepared ahead and refrigerated. MAKES 6 SERVINGS (ABOUT 1½ CUPS)

2 medium avocados, peeled, pitted, and sliced

¼ cup diced red onion

¼ cup diced tomato

1 tablespoon fresh lime juice

1 tablespoon Taco Seasoning (page 333)

Put the avocados, onion, tomato, lime juice, and taco seasoning in a bowl and mash with a fork until creamy.

CALORIES: 99 | PROTEIN: 1G | FAT: 9G | CARBS: 6G | FIBER: 4G | NET CARBS: 2G

BUFFALO WING SAUCE

There are several brands of wing sauce on the market, but most of them are processed, and some may contain corn syrup or other unnecessary ingredients. It's easy to make your own delicious sauce to smear on chicken and sweet potatoes before cooking. MAKES 14 SERVINGS (ABOUT ¾ CUP)

½ cup ghee

⅓ cup hot sauce

1 teaspoon ground ginger

½ teaspoon garlic powder

½ teaspoon sea salt

Melt the ghee in a medium saucepan over low heat. Add the hot sauce, ginger, garlic powder, and salt. Cook, stirring occasionally, for 5 minutes. If not using immediately, refrigerate in a glass jar for up to 1 week. Reheat before using, as this sauce will solidify at room temperature.

CALORIES: 63 | PROTEIN: 0G | FAT: 7G | CARBS: 0G | FIBER: 0G | NET CARBS: 0G

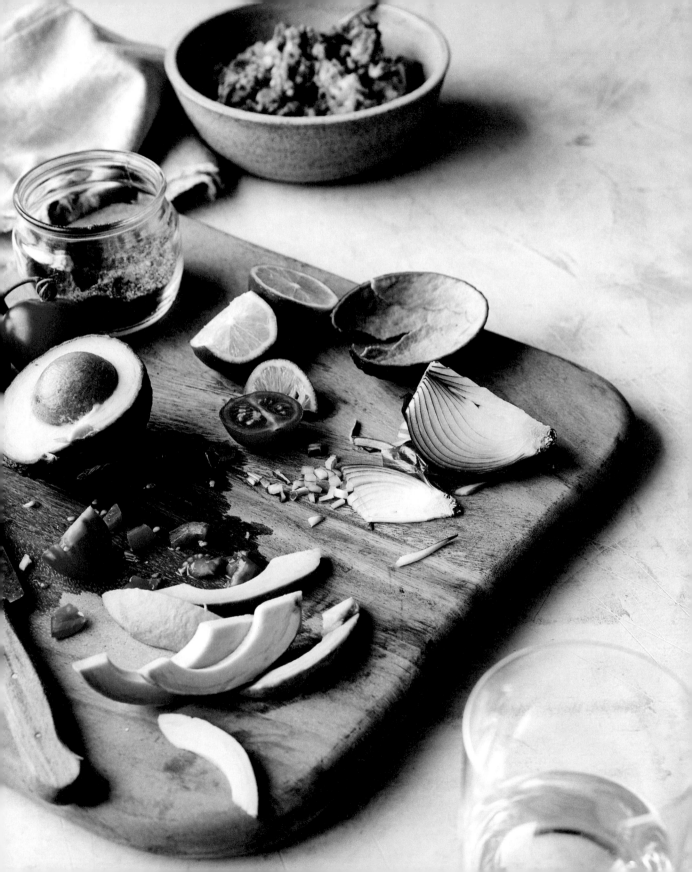

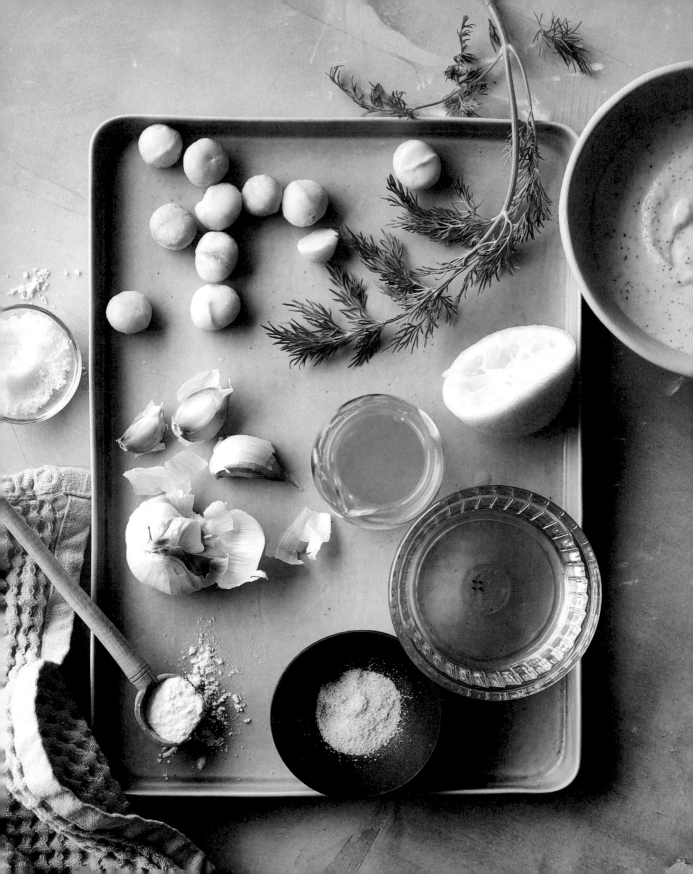

MACADAMIA RANCH DRESSING

A versatile, rich dressing that can be used on salads, with vegetables, or as a sauce with chicken or fish. The sweetener is needed to balance the acidity. Start with ½ tablespoon and then add more, if desired. MAKES ABOUT 10 SERVINGS (1⅓ CUPS)

¾ cup unsalted macadamia nuts

3 tablespoons avocado oil

2 tablespoons fresh lemon juice

2 tablespoons apple cider vinegar

½ to 1 tablespoon Swerve Sweetener Confectioners

1 garlic clove

2 teaspoons onion powder

1 teaspoon sea salt

3 sprigs fresh dill

Put the nuts, oil, lemon juice, vinegar, Swerve, garlic, onion powder, and salt in a blender with ½ cup water and blend on high until creamy and smooth. Add the dill and pulse to combine. Use immediately or refrigerate for up to 2 days.

CALORIES: 114 | PROTEIN: 0.8G | FAT: 11G | CARBS: 2G | FIBER: 1G | NET CARBS: 1G

PESTO

Nutritional yeast is used in place of cheese in my version of pesto. Toss with spiral-cut vegetable noodles or cauliflower rice for a side or main dish. MAKES ABOUT 10 1-TABLESPOON SERVINGS (⅔ CUP)

2 cups packed basil leaves

½ cup extra-virgin olive oil

½ cup walnuts

2 tablespoons nutritional yeast

2 garlic cloves, chopped

1 tablespoon lemon juice

½ teaspoon fine sea salt

¼ teaspoon freshly ground black pepper

Put the basil, oil, walnuts, nutritional yeast, garlic, lemon juice, salt, and pepper into a mini food processor. Process until nearly smooth, with some texture remaining from the walnuts.

Store in a glass jar for up to 3 days in the refrigerator.

CALORIES: 147 | PROTEIN: 1.5G | FAT: 15G | CARBS: 1.5G | FIBER: 0.5G | NET CARBS: 1G

LOW-CARB BARBECUE SAUCE

If you prefer a thinner sauce, add an additional ¼ cup water while the sauce is simmering. MAKES 16 SERVINGS (2 CUPS)

¼ cup apple cider vinegar

¼ cup Swerve Sweetener Granular

2 tablespoons balsamic vinegar

2 tablespoons unsalted butter

1 6-ounce can tomato paste

1 teaspoon garlic powder

1 teaspoon onion powder

1 teaspoon dried mustard

1 teaspoon smoked paprika

1 teaspoon sea salt

¼ teaspoon liquid smoke, optional

¼ teaspoon cayenne pepper, optional

Whisk together all the ingredients plus ½ cup water in a saucepan over medium-low heat. Once the butter has melted, bring to a low boil, then immediately reduce heat and simmer for about 10 minutes, until thickened. Use immediately or refrigerate for up to 5 days.

CALORIES: 24 | PROTEIN: 0.75G | FAT: 1G | CARBS: 2.5G | FIBER: 0G | NET CARBS: 2.5G

BETTER THAN KETCHUP

My ketchup is simple to put together and goes with all kinds of dishes, including burgers, Chicken Tenders (page 225), and Herbed Potato Wedges (page 311). MAKES 24 SERVINGS (1½ CUPS)

4 ounces (85 g) sun-dried tomatoes, not packed in oil

⅔ cup Garlic-Infused Olive Oil (page 324)

2 tablespoons apple cider vinegar

½ teaspoon fine sea salt

½ teaspoon ground black pepper

¼ teaspoon ground cloves

5 drops liquid stevia

Put ¾ cup water in a saucepan and bring to a boil. Put the tomatoes in a heat-safe bowl and cover with the boiling water. Let sit for 10 minutes.

Put the oil, vinegar, salt, pepper, cloves, and stevia into a blender. Pour ½ cup of the tomato soaking liquid into the blender, then strain the tomatoes and discard the remaining liquid. Put the tomatoes into the blender. Blend the mixture until smooth, about 1 minute.

Refrigerate in an airtight container for up to 5 days.

CALORIES: 63 | PROTEIN: 0G | FAT: 6G | CARBS: 2G | FIBER: 0G | NET CARBS: 2G

TACO SEASONING

Most packaged taco seasonings contain MSG and other chemicals that can cause inflammation. But you can make your own using the many organic herbs and spices available in health food stores and online. Spices lose their potency after 6 months; if any of your spices are that old, toss and replace them with fresh ones. Keep this spice blend on hand to use with all kinds of dishes when you want a flavor kick. MAKES ABOUT 1½ CUPS

5 tablespoons chili powder

3 tablespoons ground cumin

2½ tablespoons garlic powder

2 tablespoons sea salt

2 tablespoons paprika

2 tablespoons black pepper

2 tablespoons onion powder

2 tablespoons oregano

1 tablespoon ground turmeric

1½ teaspoons Swerve Sweetener Granular

¼ teaspoon cayenne pepper, optional

Combine all of the ingredients in a large glass jar. Cover and shake well to combine. This seasoning will keep at room temperature for several months. Be sure to shake the jar before using.

CALORIES: 6 | PROTEIN: 0G | FAT: 0G | CARBS: 0G | FIBER: 0G | NET CARBS: 0G

AVOCADO-BASIL SPREAD

Spoon some of this on chicken or scrambled eggs. The spread is used instead of mayonnaise in the Avocado-Basil Deviled Eggs on page 211. MAKES 8 SERVINGS (1 CUP)

2 small avocados, peeled and pitted

½ cup fresh basil leaves

¼ cup MCT oil

¼ cup hulled hemp seeds

2 tablespoons white balsamic vinegar

1½ teaspoons onion powder

½ teaspoon garlic powder

½ teaspoon fine sea salt

¼ teaspoon ground black pepper

Put all of the ingredients in a blender. Process on medium speed until the mixture is thick and smooth, about 20 seconds. If not using immediately, refrigerate in a glass jar for up to 1 day, stirring well before serving.

CALORIES: 129 | PROTEIN: 2G | FAT: 12G | CARBS: 4G | FIBER: 1.5G | NET CARBS: 2.5G

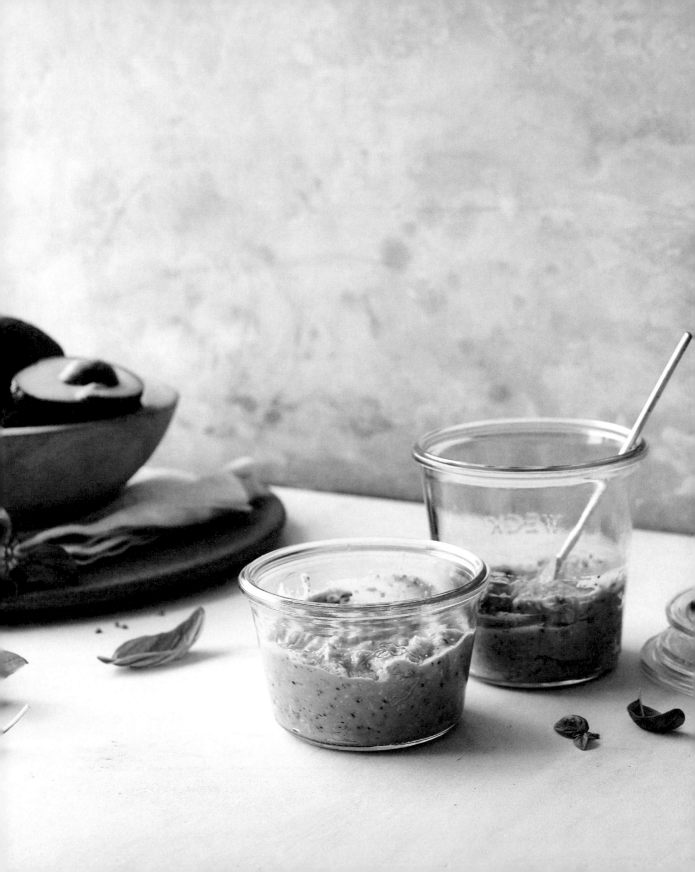

SMART ALMOND BUTTER

Vanilla beans come from a specific variety of orchid. Because growing them requires care and time, the beans are the world's second-most expensive spice after saffron. Like saffron, the beans vary in quality and price, so choose wisely. Each bean contains more than 2,000 flavorful little seeds. To collect those seeds, place the bean on a cutting surface. Use the tip of a paring knife to cut the bean lengthwise. Use the knife's tip to scrape the seeds loose from the pod. Discard the pod. MAKES 12 SERVINGS

2 cups raw almonds

½ cup MCT oil

1 tablespoon Swerve Sweetener Confectioners

2 teaspoons ground cinnamon

1 vanilla bean pod, scraped

Pinch fine sea salt

Put the almonds in a food processor and process until smooth and the consistency of nut butter, about 5 minutes. Add the MCT oil, Swerve, cinnamon, vanilla bean seeds, and sea salt and process for 1 minute. Serve immediately, or refrigerate in an airtight container.

CALORIES: 203 | PROTEIN: 4G | FAT: 19G | CARBS: 4G | FIBER: 3G | NET CARBS: 1G

LOW-CARB PIZZA CRUST

Try my Low-Carb Barbecued Chicken Pizza recipe on page 222.

MAKES 8 SERVINGS

2¼ cups almond flour

2 tablespoons Garlic-Infused Olive Oil (page 324)

2 large organic eggs

1 teaspoon garlic powder

1 teaspoon dried basil

½ teaspoon sea salt

Coconut oil cooking spray

Heat the oven to 350°F. Line a sheet pan with parchment paper.

Put the flour, oil, eggs, garlic powder, basil, and salt in a large bowl. Stir until the mixture holds together and a dough forms. The dough should be firm, yet easy to roll out. If the dough is too soft, wrap in plastic wrap and place it in the freezer for 10 minutes.

Spray 2 pieces of waxed paper with cooking spray. Place the dough in the center of one piece of paper and cover with the other. Using a rolling pin, roll the dough into an 11-to-12-inch circle.

Turn the dough onto the prepared sheet pan. Use a fork to poke some holes in the dough.

Bake for 15 to 17 minutes, until dough is cooked through and the edges are light brown.

CALORIES: 227 | PROTEIN: 8G | FAT: 20G | CARBS: 7G | FIBER: 3G | NET CARBS: 4G

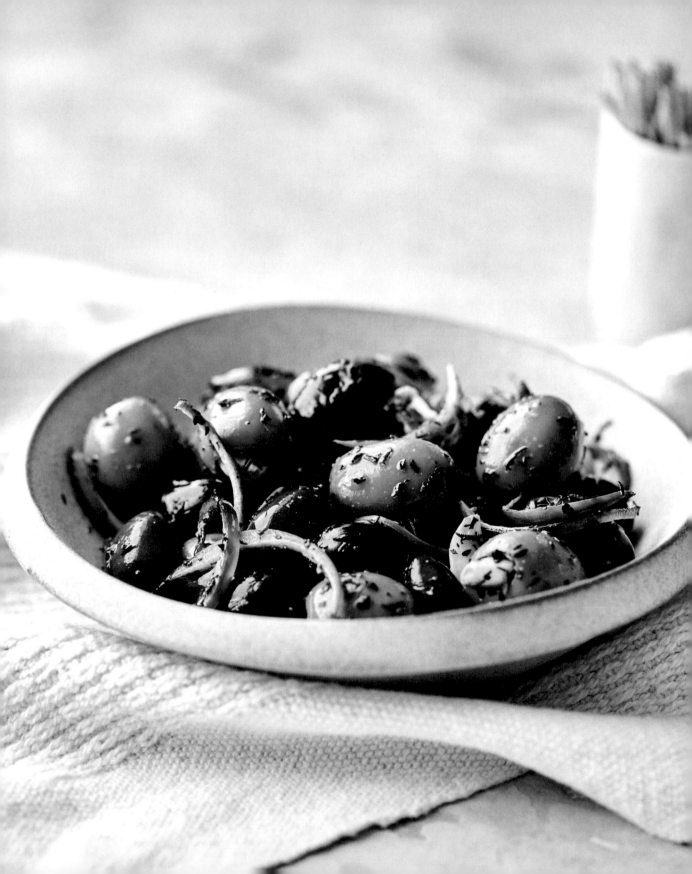

ROASTED OLIVES

The range in color of the olives, from pale green to deep purple to dark brown, makes this snack visually appealing. The color of the olives depends on how ripe they were when picked and how they were cured. Green olives are picked before ripening, and black olives are picked once ripe. All raw olives are bitter and inedible. Once cured, they are packed in salt, water, or brine. Serve these olives in your most beautiful bowl. MAKES 8 SERVINGS

2 cups pitted kalamata olives

1 cup pimento-stuffed green olives

1 cup garlic-stuffed green olives

1 cup black olives

¼ cup extra-virgin olive oil

4 garlic cloves, cut into slivers

1 medium red onion, thinly sliced

1 tablespoon dried basil

1 tablespoon dried thyme

¼ teaspoon freshly ground black pepper

Heat the oven to 425°F. Line a sheet pan with parchment paper.

Put the olives, oil, garlic, onion, basil, thyme, and pepper in a bowl and toss to combine.

Arrange the olives in a single layer on the prepared pan and roast for 10 minutes. Toss, then roast for another 10 minutes. Serve warm or at room temperature. Refrigerate any leftovers in a covered dish for up to 3 days. Bring the olives to room temperature before serving.

CALORIES: 290 | PROTEIN: 0G | FAT: 29G | CARBS: 6G | FIBER: 2G | NET CARBS: 4G

ALMOND FLOUR TORTILLAS

Light, airy, and flexible, these tortillas make great wraps or can be filled with eggs for breakfast burritos. MAKES 10 SERVINGS

10 large organic eggs

⅓ cup almond flour

3 tablespoons tapioca starch

1½ tablespoons coconut flour

1 teaspoon garlic powder

½ teaspoon fine sea salt

5 teaspoons ghee

Put the eggs, almond flour, tapioca starch, coconut flour, garlic powder, and sea salt in a blender and process for 10 seconds.

Heat a medium skillet over medium heat. Add ½ teaspoon of the ghee and swirl to coat the pan as the ghee melts.

Pour ⅓ cup of batter into the skillet and swirl to cover about ¾ of the bottom, as if you were making a crepe. Cook for about 2 minutes, until the edges begin to pull away from the sides of the skillet. Using a spatula, flip the tortilla and cook for about 1 minute, until golden. Transfer to a sheet of waxed paper. Repeat with ghee and batter until all of the batter is used up. About every third tortilla, blend the batter again for 5 seconds so the coconut flour doesn't sink to the bottom.

To store the tortillas, put them between sheets of waxed paper in a plastic bag. Seal the bag and refrigerate up to 3 days.

CALORIES: 130 | PROTEIN: 7G | FAT: 9.5G | CARBS: 4G | FIBER: 1G | NET CARBS: 3G

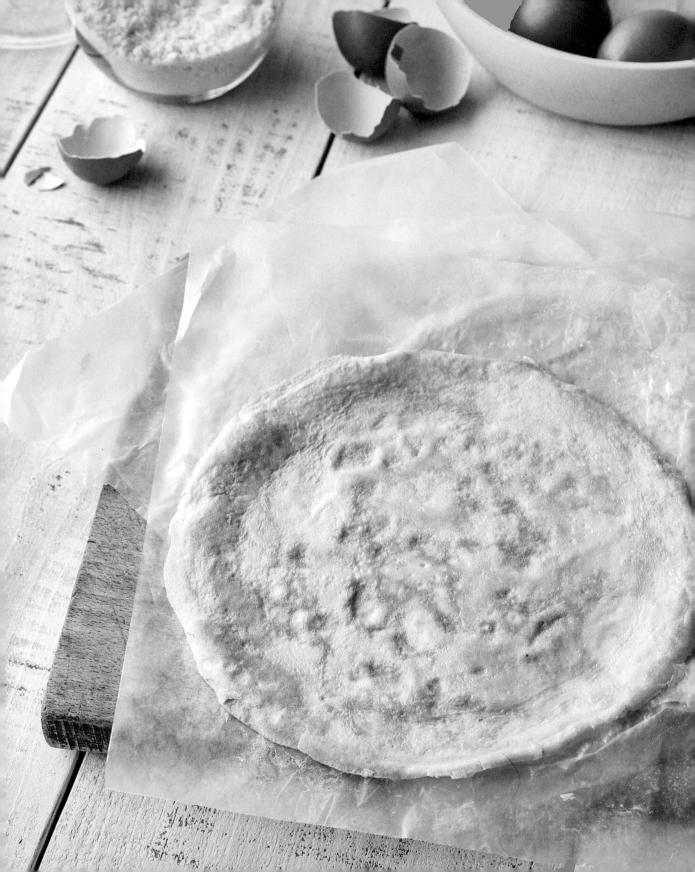

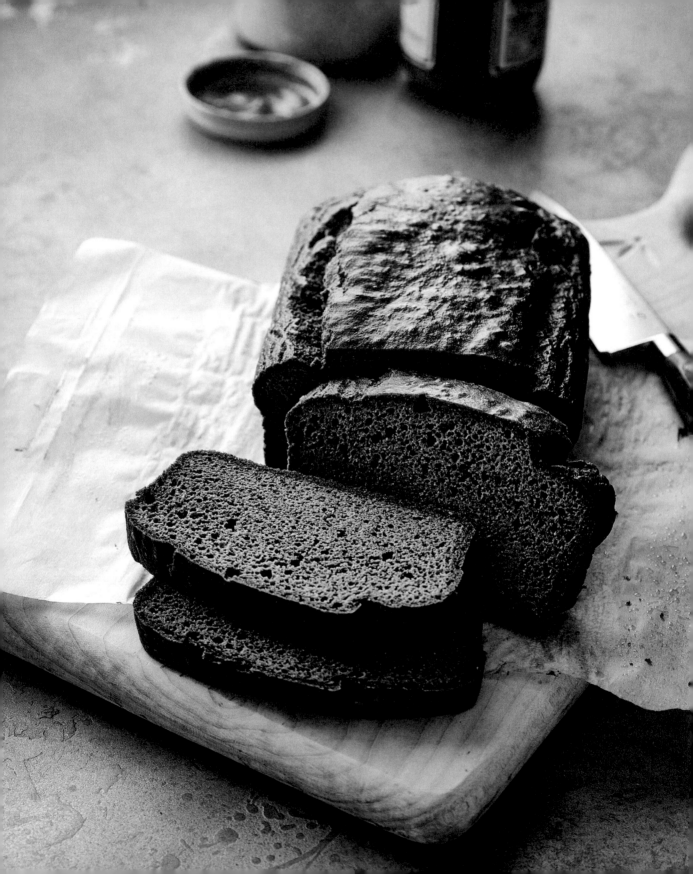

BLENDER BREAD

Once baked and sliced, this gluten-free bread can be toasted for breakfast and sandwiches. It's all put together in a blender, and you don't have to wait for the bread to rise. MAKES ABOUT 18 SERVINGS

Coconut oil cooking spray

4 large organic eggs

1 cup liquid organic egg whites

1 cup natural roasted-almond butter

½ cup coconut flour

2 tablespoons nondairy milk

1½ tablespoons apple cider vinegar

2 teaspoons baking soda

8 drops liquid vanilla stevia

¼ teaspoon sea salt

Heat the oven to 325°F. Line a 9x5-inch loaf pan with parchment paper. Spray the parchment paper with cooking oil.

Place the eggs, egg whites, and almond butter in a blender. Process on low, then turn up the speed to medium until the mixture is combined, about 1 minute. Add the coconut flour, milk, apple cider vinegar, baking soda, liquid stevia, and salt and process for 20 seconds.

Pour the batter into the prepared loaf pan. Bake for 50 to 55 minutes, until a toothpick inserted in several places comes out clean. Cool on a wire rack for 5 to 10 minutes, then turn the loaf out of the pan and cool on the rack.

CALORIES: 123 | PROTEIN: 6.5G | FAT: 9G | CARBS: 6G | FIBER: 3G | NET CARBS: 3G

CAULIFLOWER RICE

What did we eat before there was cauliflower rice? While it can now be found in markets everywhere, it's super easy to make at home. MAKES ABOUT 3¾ CUPS, 4 SERVINGS

1 large head cauliflower

1 teaspoon fine sea salt

½ teaspoon freshly ground black pepper

½ teaspoon garlic powder, optional

Heat oven to 400°F.

Separate cauliflower florets and remove large stems. Chop florets into 1-inch pieces and add to a large food processor. Pulse until it resembles long-grain rice. Spread onto a large sheet pan. Season with salt, pepper, and garlic powder, if using. Roast for 10 to 12 minutes, until cauliflower is tender and some pieces have begun to lightly brown.

Alternatively, add raw cauliflower rice and seasonings to a large, dry skillet and sauté over medium heat for 7 to 8 minutes, until tender.

CALORIES: 53 | PROTEIN: 4G | FAT: 0G | CARBS: 10G | FIBER: 4G | NET CARBS: 6G

CHICKEN BROTH

Whether you roast a chicken at home or buy a rotisserie chicken at your local market, save those nutrient-rich bones to make broth. It's easy, and the results are so nourishing. Once the broth is cooled, portion it out into individual containers and freeze. You can also freeze leftover bones from several chickens for a richer broth. MAKES 8 SERVINGS (ABOUT 8 CUPS)

1 organic rotisserie chicken carcass

1 medium yellow onion, quartered

2 stalks celery, cut into 3-inch pieces

2 carrots, peeled and cut into 3-inch pieces

1 tablespoon apple cider vinegar

10 garlic cloves, sliced in half

15 whole black peppercorns

1 teaspoon fine sea salt

Place the carcass, onion, celery, carrots, vinegar, garlic, peppercorns, and salt in a large pot. Add about 8½ cups water, adjusting the amount to cover the ingredients by 1 inch. Bring to a boil, then reduce to a low simmer and cook for 4 hours.

Set a fine-mesh strainer over a large bowl. Pour the stock through the strainer. Discard the vegetables and bones in the strainer. Once the broth is cool, ladle it into glass jars. Cover and refrigerate for up to 1 week, or freeze for up to several months. Use a spoon to skim and discard any fat off the top before reheating.

CALORIES: 10 | PROTEIN: 0G | FAT: 0G | CARBS: 0G | FIBER: 0G | NET CARBS: 0G

VEGETABLE BROTH

If you'd rather not use chicken or bone broth, use this all-vegetable version in salads or enjoy it as a tonic. MAKES 12 SERVINGS (ABOUT 12 CUPS)

1 tablespoon
avocado oil

4 garlic cloves, minced

2 celery stalks,
chopped

2 cups chopped
carrots

½ large onion,
chopped

2-inch piece of fresh
ginger, peeled

2-inch turmeric,
peeled

¾ cup seaweed
(dried wakame)

2 cups chopped
mushrooms

½ tablespoon black
peppercorns

½ teaspoon sea salt

Heat the oil in a large stock pot. Add the garlic, celery, carrots, and onion and sauté until the vegetables are fragrant and the onion is translucent, about 5 minutes.

Add all other ingredients and 12 cups water on low-medium heat. Simmer for at least 1 hour. Turn off the heat and let the broth sit until cooled.

CALORIES: 10 | PROTEIN: 0G | FAT: 0G | CARBS: 2G | FIBER: 0G | NET CARBS: 2G

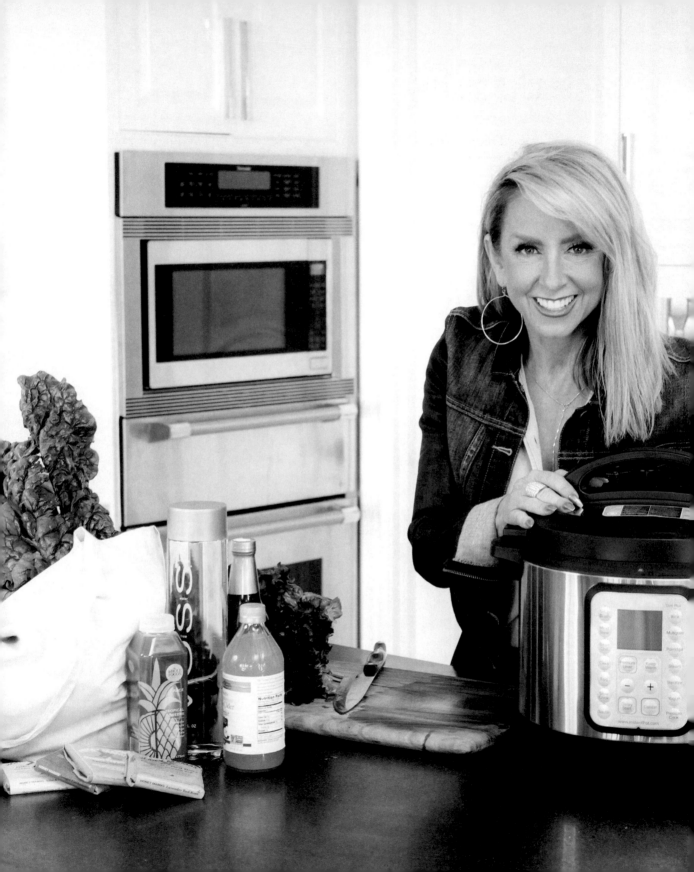

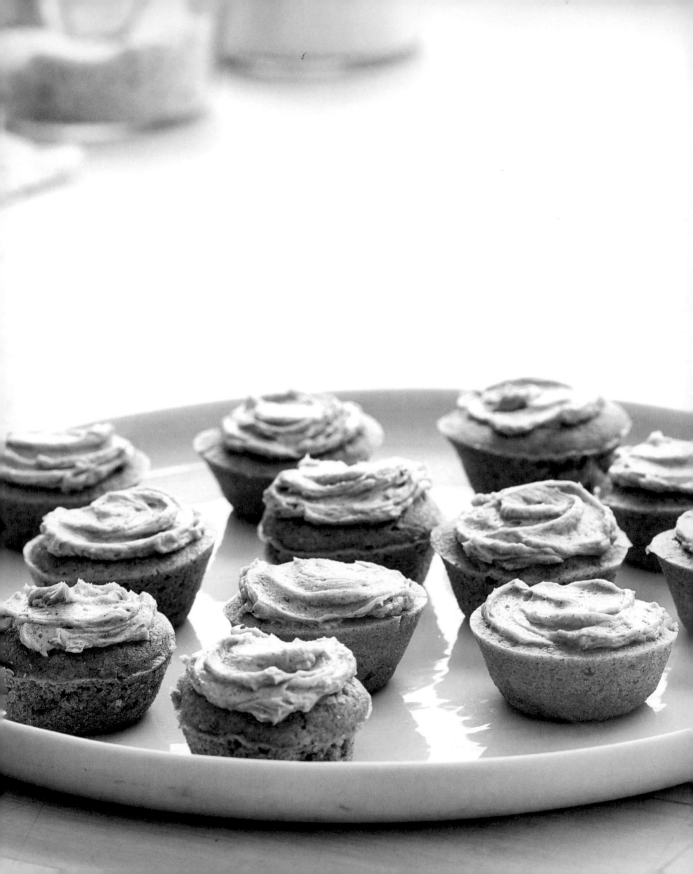

SWEET TREATS

BRAIN BOMBS FIVE WAYS

Brain Bombs are delicious high-fat, low-carb, and low-protein treats and a convenient source of those healthy fats you need to meet your macronutrient targets. Below you'll find a basic recipe that makes 10 Brain Bombs followed by 5 flavorful variations. Keep these frozen goodies on hand to enjoy when your fat amounts are too low, or when you want a sweet treat after dinner or a pick-me-up during an afternoon slump. Grab 2 or 3 Mexican Hot Chocolate Brain Bombs for breakfast on the go. Individual silicone candy molds come in many shapes and sizes. Look for them online or in housewares stores.

½ cup softened coconut butter

¼ cup MCT oil

2 tablespoons Swerve Sweetener Confectioners

⅛ teaspoon fine sea salt

BASIC BRAIN BOMBS MAKES 10 SERVINGS

Put the coconut butter, MCT oil, Swerve, and salt in a saucepan. Stir for 2 minutes over low heat until everything is melted. Using a tablespoon, divide the mixture into 10 silicone molds or mini-muffin tins. Freeze the Brain Bombs until they are hard, about 30 minutes. Remove them from the molds and store them in a sealed container in the freezer.

Ginger–Coconut Brain Bombs: Add 2 teaspoons freshly grated ginger to the other ingredients in the saucepan. Distribute the mixture among the molds, then sprinkle each with ½ teaspoon unsweetened shredded coconut. Proceed as directed.

CALORIES: 137 | PROTEIN: 1G | FAT: 13G | CARBS: 3G | FIBER: 2G | NET CARBS: 1G

Chocolate–Peanut Butter Brain Bombs: Add 1½ tablespoons natural peanut butter and 1½ tablespoons sugar-free chocolate chips to the ingredients in the saucepan. Proceed as directed.

CALORIES: 150 | PROTEIN: 1.5G | FAT: 15.7G | CARBS: 5.0G | FIBER: 2.3G | NET CARBS: 2.7G

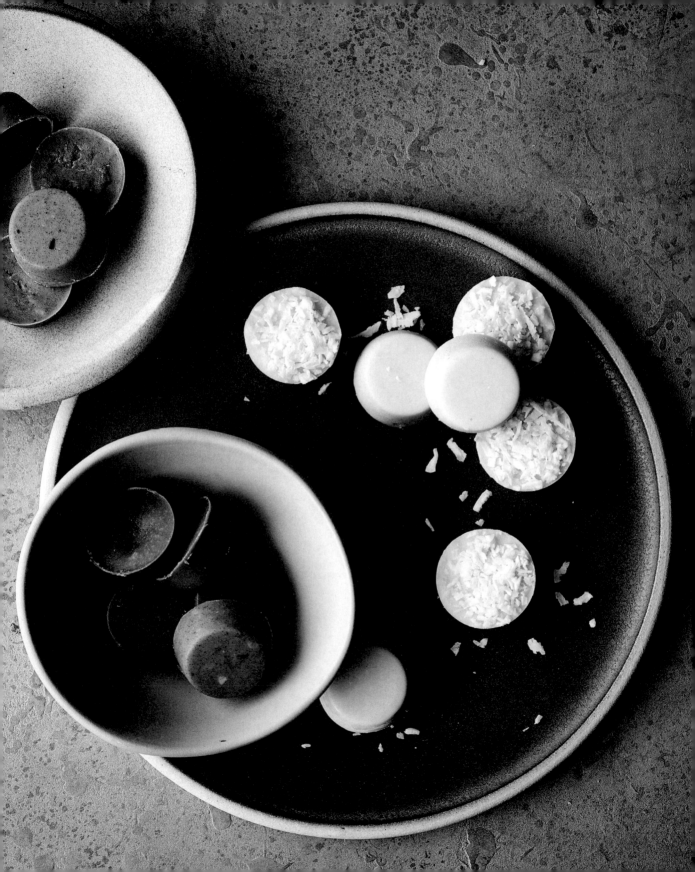

Mexican Hot Chocolate Brain Bombs: Add 1 tablespoon cacao powder, ¾ teaspoon ground cinnamon, ¾ teaspoon ground nutmeg, ½ teaspoon chili powder, and a pinch of cayenne to the ingredients in the saucepan. Proceed as directed.

CALORIES: 135 | PROTEIN: 1G | FAT: 13G | CARBS: 3G | FIBER: 2G | NET CARBS: 1G

Cinnamon–Almond Crunch Brain Bombs: Add 1 tablespoon crunchy, salted almond butter, 1 teaspoon ground cinnamon, and ½ teaspoon almond extract to the ingredients in the saucepan. Proceed as directed.

CALORIES: 141 | PROTEIN: 1G | FAT: 14G | CARBS: 3G | FIBER: 2G | NET CARBS: 1G

Chocolate-Peppermint Brain Bombs: Add 2 teaspoons cacao powder and ½ teaspoon peppermint extract to the ingredients in the saucepan. Proceed as directed.

CALORIES: 133 | PROTEIN: 1G | FAT: 13G | CARBS: 3G | FIBER: 2G | NET CARBS: 1G

SWEET AND SALTY MACADAMIA NUTS

Among all types of nuts, rich macadamias are among the highest in fats and lowest in carbs. One-quarter cup of these makes a satisfying snack. MAKES 16 SERVINGS (4 CUPS)

4 cups (1.2 pounds) macadamia nuts

2 tablespoons coconut oil, melted

¼ cup Swerve Sweetener Confectioners

1 teaspoon pure vanilla extract

1 teaspoon ground cinnamon

½ teaspoon ground nutmeg

½ teaspoon fine sea salt

Heat the oven to 250°F. Combine all of the ingredients in a large bowl and mix well. Arrange the nuts on a sheet pan in a single layer. Roast the nuts for 15 minutes; then give the pan a shake. Roast for another 10 minutes, until the nuts are golden.

CALORIES: 260 | PROTEIN: 3G | FAT: 28G | CARBS: 5G | FIBER: 3G | NET CARBS: 2G

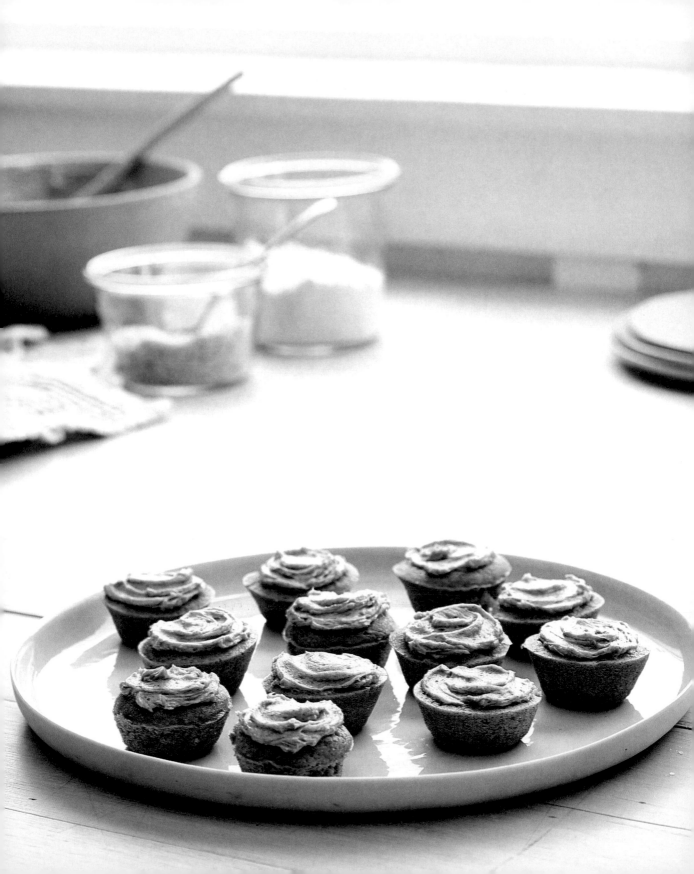

CINNAMON MUFFINS WITH VANILLA ICING

A cross between a muffin and a cupcake, these treats satisfy carb cravings and are just the right size to have 1 or 2 and still stay on track. MAKES 12 SERVINGS

MUFFINS:

Coconut oil cooking spray

½ cup almond flour

¼ cup Swerve Sweetener Confectioners

1 tablespoon coconut flour

½ teaspoon aluminum-free baking powder

⅓ cup coconut cream

1 large egg

1 teaspoon pure vanilla extract

1 teaspoon ground cinnamon

ICING:

3 tablespoons unsalted butter, softened

1½ tablespoons Swerve Sweetener Confectioners

1 teaspoon pure vanilla extract

¼ teaspoon ground cinnamon

Heat oven to 350°F. Coat a mini-muffin tin with coconut oil cooking spray, or use mini silicone muffin cups.

To make the muffins: Whisk together the almond flour, Swerve, coconut flour, and baking powder in a bowl.

Put the coconut cream, egg, vanilla, and cinnamon in another bowl and mix with a hand mixer until well blended. Add the dry ingredients to the bowl and continue mixing to combine. Divide the batter among the 12 muffin cups. Bake for 12 to 14 minutes, until a toothpick inserted in the center of the muffins comes out clean. Turn the muffins onto a wire rack and let cool completely.

To make the icing: Combine the butter, Swerve, vanilla extract, and cinnamon in a bowl. Whisk vigorously until fluffy.

When the muffins are cool, spread the icing on top of each one. Cover the iced muffins and store in the refrigerator for up to 3 days.

CALORIES: 77 | PROTEIN: 2G | FAT: 7G | CARBS: 2G | FIBER: 0.5G | NET CARBS: 1.5G

CHOCOLATE–MINT CHIP ICE CREAM

When making this frozen treat, freeze the serving bowls so the ice cream doesn't melt too quickly. The avocado adds creaminess and a boost of fiber. Start with just 1 teaspoon of peppermint extract, since different brands are more intense than others. Taste the mixture and add more extract if necessary.

MAKES 4 SERVINGS

1 avocado, peeled, pitted, and cut up

One 13.5-ounce can full-fat coconut milk

½ cup coconut oil, melted

5 tablespoons Swerve Sweetener Confectioners

2 tablespoons cacao powder

1 to 1¼ teaspoons peppermint extract

Pinch fine sea salt

¼ cup sugar-free chocolate chips

Put the avocado, coconut milk, coconut oil, Swerve, cacao powder, peppermint extract, and salt in a blender and process for about 20 seconds, until the mixture is smooth and fluffy.

Pour the mixture into a lidded glass bowl and freeze for 2 hours or longer, if necessary. Spoon into serving bowls and top with chocolate chips.

CALORIES: 520 | PROTEIN: 4G | FAT: 53G | CARBS: 13G | FIBER: 6G | NET CARBS: 7G

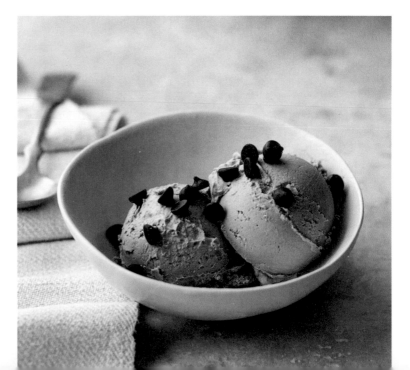

CHOCOLATE SILK PUDDING

Avocado and coconut cream make this fat-burning dessert smooth and silky—and there's a whopping 8 grams of fiber in each serving. If you have the carbs to spare, don't be afraid of a dessert that contains healthy fiber.

MAKES 2 SERVINGS

1 large avocado, soft but not too ripe, peeled and pitted

¼ cup canned coconut cream

⅓ cup Swerve Sweetener Confectioners

2½ tablespoons cacao powder

2 teaspoons MCT oil

1 teaspoon pure vanilla extract

Pinch fine sea salt

Put all ingredients in a blender and process for about 20 seconds, until smooth. Spoon into 2 small bowls and refrigerate for at least 1 hour before serving.

CALORIES: 231 | PROTEIN: 3G | FAT: 22G | CARBS: 11G | FIBER: 8G | NET CARBS: 3G

GLOSSARY

Adrenal Fatigue/Adrenal Dysfunction An imbalance in the system that supports and communicates to the adrenal glands. The scientific term for this is *HPA axis dysfunction*.

Amino Acids The building blocks of protein. Protein is composed of both essential and nonessential amino acids. There are nine essential amino acids that we must get from food because our body cannot make them. The rest are nonessential amino acids that can be synthesized or produced by our body.

Autoimmune Disease Various conditions that cause the immune system to attack the body instead of a foreign invader. Examples include psoriasis, Hashimoto's disease, lupus, celiac disease, multiple sclerosis, Crohn's disease, and others.

Autophagy The destruction and recycling of cells, from *auto* ("self") + *phagy* ("eating").

Bone Broth A broth made by simmering bones for a long time (8–48 hours) to extract the gelatin, collagen, and other minerals. This is different from regular broths and stocks purchased in grocery stores, which rarely use bones or are not simmered for long periods to extract the nutrients.

Brain Fog A nonmedical term used to describe a cognitive state that includes an inability to focus, lack of clarity, disorganization, poor concentration, mild confusion, and poor memory.

Breaking a Fast Any calories consumed (regardless of the source) after a period of not eating. Technically *any* calorie will break a fast. If you are doing intermittent fasting in the 131 Method, what "breaks" your fast is something that will spike your blood sugar, so keep sugars and carbs as minimal as possible when doing intermittent fasting.

Carbohydrate A macronutrient that provides glucose for the body to use or store for use later.

Celiac Disease An autoimmune condition affecting gut health that requires a person to completely eliminate gluten from their diet.

Cortisol The fight-or-flight stress hormone released by the adrenal glands.

Dysbiosis A change or imbalance of normal bacteria in a certain area of the body (e.g., the gut).

Electrolytes Naturally occurring elements that are vital to our health, including cellular hydration. The body cannot be truly hydrated without electrolytes, which include sodium, potassium, chloride, magnesium, calcium, phosphate, and bicarbonate.

Epigenetics Lifestyle and environmental factors that impact genetic expression.

Exogenous Ketones Dietary supplements taken in supplemental form, usually as a powder or liquid, that raise the body's ketone levels. *Exogenous* means it is not created by the body.

Fat A vital and essential macronutrient found in food sources like oils, nuts and seeds, avocados, etc. There are many forms of fat in our diet, such as saturated, unsaturated, polyunsaturated, monounsaturated, and trans fats.

Fat Adaptation The body's transition to burning ketones (from fat) for energy, rather than primarily burning glucose.

FODMAP A term for a class of carbohydrates that are fermentable sugars from commonly consumed foods; the acronym stands for fermentable oligosaccharides, disaccharides, monosaccharides, and polyols. Those with IBS commonly find high-FODMAP foods to be a trigger for their IBS and may need to stop eating them temporarily as their gut heals.

Ghrelin A hunger hormone that makes us want to eat more.

Gluconeogenesis Glucose formation from a non-carbohydrate source (like protein).

Glucose The term used for blood sugars. When glucose is present in the body, it is the main source of fuel used.

Gluten A protein found in wheat, barley, and rye.

Glycemic Index (GI) A scale from 1 to 100 indicating how quickly a specific food impacts blood sugar.

Glycemic Load (GL) A number indicating how much and how quickly one serving of a specific food impacts blood sugar.

Glycogen Excess glucose stored in the liver and muscles.

Hashimoto's Disease An autoimmune condition that affects the function of the thyroid gland.

Human Growth Hormone (HGH) A peptide hormone produced by the body that stimulates growth, cell reproduction, and cell regeneration. It contributes to a youthful look and feeling.

IBS Irritable bowel syndrome. A term used to name unexplained digestive issues like bloating, constipation, diarrhea, or pain.

IBD Inflammatory bowel disease. It includes conditions, like Crohn's disease and ulcerative colitis, that cause inflammation in the gut.

Insoluble Fiber A type of fiber that is not dissolved in the gut and passes through the digestive system. This fiber is usually a "bulking" agent to aid digestion.

Insulin A hormone produced by the pancreas important for many functions of metabolism. One of its primary roles is to regulate glucose (blood sugar) levels.

Integrative/Functional Medicine/Health Evidence-based care focused on the patient as a whole and looking at the root cause of symptoms.

Intermittent Fasting A style of eating in which the eating window is monitored and adjusted. Also called time-restricted eating, it is a pattern of eating with many health benefits. An example of intermittent fasting is eating only within an eight-hour period, say from 10 A.M. to 6 P.M.

Intuitive Eating A way of eating that involves being tuned in to one's hunger signals as opposed to counting calories and macronutrients. It means listening to your body, listening to personal cues, and not watching the clock to decide when to eat. It's possible—and important—to eat intuitively and still eat healthy while following the 131. It may take practice until you learn what your body responds to best, but once you do, eating intuitively is great for your mind-set and health.

Keto Flu/Carb Flu Symptoms including (but not limited to) nausea, brain fog, and headaches that typically develop in the first few days of transition from burning glucose to burning fat.

Ketones A fuel produced from fat when the body has depleted its sources of carbohydrates and is no longer running on glucose. When someone is burning primarily ketones for energy, they are in a state of ketosis. Scientifically, ketones are an organic compound containing a carbonyl group C=O bonded to two hydrocarbon groups. There are three forms of ketones: beta-hydroxybutyrate, acetone, and acetoacetate.

Ketosis A metabolic state in which the body burns ketones (a type of fat) for energy.

Krebs Cycle A cycle of reactions in living cells that results in energy. It's the final step after metabolism of carbohydrates, proteins, and fatty acids.

Leaky Gut A common term for intestinal permeability—unwanted gaps in the lining of the gut that protects us from foreign invaders like bacteria.

Leptin A satiety hormone that limits our desire to eat.

Macronutrients The large components of foods that provide calories: our proteins, fats, and carbohydrates. Often referred to as macros.

Macrophasing A method of phasing macronutrient intake to maintain metabolic flexibility. This is the cornerstone of Renew.

MCT Oil Medium-chain triglycerides. MCTs are quickly and efficiently broken down by the body and used as a quick source of energy, as opposed to being stored as fat.

Melatonin Hormone that helps regulate sleep.

Metabolic Adaptation The body's necessary adjustments to maintain internal stability (homeostasis) and decrease energy expenditure.

Metabolic Flexibility The body's ability to easily switch between fat (ketones) and sugar (glucose) for fuel.

Metabolism The chemical changes in living cells by which energy is provided for vital processes and activities and new material is taken in.

Microbiome The trillions of microorganisms and bacteria living in the human body, primarily in the gut. The microbiome refers to the organisms as well as their genes. Every individual has a different microbiome.

Micronutrients The non-calorie-providing components of foods including vitamins, minerals, antioxidants, phytonutrients, and more.

Net Carbs A term used to describe the impact of carbohydrates after subtracting the grams of fiber per serving from the total carbohydrates per serving.

Nightshade Vegetables Foods belonging to the Solanaceae plant family, including eggplant, tomatoes, white potatoes, okra, peppers, paprika, and a wide variety of other foods. Some people find these foods produce inflammation in the body.

Nitrites/Nitrates Preservatives added to many products such as meat to extend shelf life. Natural nitrates are also found in foods like celery and spinach.

Plant Based A style of eating that includes meals rich in and mostly from all plant sources.

Prebiotics Nutrients that support probiotics (see below), found in the fiber of many fruits, vegetables, beans, and more.

Probiotics Living beneficial bacteria found in fermented foods and supplements.

Protein A macronutrient made up of amino acids. Protein is essential to our health for various structures, functions, and reactions.

Refined Carbohydrates Processed carbs that have been stripped of fiber, vitamins, and minerals.

Refueling The process of reintroducing foods or calories after a period of fasting.

Registered Dietitian A leading nutrition expert who has received at a minimum a bachelor's degree, completed an accredited internship, and maintains continuing education on current science. The 131 Method dietitians have additional years of education, training, and experience in integrative and functional nutrition.

Saturated Fat A type of fatty acid found in coconut oil, butter, and many animal products.

SIBO Small Intestinal Bacterial Overgrowth. A condition in which the bacteria that are meant to be in the large intestine have moved into the small intestine.

Soluble Fiber Fiber that dissolves in water. This type of fiber creates a gel-like substance and helps nutrients and waste to smoothly pass through the digestive tract.

Thermogenics The production of heat. It commonly refers to drugs or compounds that increase or speed up metabolism.

Trans Fat A type of fatty acid to which hydrogen has been added. Often found in processed and packaged food, it is the most dangerous of all types of fat because it is chemically altered.

Vegetarian Someone whose style of eating does not include any animal protein.

Vegan Someone whose style of eating omits animal protein and products produced from animals, such as milk, cheese, honey, and eggs.

APPENDIX

MACRO TRACKING 3 PHASE CHEAT SHEET:

Ideal ranges of macronutrients for each phase:

IGNITE:

Carbohydrates: 5-10%
Fat: 70-80%
Protein: 10-20%

NOURISH:

Carbohydrates: 10-30%
Fat: 50-80%
Protein: 10-20%

*In Nourish Week 3, prior
to your fast if you are fasting, decrease your carb intake
to 5-15% to prepare for
your fast.

RENEW:

Lean Green:
Carbohydrate: 20-40% (low-moderate)
Fat: 10-15% fat (low)
Protein: 30-50% (high)

Carb Charge:
Carbohydrate: 55-70% (high)
Fat: 15-20% (low-moderate)
Protein: 15-25% (moderate)

Fat Burning:
Carbohydrates: 5-10%
Fat: 70-80%
Protein: 10-20%

HOW TO USE YOUR MYFITNESSPAL TRACKING APP:

• Download a free app such as MyFitnessPal, Lose It, MyNetDiary, MyPlate, or MyMacros. (My Fitness Pal is my favorite.)

• Create an account.

• Go to "Goals" and customize your default or daily goals, with macros as your main focus.

• Set your percentages to match the goals depending on which phase you are doing

• Enter all foods for the day into "Diary." It's ideal to enter food as you go, as opposed to the end of the day so as to have a better idea of how to adjust your menu as needed.

• Record everything you eat or drink to provide a clear picture of your macronutrient ratio.

• Suggested ranges for each phase relate to your intake for the day (not each specific meal).

• Once you've entered all your foods, check the percentage of the total day. On MyFitnessPal, go to Diary, then at the bottom click Nutrition, then go to Macros to view your daily summary.

CARB COUNT IN EVERYDAY FOODS

As you're learning about the nutritional makeup of your favorite foods, you can use this list to help you identify which foods are highest (or lowest) in carbohydrates:

VEGETABLES:

Asparagus, 5 spears: 4g carb, 1g fiber

Artichoke hearts, 2 pieces: 5g carb, 2g fiber

Beets, ¼ cup: 3g carb, 1g fiber

Bell pepper, 1 medium: 6g carb, 2g fiber

Bok choy, 1 cup: 4g carb, 1g fiber

Broccoli, 1 medium stalk: 8g carb, 3g fiber

Broccoli slaw, ½ cup: 3g carb, 1g fiber

Brussels sprouts, ½ cup: 4g carb, 2g fiber

Butternut squash, ½ cup: 11g carb, 3g fiber

Carrot, 1 large: 7g carb, 2g fiber

Cauliflower, ⅙ medium head: 5g carb, 2g fiber

Celery, 2 medium stalks: 4g carb, 1g fiber

Collard greens, ½ cup: 5g carb, 2g fiber

Cucumber, ⅓ medium: 2g carb, 1g fiber

Eggplant, ½ cup: 4g carb, 1g fiber

Green (snap) beans, ¾ cup cut: 5g carb, 2g fiber

Green cabbage 1⁄12 medium head: 5g carb, 2g fiber

Kale, 1 cup: 9g carb, 6g fiber

Lettuce, 1½ cup: 2g carb, 1g fiber

Mushrooms, 5: 3g carb, 1g fiber

Mustard greens, ½ cup: 4g carb, 2g fiber

Okra, ½ cup: 4g carb, 2g fiber

Onion, 1 medium: 11g carb, 4g fiber

Portobello mushroom, ½ cup: 3g carb, 1g fiber

Potato, 1 medium: 26g carb, 9g fiber

Radish, 7: 3g carb, 1g fiber

Rhubarb, 1 stalk: 2g carb, 1g fiber

Rutabaga, ½ cup: 6g carb, 2g fiber

Salsa, 2 Tbsp: 4g carb, 1g fiber

Spaghetti squash, 1 cup: 10g carb, 2g fiber

Spinach, 1 cup: 1g carb, 1g fiber

Sweet potato, 1 medium: 23g carb, 8g fiber

Swiss chard, ½ cup: 4g carb, 2g fiber

Tomato, 1 medium: 5g carb, 2g fiber

Turnip, 1 small: 4g carb, 1g fiber

Water chestnuts, ¼ cup: 4g carb, 1g fiber

Zucchini, ½ medium: 4g carb, 1g fiber

FRUITS:

Apple, 1 large: 34g carb, 11g fiber

Avocado, ⅕ medium: 3g carb, 1g fiber

Banana, 1 medium: 30 g carb, 10g fiber

Blueberries, ½ cup: 10g carb, 2g fiber

Blackberries, ½ cup: 7g carb, 4g fiber

Cantaloupe, ¼ medium: 12g carb, 4g fiber

Cherries, ¼ cup: 32g carb, 2g fiber

Figs, ¼ cup: 26g carb, 5g fiber

Grapefruit, ½ medium: 15g carb, 5g fiber

Grapes, ¾ cup: 23g carb, 8g fiber

Honeydew melon, 1⁄10 medium: 12g carb, 4g fiber

Kiwi fruit, 2 medium: 20g carb, 7g fiber

Mango, 1 cup, 1"pieces: 27g carb, 3g fiber

Nectarine, 1 raw: 15g carb, 2g fiber

Orange, 1 medium: 19g carb, 6g fiber

Papaya, 1 cup, 1"pieces: 16g carb, 3g fiber

Peach, 1 medium: 15g carb, 5g fiber

Pear halves, ½ cup: 14g carb, 2g fiber

Pineapple, 1 cup, 1"pieces: 22g carb, 2g fiber

Pomegranate, ½ whole: 26g carb, 6g fiber

Plum, 1 whole: 8g carb, 1g fiber

Raspberries, ½ cup: 7g carb, 4g fiber

Strawberries, 8 medium: 11g carb, 4g fiber

Tangerine, 1 small: 10g carb, 1g fiber

Watermelon, 2 cups diced: 21g carb, 7g fiber

DRIED FRUITS:

Dried dates, 6 dates: 30g carb, 3g fiber

Prunes, ¼ cup: 26g carb, 3g fiber

Raisins, ¼ cup: 28g carb, 2g fiber

Craisins, ¼ cup: 33g carb, 3g fiber

Mango, 1oz/~4 pieces: 21g carb, 1g fiber

Banana chips, ¼ cup: 17g carb, 2g fiber

HEALTHY FATS:

Almonds, 1 oz: 6g carb, 3.5g fiber

Almond butter, 1 Tbsp: 3g carb, 1.5g fiber

Brazil nuts, 1 oz: 3.5g carb, 2g fiber

Cashews, 1 oz: 9g carb, 1g fiber

Chia seeds, 2 Tbsp: 10g carb, 9g fiber

Cheese, full-fat, 1 oz: 0g carb, 0g fiber

Coconut milk, full fat: 4 carb, 0g fiber

Egg, 1 large: 0 g carb, 0 fiber

Flax seeds, ground, 2 Tbsp: 3g carb, 2g fiber

Hazelnuts, 1 oz: 5g carb, 3g fiber

Hemp seeds, shelled, 2 Tbsp: 0g carb, 3g fiber

Kalamata olives, 3 pieces: 2g carb, 1g fiber

Macadamia nuts, 1 oz: 4g carb, 2.5g fiber

Pecans, 1 oz: 4g carb, 2.5g fiber

Peanuts, 25: 8g carb, 4g fiber

Pistachios, shelled, 1 oz: 8g carb, 3g fiber

Pine nuts, 3 Tbsp: 7g carb, 3g fiber

Pumpkin seeds, 1 oz: 15g carb, 5g fiber

Sesame seeds, 1 Tbsp: 2g carb, 1g fiber

Sunflower butter, 1 Tbsp: 3.5g carb, 2g fiber

Walnuts, 1 oz: 4g carb, 2g fiber

Whole milk (organic), 1 cup: 12g carb, 0g fiber

Whole plain organic yogurt, 1 cup: 12g carb, 0g fiber

BEANS/LEGUMES

Black beans, ½ cup cooked: 27g carb, 7g fiber

Pinto beans, ½ cup cooked: 22g carb, 8 g fiber

Red kidney beans, ½ cup cooked: 20g carb, 7g fiber

Fava beans, ½ cup cooked: 17g carb, 5g fiber

Refried beans (vegetarian), ½ cup cooked: 16g carb, 6g fiber

Garbanzo beans, ½ cup cooked: 23g carb, 6g fiber

Lentils, ½ cup cooked: 20g carb, 8g fiber

Tempeh, 4 oz: 7g carb, 5g fiber

Edamame, ½ cup: 32g carb, 10g fiber

PROTEINS

Beef, ground, tips, steak, etc., 4 oz: 0g carb, 0g fiber

Chicken breast, grilled, 4 oz: 0g carb, 0g fiber

Chicken breast, grilled, breaded, 4 oz: 11g carb, 0g fiber

Cod, 4 oz: 0g carb, 0g fiber

Eggs Whole, 1 egg: 0g carb, 0g fiber

Egg Yolks, 1 yolk: 0g carb, 0g fiber

Pork Tenderloin, 4 oz: 2g carb, 0g fiber

Salmon, 4 oz: 0g carb, 0g fiber

Shrimp, 4 oz: 0g carb, 0g fiber

Turkey, ground, 4 oz: 0g carb, 0g fiber

GRAINS

Corn, 1 large ear: 25g carb, 3g fiber

Basmati rice, ½ cup cooked: 20g carb, 0g fiber

Brown rice, ½ cup cooked: 26g carb, 2g fiber

Quinoa, ½ cup cooked: 20g carb, 3g fiber

Spelt, ½ cup cooked: 26g carb, 4g fiber

Sprouted bread, 1 slice: 16g carb, 2g fiber

Steel cut oats, ½ cup cooked: 27g carb, 4g fiber

Wild rice, ½ cup cooked: 18g carb, 2g fiber

POPULAR ITEMS

Tall Starbucks Latte, 12 oz non-fat: 15g carb, 0g fiber

Tall Iced Vanilla Starbucks Latte, 12 oz non-fat: 24g carb, 0g fiber

Coffee, black, 12 oz: 0g carb, 0g fiber

Fiber One Bar (90 cal Chewy Bar): 17g carb, 5g fiber

Rx Bar (Chocolate Sea Salt), 1 bar: 24g carb, 6g fiber

Lara Bar (Cashew Cookie), 1 bar: 23g carb, 3g fiber

Epic Bar (Beef- Apple): 4g carb, 0g fiber

Mini Pretzels, 20: 25g carb, 1g fiber

Gluten Free Mini Pretzels, 25 sticks: 25g carb, 1g fiber

Miracle Noodle, 6 oz: 1g carb, 1g fiber

Avocado Oil-Based Mayo, 1 tbsp: 0g carb, 0g fiber

Tortilla Chips, 1 oz/~12 chips; 17g carb, 1g fiber

Siete/Grain Free Chips. 1 oz/ ~9 chips: 19g carb, 2g fiber

Almond Flour Crackers (Simple Mills), 17 crackers: 17g carb, 2g fiber

ENDNOTES

INTRODUCTION
1. Centers for Disease Control and Prevention, "National Center for Health Statistics 2017, Table 53," U.S. Department of Health & Human Services, last modified May 3, 2017, https://www.cdc.gov/nchs/fastats/obesity -overweight.htm.

2. Eric A. Finkelstein, Ian C. Fiebelkorn, and Guijing Wang. "National Medical Spending Attributable To Overweight And Obesity: How Much, And Who's Paying?," *Health Affairs* W3 (2003): 219–226. https://pdfs. semanticscholar.org/4c23/ ce797a03e7a0b5d62752992592660f915c67 .pdf.

3. "Why Good Nutrition is Important," Center for Science in the Public Interest, accessed November 15, 2018, https://cspinet.org/ eating-healthy/why-good-nutrition-important.

CHAPTER 3
1. Uffe Ravnskov et al., "Lack of an association or an inverse association between low-density-lipoprotein cholesterol and mortality in the elderly: a systematic review," *BMJ Open* 2016;6:e010401, doi: 10.1136/ bmjopen-2015-010401.

CHAPTER 4
1. Michael Boschmann et al., "Water-Induced Thermogenesis," *The Journal of Clinical Endocrinology & Metabolism* 88, no. 12 (December 1, 2003): 6015–6019. https://doi .org/10.1210/jc.2003-030780.

2. Rachel R. Markwald et al., "Impact of insufficient sleep on total daily energy expenditure, food intake, and weight gain," Proceedings of the National Academy of Sciences of the United States of America 110, no. 14 (April 2, 2013): 5695-5700, doi: 10.1073/ pnas.1216951110.

3. Uwe Gröber, Joachim Schmidt, and Klaus Kisters, "Magnesium in Prevention and Therapy," *Nutrients* 7, no. 9 (September 2015): 8199–8226, doi:10.3390/nu7095388.

4. Scott A. Lear, Ph.D. et al., "The effect of physical activity on mortality and cardiovascular disease in 130,000 people from 17 high-income, middle-income, and low-income countries: the PURE study," *The Lancet* 390, no. 10113 (September 21, 2017):2643–2654, doi: https://doi.org/10.1016/ S0140-6736(17)31634-3.

CHAPTER 5
1.Simon Ingves, et al., "A randomized cross-over study of the effects of macronutrient composition and meal frequency on GLP-1, ghrelin and energy expenditure in humans," *Peptides* 93 (July 2017):20-26, doi: 10.1016/j .peptides.2017.04.011.

2. Enhad A. Chowdhury et al., "Carbohydrate-rich breakfast attenuates glycaemic, insulinaemic and ghrelin response to ad libitum lunch relative to morning fasting in lean adults," *British Journal of Nutrition* 114, no. 1 (July 14, 2015): 98-107, doi: 10.1017/ S0007114515001506.

3. Tatiana Moro et. al., "Effects of eight weeks of time-restricted feeding (16/8) on basal metabolism, maximal strength, body composition, inflammation, and cardiovascular risk factors in resistance-trained males," *Journal of Translational Medicine* 14, no. 290 (October 12, 2016), doi: https://doi.org/10.1186/s12967-016-1044-0.

CHAPTER 7
1. Adam I. Orr, "How Cows Eat Grass," U.S. Food and Drug Administration, last modified November 13, 2017, accessed November 15, 2018, https://www.fda.gov/AnimalVeterinary/ ResourcesforYou/AnimalHealthLiteracy/ ucm255500.htm.

2. Cynthia Daley et al., "A review of fatty acid profiles and antioxidant content in grass-fed and grain-fed beef," *Nutrition Journal* 9, no. 10 (Mach 10, 2010), doi: 10.1186/1475-2891-9-10.

BIBLIOGRAPHY

Amen, Daniel G., MD. *Change Your Brain, Change Your Body: Use Your Brain to Get and Keep the Body You Have Always Wanted*. New York: Crown Publishing Group, 2010.

Avedon, Gregg. Men's Health *Muscle Chow: More Than 150 Easy-to-Follow Recipes to Burn Fat and Feed Your Muscles*. New York: Rodale, Inc., 2017.

Bailey, Claire. *The Clever Guts Diet Recipe Book: 150 Delicious Recipes to Mend Your Gut and Boost Your Health and Wellbeing*. Short Books, 2017.

Barber, Dan. *The Third Plate: Field Notes on the Future of Food*. New York: Penguin Press, 2014.

Beck, Judith S., PhD. *The Beck Diet Solution: Train Your Brain to Think Like a Thin Person*. Birmingham, AL: Oxmoor House, Inc., 2008.

Beck, Judith S., PhD. *The Beck Diet Solution Weight Loss Workbook: The 6-Week Plan to Train Your Brain to Think Like a Thin Person*. Birmingham, AL: Oxmoor House, Inc., 2007.

Berg, Frances M., MS, LN and Stacy Debroff. *Underage and Overweight: America's Childhood Obesity Epidemic—What Every Parent Needs to Know*. New York: Hatherleigh Press, 2004.

Blatner, Dawn Jackson. *The Flexitarian Diet: The Mostly Vegetarian Way to Lose Weight, Be Healthier, Prevent Disease, and Add Years to Your Life*. New York: McGraw Hill, 2009.

Campbell, Jay. *The Definitive Testosterone Replacement Therapy MANual: How to Optimize Your Testosterone for Lifelong Health and Happiness*. San Bernardino, CA: Archangel Ink, 2015.

Ciuciu, Asheritah and Linda Dillow. *Full: Food, Jesus, and the Battle for Satisfaction*. Chicago: Moody Publishers, 2017.

Fung, Jason, MD. *The Obesity Code: Unlocking the Secrets of Weight Loss*. Vancouver, BC: Greystone Books, 2016.

Fung, Jason, MD and Jimmy Moore. *The Complete Guide to Fasting: Heal Your Body Through Intermittent, Alternate-Day, and Extended Fasting*. Las Vegas, NV: Victory Belt Publishing Inc., 2016.

Gedgaudas, Nora T. *Primal Body, Primal Mind: Empower Your Total Health the Way Evolution Intended (...And Didn't)*. Rochester, VT: Healing Arts Press, 2009.

Gorman, John. *The Flexible Fat Loss Solution: The Fat Loss System that is Sustainable for Life (The Physique Enhancement Series) (Volume 2)*. San Bernardino, CA: Team Gorman LLC, 2016.

Gottfried, Sara, MD. *The Hormone Cure: Reclaim Balance, Sleep and Sex Drive; Lose Weight; Feel Focused, Vital, and Energized Naturally with the Gottfried Protocol*. New York: Scribner, 2013.

Greger, Michael, MD and Gene Stone. *How Not to Die: Discover the Foods Scientifically Proven to Prevent and Reverse Disease*. New York: Flatiron Books, 2015.

Greger, Michael, MD and Gene Stone. *How Not to Die Cookbook: 100+ Recipes to Help Prevent and Reverse Disease*. London: Flatiron Books, 2017.

Gundry, Steven R., MD. *The Plant Paradox: The Hidden Dangers in "Healthy" Foods That Cause Disease and Weight Gain*. New York: HarperCollins Publishers, 2017.

Hartwig, Melissa and Dallas Hartwig. *Whole30: The 30-Day Guide to Total Health and Food Freedom*. New York: Houghton Mifflin Harcourt, 2015.

Holmes, Lee. *Heal Your Gut: A Healing Protocol and Step-by-Step Program with More Than 90 Recipes to Cleanse, Restore, and Nourish (Supercharge)*. Beverly, MA: Fair Winds Press, 2016.

Holmes, Lee. *Supercharge Your Gut: Supercharged Food*. Crows Nest, NSW Australia: Murdoch Books, 2018.

Kessler, David A. *The End of Overeating: Taking Control of the Insatiable American Appetite*. New York: Rodale, Inc., 2009.

Longo, Valter, PhD. *The Longevity Diet: Discover the New Science to Slow Ageing, Fight Disease and Manage Your Weight*. New York: Penguin Random House, LLC, 2018.

Masley, Steven, MD and Jonny Bowden, PhD. *Smart Fat: Eat More Fat. Lose More Weight. Get Healthy Now*. New York: Harper One, 2016.

Mercola, Joseph, MD. *Fat for Fuel: A Revolutionary Diet to Combat Cancer, Boost Brain Power, and Increase Your Energy*. Carlsbad, CA: Hay House Inc., 2017.

Mercola, Joseph, MD. *Fat for Fuel Cookbook: Recipes and Ketogenic Keys to Health from a World-Class Doctor and an Internationally Renowned Chef*. Carlsbad, CA: Hay House, Inc., 2017.

Nichols, Lily. *Real Food for Pregnancy: The Science and Wisdom of Optimal Prenatal Nutrition*. Lily Nichols, 2018.

Niman, Nicolette Hahn. *Defending Beef: The Case for Sustainable Meat Production*. White River Junction, VT: Chelsea Green Publishing, 2014.

Obermeder, Sally and Maha Koraiem. *Super Green—Simple and Lean: 140 Smoothies, Salad & Bowl Recipes*. Crows Nest, NSW Australia: Allen & Unwin, 2017.

Oz, Mehmet, MD. *Food Can Fix It: The Superfood Switch to Fight Fat, Defy Aging, and Eat Your Way Healthy*. New York: Scribner, 2017.

Pasternak, Harley and Myatt Murphy. *The 5-Factor Diet: The Diet and Fitness Secret of Hollywood's A-List*. Des Moines, IA: Meredith Books, 2006.

Ruhlman, Michael. *Grocery: The Buying and Selling of Food in America*. New York: Abrams Press, 2017.

Swanhart, Kenzie. *Clean Eating Bowls: 100 Real Food Recipes of Eating Clean*. Berkeley: Rockridge Press, 2016.

Teta, Jade and Keoni Teta. *The Metabolic Effect Diet: Eat More. Work Out Less, and Actually Lose Weight While You Rest*. New York: HarperCollins Publishers, 2010.

Wicks, Joe. *The Fat-Loss Plan: 100 Quick and Easy Recipes with Workouts*. Bluebird Books for Life, 2017.

Wilson, Sarah. *I Quit Sugar: Simplicious*. Sydney, Australia: Pan Macmillan, 2015.

Wolf, Robb. *Wired to Eat: Turn Off Cravings, Rewire Your Appetite for Weight Loss, and Determine the Foods That Work for You*. New York: Harmony Books, 2017.

INDEX

ACKNOWLEDGMENTS

Special thanks to the many esteemed professionals who kindly shared their time, research, studies, opinions, and expertise with me:

Bert Herring, MD

Daniel Amen, MD

Dan Witkowski, MD

Dominic D'Agostino, PhD

Eric Battersby

Jason Fung, MD

Jimmy Moore

Michael Breus, PhD

Michael Ruscio, DC

Neil Thanedar

Shawn Stevenson

Steve Savage, PhD

Valter Longo, PhD

Zach Bush, MD

Dawn DeSylvia, MD

In recognition of the dedicated professionals who contributed to the testing and development of the 131 Method:

Mcayla Sarno, PsyD, MFT

Paul Garcia, DC

Ashley Sweeney, MS, RD, 131 Method Program Director

Ana Cristina Jurczyk, MS, RD

Christa Biegler, RD

Leigh Wagner, PhD, MS, RD

Sarah Rainey, RD, LD

Taryn Sutterfield, RD

Whitney Crouch, RDN, CLT

Erin Woodbury, 131 Method Media Chef

ABOUT THE AUTHOR

Chalene Johnson is a world-renowned motivational speaker with more than 30 years as a health expert. She is a *New York Times* best-selling author, health and lifestyle expert, and top health podcaster with more than 30 million downloads of her shows. Millions of people around the globe have transformed their bodies and their lives with her help. Her fitness programs have been featured in gyms and on TV for more than 12 years. She and Bret, her husband of more than 20 years, are the founders of the 131 Method. They have built and sold several multimillion-dollar lifestyle companies and helped countless heart-centered entrepreneurs to bring their ideas to market. Despite their accomplishments, Chalene and Bret say their number one priority and greatest achievement has been to raise their two children, Brock and Cierra.

Website: chalenejohnson.com and 131method.com

HAY HOUSE TITLES OF RELATED INTEREST

YOU CAN HEAL YOUR LIFE,
the movie, starring Louise Hay & Friends
(available as a 1-DVD program, an expanded 2-DVD set,
and an online streaming video)
Learn more at www.hayhouse.com/louise-movie

THE SHIFT, the movie,
starring Dr. Wayne W. Dyer
(available as a 1-DVD program, an expanded 2-DVD set,
and an online streaming video)
Learn more at www.hayhouse.com/the-shift-movie

***

BRIGHT LINE EATING: The Science of Living Happy, Thin,
and Free, by Susan Peirce Thompson, Ph.D.

COMPLETE KETO: A Guide to Transforming Your Body and
Your Mind for Life, by Drew Manning

JOY'S SIMPLE FOOD REMEDIES: Tasty Cures for
Whatever's Ailing You, by Joy Bauer

MAKE YOUR OWN RULES DIET, by Tara Stiles

All of the above are available at your local bookstore,
or may be ordered by contacting Hay House
(see next page).

***

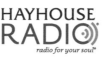

We hope you enjoyed this Hay House book. If you'd like to receive our online catalog featuring additional information on Hay House books and products, or if you'd like to find out more about the Hay Foundation, please contact:

Hay House, Inc., P.O. Box 5100, Carlsbad, CA 92018-5100
(760) 431-7695 or (800) 654-5126
(760) 431-6948 (fax) or (800) 650-5115 (fax)
www.hayhouse.com® • www.hayfoundation.org

———

Published in Australia by:
Hay House Australia Pty. Ltd., 18/36 Ralph St., Alexandria NSW 2015
Phone: 612-9669-4299 • *Fax:* 612-9669-4144 • www.hayhouse.com.au

Published in the United Kingdom by:
Hay House UK, Ltd., Astley House, 33 Notting Hill Gate, London W11 3JQ
Phone: 44-20-3675-2450 • *Fax:* 44-20-3675-2451 • www.hayhouse.co.uk

Published in India by: Hay House Publishers India,
Muskaan Complex, Plot No. 3, B-2, Vasant Kunj, New Delhi 110 070
Phone: 91-11-4176-1620 • *Fax:* 91-11-4176-1630 • www.hayhouse.co.in

———

Access New Knowledge.
Anytime. Anywhere.

Learn and evolve at your own pace
with the world's leading experts.

www.hayhouseU.com